Adult Congenital Heart Disease

Editor

CURT J. DANIELS

CARDIOLOGY CLINICS

www.cardiology.theclinics.com

August 2020 • Volume 38 • Number 3

ELSEVIER

1600 John F. Kennedy Boulevard • Suite 1800 • Philadelphia, Pennsylvania, 19103-2899

http://www.theclinics.com

CARDIOLOGY CLINICS Volume 38, Number 3
August 2020 ISSN 0733-8651, ISBN-13: 978-0-323-76120-8

Editor: Stacy Eastman
Developmental Editor: Donald Mumford

Cardiology Clinics (ISSN 0733-8651) is published quarterly by Elsevier Inc., 360 Park Avenue South, New York, NY 10010-1710. Months of issue are February, May, August, and November. Business and Editorial Offices: 1600 John F. Kennedy Blvd., Ste. 1800, Philadelphia, PA 19103-2899. Customer Service Office: 3251 Riverport Lane, Maryland Heights, MO 63043. Periodicals post-age paid at New York, NY and additional mailing offices. Subscription prices are $352.00 per year for US individuals, $706.00 per year for US institutions, $100.00 per year for US students and residents, $432.00 per year for Canadian individuals, $885.00 per year for Canadian institutions, $466.00 per year for international individuals, $885.00 per year for international institutions, $100.00 per year for Canadian students/residents and $220.00 per year for international students/residents.To receive student/resident rate, orders must be accompanied by name of affiliated institution, data of term, and the *signature* of program/residency coordinator on institution letterhead. Orders will be billed at individual rate until proof of status is received. Foreign air speed delivery is included in all *Clinics* subscription prices. All prices are subject to change without notice. **POSTMASTER:** Send address changes to *Cardiology Clinics*, Elsevier Health Sciences Division, Subscription Customer Service, 3251 Riverport Lane, Maryland Heights, MO 63043. **Customer Service: 1-800-654-2452 (U.S. and Canada); 314-447-8871 (outside U.S. and Canada). Fax: 314-447-8029. E-mail: journalscus-tomerservice-usa@elsevier.com (for print support); journalsonlinesupport-usa@elsevier.com (for online support).**

Reprints. For copies of 100 or more, of articles in this publication, please contact the Commercial Reprints Department, Elsevier Inc., 360 Park Avenue South, New York, NY 10010-1710. Tel.: 212-633-3874; Fax: 212-633-3820; E-mail: reprints@elsevier.com.

Cardiology Clinics is also published in Spanish by McGraw-Hill Interamericana Editores S. A., P.O. Box 5-237, 06500, Mexico D. F., Mexico; in Portuguese by Reichmann and Alfonso Editores Rio de Janeiro, Brazil; and in Greek by Dimitrios P. Lagos, 8 Pondon Street, GR115-28 Ilissia, Greece.

Cardiology Clinics is covered in *MEDLINE/PubMed (Index Medicus), Excerpta Medica, The Cumulative Index to Nursing and Allied Health Literature* (CINAHL).

Contributors

LAUREN ANDRADE, MD
Adult Congenital Heart Disease Fellow, Philadelphia Adult Congenital Heart Center, Perelman School of Medicine, University of Pennsylvania, Penn Medicine and Children's Hospital of Philadelphia, Perelman Center for Advanced Medicine, Philadelphia, Pennsylvania, USA

ELISA A. BRADLEY, MD
Department of Internal Medicine, Division of Cardiovascular Medicine, The Ohio State University, Columbus, Ohio, USA

LUKE J. BURCHILL, MBBS, PhD
Department of Cardiology, The Royal Melbourne Hospital, Department of Medicine, The University of Melbourne, Melbourne, Victoria, Australia

HEIDI M. CONNOLLY, MD
Department of Cardiovascular Medicine, Mayo Clinic, Rochester, Minnesota, USA

ANDREW CONSTANTINE, MBBS, MA, MRCP
ACHD Sub-Speciality Trainee, Royal Brompton Hospital, Royal Brompton & Harefield NHS Foundation Trust, PhD Research Fellow, The National Heart & Lung Institute, Imperial College London, London, United Kingdom

STEPHEN C. COOK, MD, FACC
Director, Adult Congenital Heart Disease Program, Congenital Heart Center, Helen DeVos Children's Hospital, Frederik Meijer Heart & Vascular Institute, Clinical Professor, Pediatrics and Human Development, Michigan State University, Grand Rapids, Michigan, USA

TIMOTHY B. COTTS, MD
Associate Professor, Internal Medicine and Pediatrics, University of Michigan, Michigan Congenital Heart Center, Ann Arbor, Michigan, USA

CURT J. DANIELS, MD
Director, COACH Program: Columbus Ohio Adult Congenital Heart Disease Program, Dottie Dohan Shepard Professor in Cardiovascular Medicine, Department of Internal Medicine and Pediatrics, The Ohio State University College of Medicine,

Nationwide Children's Hospital, Columbus, Ohio, USA

KONSTANTINOS DIMOPOULOS, MD, MSc, PhD, FESC
Consultant Cardiologist, Royal Brompton Hospital, Royal Brompton & Harefield NHS Foundation Trust, Professor of Practice in Adult Congenital Heart Disease and Pulmonary Hypertension, The National Heart & Lung Institute, Imperial College London, London, United Kingdom

SUSAN M. FERNANDES, LPD, PA-C
Adult Congenital Heart Program Stanford, Stanford Health Care, Lucile Packard Children's Hospital Stanford, Stanford University, School of Medicine, Stanford, California, USA

KRISTEN R. FOX, PhD
Center for Biobehavioral Health, Abigail Wexner Research Institute, Nationwide Children's Hospital, Columbus, Ohio, USA

MARGARET M. FUCHS, MD
Department of Cardiovascular Medicine, Mayo Clinic, Rochester, Minnesota, USA

STEPHANIE FULLER, MD, MS
Associate Professor, The Division of Cardiothoracic Surgery, Children's Hospital of Philadelphia, Perelman School of Medicine, University of Pennsylvania, Philadelphia, Pennsylvania, USA

TRACY GEOFFRION, MD, MPH
Clinical Instructor, The Division of Cardiothoracic Surgery, Children's Hospital of Philadelphia, Philadelphia, Pennsylvania, USA

MICHELLE GURVITZ, MD, MS
Assistant Professor, Pediatrics/Cardiology, Boston Children's Hospital, Harvard Medical School, Boston, Massachusetts, USA

ZIYAD M. HIJAZI, MD, MPH
Sidra Heart Center, Sidra Medicine, Doha, Qatar; Weill Cornell Medicine, Cornell University, New York, New York, USA

DANIELLE M. HILE, BS
Adult Congenital Heart Association, Media, Pennsylvania, USA

JAMIE L. JACKSON, PhD
Center for Biobehavioral Health, Abigail Wexner Research Institute, Nationwide Children's Hospital, Columbus, Ohio, USA

PAUL KHAIRY, MD, PhD
Professor of Medicine and André Chagnon Research Chair, Electrophysiology and Congenital Heart Disease, Department of Medicine, Montreal Heart Institute, Université de Montreal, Montreal, Quebec, Canada

YULI Y. KIM, MD, FACC
Medical Director, Philadelphia Adult Congenital Heart Center, Assistant Professor of Medicine, Perelman School of Medicine, University of Pennsylvania, Penn Medicine and Children's Hospital of Philadelphia, Perelman Center for Advanced Medicine, Philadelphia, Pennsylvania, USA

ADRIENNE H. KOVACS, PhD
Oregon Health & Science University, Knight Cardiovascular Institute, Portland, Oregon, USA

ERIC V. KRIEGER, MD
Associate Professor, Department of Medicine, Division of Cardiology, University of Washington School of Medicine, University of Washington Medical Center, Seattle, Washington, USA

AHMED KRIMLY, MBChB, FRCPC, ABIM
Department of Cardiology, King Faisal Cardiac Center, King Abdulaziz Medical City, Ministry of National Guard Health Affairs, Department of Medical Research, King Abdullah International Medical Research Center, Department of Medical Research, King Saud Bin Abdulaziz University for Health Science, Jeddah, Saudi Arabia

MELISSA G.Y. LEE, MBBS, PhD
Department of Cardiology, The Royal Melbourne Hospital, Heart Research, Clinical Sciences, Murdoch Children's Research Institute, Department of Paediatrics, The

University of Melbourne, Melbourne, Victoria, Australia

GEORGE K. LUI, MD
Clinical Associate Professor, Medicine, Cardiovascular Medicine Clinical Associate Professor, Pediatrics - Cardiology, The Adult Congenital Heart Program, Stanford University School of Medicine, Stanford, California, USA

ARIANE MARELLI, MD, MPH
Founder, McGill Adult Unit for Congenital Heart Disease Excellence, Professor of Medicine, Director of Cardiovascular Research, McGill University Health Center, RVH/Glen site, Montreal, Quebec, Canada

JEREMY P. MOORE, MD, MS
Associate Professor, Director, Adult Congenital Electrophysiology Program, Ahmanson-UCLA/Adult Congenital Heart Disease Center, Department of Medicine, UCLA Medical Center, Los Angeles, California, USA

VIDANG P. NGUYEN, MD
Department of Cardiology, Cedars-Sinai Heart Institute, Los Angeles, California, USA

ALEXANDER R. OPOTOWSKY, MD, MPH, MMSc
Professor, Department of Pediatrics, The Heart Institute, Cincinnati Children's Hospital, University of Cincinnati College of Medicine, Cincinnati, Ohio, USA

RAHUL RATHOD, MD
Department of Pediatrics, Harvard Medical School, Boston Children's Hospital, Boston, Massachusetts, USA

YEZAN SALAM, MBBS
College of Medicine, Alfaisal University, Riyadh, Saudi Arabia

KATHERINE B. SALCICCIOLI, MD
Adult Congenital Heart Disease Fellow, University of Michigan, Michigan Congenital Heart Center, Ann Arbor, Michigan, USA

KAREN K. STOUT, MD, FACC
Division of Cardiology, Department of
Medicine, University of Washington, Seattle,
Washington, USA

SARA K. SWANSON, MD, PhD
Assistant Professor, Pediatrics, University of
Nebraska Medical Center, Children's Hospital
& Medical Center, Nebraska Medicine, Omaha,
Nebraska, USA

ANNE MARIE VALENTE, MD
Associate Professor, Medicine and Pediatrics,
Harvard Medical School, Staff Cardiologist,
Pediatric Cardiology, Boston Children's
Hospital, Staff Cardiologist, Internal Medicine,
Division of Cardiology, Department of
Medicine, Brigham and Women's Hospital,
Boston, Massachusetts, USA

GRUSCHEN R. VELDTMAN, MBChB, FRCP
Adult Congenital Heart Disease, Heart
Centre, King Faisal Specialist Hospital
and Research Centre, Riyadh,
Saudi Arabia

ANJI T. YETMAN, MD
Professor, Pediatrics and Medicine, Director,
Aortopathy Program, University of Nebraska
Medical Center, Children's Hospital & Medical
Center, Nebraska Medicine, Omaha,
Nebraska, USA

ALI N. ZAIDI, MD
Mount Sinai Cardiovascular Institute,
The Children's Heart Center, Kravis
Children's Hospital, Icahn School of Medicine
at Mount Sinai, New York, New York,
USA

Contents

This volume is dedicated to advances in the care of adults with congenital heart disease (CHD). In this chapter the authors review the data cornerstone to the growing workforce needs. This first chapter serves as a backdrop to the second chapter that applies these observations to the planning of health care services delivery in the United States accounting for the definition and organization of multisystem expertise and centers for adults with CHD at a health systems level.

The landscape of congenital heart disease has changed rapidly over the past few decades. The shift from pediatric to adult congenital heart disease care has stretched resources and the ability to provide high-quality access and delivery of care for the more than 1.5 million adults with congenital heart disease in the United States. Meeting the demand for delivering high-quality care requires a team-based approach, with each member highly specialized. This review describes the deficits and deficiencies in providing care for adults with congenital heart disease in the United States and a team-based approach to improving access and delivery of care.

Although the majority of congenital heart disease survivors are thriving, many are at risk for declining emotional well-being as they age. Emotional distress is a risk factor for poorer health outcomes and must be addressed. Primary care and cardiology teams may be the first line of defense in identifying and providing referral resources for symptoms of depression, anxiety, and medical trauma. The current review provides information about commonly used self-report measures of emotional distress to identify symptoms that warrant referral and describes multiple options for addressing these symptoms.

 Video content accompanies this article at http://www.cardiology.theclinics.com.

Atrial septal defects are common congenital heart defects, characterized by insufficient/absent tissue at the interatrial septum. An unrepaired defect may be associated with right heart volume overload, atrial arrhythmia or pulmonary arterial hypertension.

The 3 major types of atrial septal defect are: ostium secundum defect, ostium primum defect, and sinus venosus. Characteristic physical findings include a midsystolic pulmonary flow or ejection murmur, accompanied by a fixed split-second heart sound. Small defects may spontaneously close; larger defects may persist and result in hemodynamic and clinical sequelae requiring percutaneous or surgical intervention. Severe pulmonary arterial hypertension is a contraindication to closure.

Aortopathy in Congenital Heart Disease

Timothy B. Cotts, Katherine B. Salciccioli, Sara K. Swanson, and Anji T. Yetman

Aortic dilatation is common in patients with congenital heart disease and is seen in patients with bicuspid aortic valve and those with conotruncal congenital heart defects. It is important to identify patients with bicuspid aortic valve at high risk for aortic dissection. High-risk patients include those with the aortic root phenotype and those with syndromic or familial aortopathies including Marfan syndrome, Loeys-Dietz syndrome, and Turner syndrome. Aortic dilatation is common in patients with conotruncal congenital heart defects and rarely results in aortic dissection.

Aortic Coarctation

Yuli Y. Kim, Lauren Andrade, and Stephen C. Cook

Aortic coarctation is a discrete narrowing of the thoracic aorta. In addition to anatomic obstruction, it can be considered an aortopathy with abnormal vascular properties characterized by stiffness and impaired relaxation. There are surgical and transcatheter techniques to address the obstruction but, despite relief, patients with aortic coarctation are at risk for hypertension, aortic complications, and abnormalities with left ventricular performance. This review covers the etiology, pathophysiology, diagnosis, and management of adults with aortic coarctation, with emphasis on multimodality imaging characteristics and lifelong surveillance to identify long-term complications.

Ebstein Anomaly in the Adult Patient

Margaret M. Fuchs and Heidi M. Connolly

Ebstein anomaly is a congenital malformation involving primarily the tricuspid valve, with failure of delamination from the underlying myocardium and right ventricular myopathy. Echocardiography is diagnostic in most patients and demonstrates apical displacement of the septal leaflet and variable tethering of leaflet tissue to the right ventricular myocardium. Operative intervention is considered for exertional symptoms, progressive right ventricular enlargement, or right ventricular dysfunction. Tricuspid valve cone repair is the preferred surgical approach. Tricuspid valve replacement and bidirectional cavopulmonary shunt also are considered in patients with advanced disease. Pregnancy generally is well tolerated. Patients with Ebstein anomaly require lifelong follow-up.

Tetralogy of Fallot

Eric V. Krieger and Anne Marie Valente

 Video content accompanies this article at http://www.cardiology.theclinics.com.

Repaired tetralogy of Fallot is one of the most common conditions managed by adult congenital heart disease providers. Recent comprehensive review articles and book

chapters are devoted to this topic. The purpose of this article is to address several common clinical questions encountered in the management of patients with repaired tetralogy of Fallot. These answers are not intended to supplant Practice Guidelines.

The authors summarize the most important anatomic and physiologic substrates of Fontan circulation. Common anatomic substrates include hypoplastic left heart syndrome, tricuspid atresia, double inlet left ventricle, and unbalanced atrioventricular septal defects. After the Fontan operation exercise capacity is limited and the key hemodynamic drivers is limited preload due to a relatively fixed pulmonary vascular resistance. The authors provide contemporary data on survival, morbidity, and need for reintervention. Operative morality is now expected to be less than 1% and 30 year survival approximately 89%. The authors delineate potential therapeutic approaches for the potential late complications.

This article provides a detailed review of the current practices and future directions of transcatheter interventions in adults with congenital heart disease. This includes indications for intervention, risks, and potential complications, as well as a review of available devices and their performance.

 Video content accompanies this article at http://www.cardiology.theclinics.com.

Arrhythmia management in adult congenital heart disease (ACHD) encompasses a wide range of problems from bradyarrhythmia to tachyarrhythmia, sudden death, and heart failure-related electrical dyssynchrony. Major advances in the understanding of the pathophysiology and treatments of these problems over the past decade have resulted in improved therapeutic strategies and outcomes. This article attempts to define these problems and review contemporary management for the patient with ACHD presenting with cardiac arrhythmia.

Technical and medical improvements for congenital cardiac disease in children have contributed to an increasing population of patients who survive into adulthood. These patients may be prone to progression of their native palliated disease or suffer from sequelae of their childhood repair that requires repeat surgical intervention. Surgery for adult congenital cardiac disease poses unique challenges and risks.

Pulmonary hypertension (PH) is common in adults with congenital heart disease and carries fundamental implications for management and prognosis. A high index of suspicion, combined with knowledge of the pathogenesis and pathophysiology of PH, is required to achieve a timely, accurate diagnosis, and appropriate classification and treatment. This article provides a guide on how to approach the adult with congenital heart disease and suspected PH of different types, including current management.

As the population of adult congenital heart disease patients ages and grows, so too does the burden of heart failure in this population. Despite the advances in medical and surgical therapies over the last decades, heart failure in adult congenital heart disease remains a formidable complication with high morbidity and mortality. This review focuses on the challenges in determining the true burden and management of heart failure in adult congenital heart disease. There is a particular focus on the need for developing a common language for classifying and reporting heart failure in adult congenital heart disease, the clinical presentation and prognostication of heart failure in adult congenital heart disease, the application of hemodynamic evaluation, and advanced heart failure treatment. A common case study of heart failure in adult congenital heart disease is utilized to illustrate these key concepts.

CARDIOLOGY CLINICS

SERIES OF RELATED INTEREST

Cardiac Electrophysiology Clinics
https://www.cardiacep.theclinics.com/
Heart Failure Clinics
https://www.heartfailure.theclinics.com/
Interventional Cardiology Clinics
https://www.interventional.theclinics.com/

THE CLINICS ARE AVAILABLE ONLINE!
Access your subscription at:
www.theclinics.com

CARDIOLOGY CLINICS

FORTHCOMING ISSUES

November 2020
Coronary Artery Disease
Alberto Polimeni, Editor

February 2021
Pregnancy and Heart Disease
Melinda Davis and Kathryn Lindley, Editors

RECENT ISSUES

May 2020
Right Ventricular Function and Failure
Jerry D. Estep and Miriam Jacob, Editors

February 2020
Aortic Valve Disease
Marie-Annick Clavel and Philippe Pibarot,
Editors

SERIES OF RELATED INTEREST

Cardiac Electrophysiology Clinics
https://www.cardiacep.theclinics.com/
Heart Failure Clinics
https://www.heartfailure.theclinics.com/
Interventional Cardiology Clinics
https://www.interventional.theclinics.com/

Preface

Adult Congenital Heart Disease: A Population that Has Come of Age

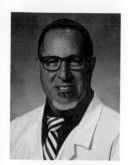

Curt J. Daniels, MD
Editor

Over the last several decades, we have witnessed a dramatic shift in the congenital heart disease population from mostly children to now adults by a two-thirds margin. The diverse anatomies and physiologies, surgical procedures, and adult co-morbidities, has created the most unique population in cardiovascular medicine - adults with congenital heart disease (ACHD). Patients with ACHD may develop complex arrhythmias, valvular heart disease, heart failure, pulmonary hypertension and require complex advanced imaging, electrophysiologic, transcatheter, and/or surgical interventions to improve their quality of life. As well, many patients with ACHD suffer from emotional distress which can affect their quality of life and place them at increased risk for cardiovascular events.

Both in the US and internationally, there has been a growing demand for a highly specialized ACHD work force, and this has led to governing bodies, professional societies, and patient advocacy organizations recognizing and partnering with providers to improve access and delivery of care. ACHD is developing as a subspecialty with specific training beyond general cardiology, board certification and ACHD program development. All of this has led to improved research efforts, care guidelines, quality metrics and measures and program criteria and accreditation.

The following issue of *Cardiology Clinics* focuses on the complexities of the ACHD population with a series of articles authored by experts from the United States and around the world. The topics include those most pertinent to understanding and caring for patients with ACHD and provide an updated resource for general cardiology and ACHD fellows, young and seasoned general cardiologists, cardiovascular subspecialists, and advanced practice providers.

Curt J. Daniels, MD
The Ohio State University
College of Medicine
Nationwide Children's Hospital
Davis Heart and Lung
Research Institute
2nd Floor Cardiology Division
473 West 12th Avenue
Columbus, OH 43210, USA

E-mail addresses:
Curt.daniels@osumc.edu
Curt.daniels@nationwidechildrens.org

Cardiol Clin 38 (2020) xiii
https://doi.org/10.1016/j.ccl.2020.05.001
0733-8651/20/© 2020 Published by Elsevier Inc.

cardiology.theclinics.com

Adult Congenital Heart Disease—Preparing for the Changing Work Force Demand

Michelle Gurvitz, MD, MS[a], George K. Lui, MD[b], Ariane Marelli, MD, MPH[c],*

KEYWORDS

• Congenital heart disease • Health care • Life course • Noncardiac surgery

KEY POINTS

- The demographics of the ACHD population continue to evolve and require a life course approach to policy and workforce planning.
- Adult congenital heart disease is a multisystem condition encompassing not only the congenital heart defect but the additional cardiac and non-cardiac morbidities that may interact with the underlying CHD.
- Establishing methods to provide, measure and improve high –quality healthcare is imperative to maintaining patient care and the appropriate workforce for adults with CHD.

INTRODUCTION

This volume is dedicated to advances in the care of adults with congenital heart disease. Scientific inquiry is new to our field relative to other forms of cardiovascular disease in adults. Non-the-less the last 2 decades have seen an exponential increase in the number of guidelines generated in several international expert groups, most recently in the US population data from a variety of jurisdictions and single center studies demonstrating the science behind the success of our field.[1] As we enter this third decade of the twenty-first century, there is a need to assemble the emerging data on several specific conditions that mandate the attention that longevity now permits. In this chapter the authors review the data cornerstone to the growing workforce needs. They first review the determinants of disease in congenital heart disease (CHD), outlining the demographic changes that underlie the growing population in terms of number of children compared with adults, the age

distribution of the population, and the emerging sex differences. They propose a life-course epidemiology framework to capture the complexity of a condition expressed variably over the stages of life. The authors then summarize the rapidly growing body of evidence that CHD in adults is a multisystemic condition with rising complication rates as patients age and develop complications at a distance from the heart. They then review quality indicators specifically developed for adults with CHD as applied to recommendations for follow-up at the patient level. This first chapter serves as a backdrop to the Susan M. Fernandes and colleagues' article, "Access and Delivery of Adult Congenital Heart Disease Care in the US: Quality Driven Team Based Care," in this issue that applies these observations to the planning of health care services delivery in the United States accounting for the definition and organization of multisystem expertise and centers for adults with CHD at a health systems level.

a Boston Adult Congenital Heart (BACH) and Pulmonary Hypertension Program, Department of Cardiology, Boston Children's Hospital, Harvard Medical School, 300 Longwood Avenue, Boston, MA 02115, USA; b Adult Congenital Heart Program Stanford, Stanford Health Care and Lucile Packard Children's Hospital Stanford, Stanford University School of Medicine, 300 Pasteur Drive, Stanford, CA 94305, USA; c McGill Adult Unit for Congenital Heart Disease Excellence (MAUDE Unit), Division of Cardiology, McGill University, RVH/Glen Site, D055108, 1001 Decarie Boulevard, Montreal, Quebec H4A3J1, Canada
* Corresponding author.
E-mail address: ariane.marelli@mcgill.ca

Cardiol Clin 38 (2020) 283–294
https://doi.org/10.1016/j.ccl.2020.04.011
0733-8651/20/© 2020 Elsevier Inc. All rights reserved.

DETERMINANTS OF HEALTH AND DISEASE IN CONGENITAL HEART DISEASE—WHAT ARE THEY?
Demographic Shifts in Age, Disease Severity, and Sex

The changing age distribution of CHD provides a powerful motivation to reorient the workforce, as demographic shifts are resulting in a growing number of adults and women with CHD. Data supporting the shift in demographics began to emerge between 2000 and 2010. On a population level, a rising prevalence of CHD in adults compared with children from 1985 to 2000 was observed, such that the number of adults and children with CHD had equalized as shown in Québec and expected to reflect national and international trends.[2] By 2010, the number of adults with severe as well as all forms of CHD exceeded the number of children, with fully two-thirds of the population being adults.[3] Using comprehensive population data sources, the life span prevalence rates of subjects with CHD were documented: 8.12 per 1000 at birth, 13.11 per 1000 in children, 6.12 per 1000 in adults, and 3.7 per 1000 in geriatric populations older than 65 years, thus warranting coining the term "Geriatric Adult Congenital Heart Disease."[4]

In the United States, working together with the Center for Disease Control and Prevention (CDC), investigators used Canadian data to estimate the magnitude of the problem, generating first-time empirical estimates. **Fig. 1** illustrates that of a total of 2.4 million subjects in the United States with CHD, 1.4 million were adults, whereas 1 million were children in 2010.[5] **Table 1** illustrates the age distribution of CHD in the United States with prevalence rates and corresponding numbers by severity of disease. Obtaining prevalence rates of 6.16 per 1000 adults older than 18 years, there were, as generated by empirical estimates in 2010, a total of 160,000 adults with severe CHD compared with 123,000 children with severe CHD underscoring the need to expand the workforce needed to care for adults with both simple and complex forms of CHD. In the United States, several methods have been and are being used to generate direct empirical measures of adult CHD (ACHD) populations.[6,7] Using capture and recapture methodology applied to 3 inpatient and outpatient data sources in 11 New York counties from 2008 to 2010, the prevalence of adolescents with CHD was 6.4 per 1000 cases.[8] Using similar methods applied to administrative records in Atlanta, Georgia counties, a prevalence rate of 6.08 per 1000 adults older than 20 years was observed in 2010.[8] Using ICD-9 codes and data sources in Atlanta, Massachusetts and New York, the proportion of patients with severe CHD seeking health care varied between 13% and 21%, which is higher than previously observed more conservative estimate of an approximate 10%.[5,7]

An important observation in population-based surveillance studies is that despite the limitations in ascertainment of gender-related health care behavior, there seems to be a predominance of women among adults with CHD, notably in the reproductive age group. **Fig. 2** illustrates a striking predominance of women compared with men in the 18- to 45-year-old age group. In 2010, there were 342,000 women compared with 236,000 men with CHD in the United States, with a higher proportion of women with severe CHD than men.[5] As part of the larger CDC surveillance initiative, 5672 pregnancies were identified in 26,655 women with CHD between the ages of 11 and 50 years. Interestingly, age-adjusted pregnancy rates did not substantially differ between women with severe and nonsevere CHD and were observed to be between 10% and 25%.[9] Moreover, pregnant women with CHD of any severity had more noncardiovascular comorbidities.[9] Sex differences in outcomes and health services utilization have been shown between men and women using the Kids Inpatients Database in the United States in children and using the Dutch CONCOR database and the Québec CHD database in adults. As where more infant men undergo high-risk cardiac procedures, surviving women have less severe forms of CHD, potentially optimizing reproductive fitness.[10] The protective effect conferred to adult women carries over into adulthood in terms of health services utilization underscoring the importance of gender-driven variations in health behavior that can affect cardiovascular disease outcomes.[11,12] Thus, there is ample empirical evidence to support the lifespan demographic framework of CHD where the same lesion expresses it differently depending on the life stage. This is so not only from childhood to adulthood but also across the developmental frames that adulthood now spans: from the young adult, to the adult of reproductive age, to middle age, and finally to advanced age.

A Life Course Epidemiology Framework

Thus, a conceptual shift is needed to consider the implications of demographic shifts in CHD across the lifespan. This poses a particular challenge on the growing workforce requirement where interdisciplinary care models need to be integrated not just vertically from primary care to specialized

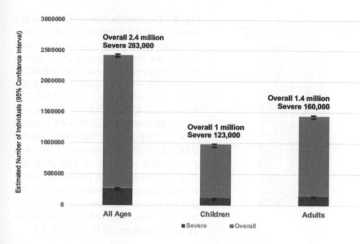

Fig. 1. The total population of CHD in the United States shown by age in children compared adults for all and for severe CHD in 2010. Corresponding prevalence rates per 1000 (CI) for all ages-overall 7.85(7.79–7.92), for all ages-severe 0.92(0.90–0.94), for children-overall 13.21(13.03–13.39), for children-severe 1.66(1.60–1.73), for adults-overall 6.16(6.10–6.22), and for adults-severe 0.68(0.66–0.70). (*Data from* Gilboa SM, Devine OJ, Kucik JE, et al. Congenital Heart Defects in the United States: Estimating the Magnitude of the Affected Population in 2010. Circulation. 2016;134:101-9.)

care but horizontally as persons with CHD progress from one life stage to another. **Fig. 3** outlines a life course epidemiology framework illustrating the developmental time frames for the expression of CHD across the lifespan.[13] Life-course epidemiology moves beyond longitudinal studies, bringing theoretic constructs that facilitate the modeling of disease events across the lifespan, improving study design and analyses.[13–15] The life course health development framework was created to shift the emphasis away from disease and toward health, with the knowledge that health is a consequence of genetic, biological, and social determinants and with the understanding that health development is an adaptive process.[14] As illustrated in **Fig. 3**, as patients with CHD move across the life stages, determinants of health include genetics, CHD severity, psychosocial health, health behavior, and the environment in addition to access to the right health care. These converge with processes of health development to determine developmental trajectories of health and expression of disease across the lifespan.[13]

Table 1
Estimated prevalence and numbers of congenital heart diseases by age, severity, and race-ethnicity in the United States in 2010

Category and Age Group	CHD Severity/ Race-Ethnicity	Estimated US Prevalence per 1000 (95% Confidence Interval) (%)	Estimated No. of Individuals (95% Confidence Interval)
CHD severity			
All ages	Overall	7.85 (7.79–7.92)	2,425,000 (2,405,000–2444 000)
	Severe	0.92 (0.90–0.94)	283000(277000–290000)
Children	Overall	13.21 (13.03–13.39)	980000 (966000–993000)
	Severe	1.66 (1.60–1.73)	123000 (119000–128000)
Adults	Overall	6.16(6.10–6.22)	1444,500 (1431,000–1459,000)
	Severe	0.68 (0.66–0.70)	160000 (155000–165000)
Race-ethnicity			
Children	Non-Hispanic white	13.31 (13.12–13.49)	620000(612000–629000)
	Non-Hispanic black	12.69 (12.50–12.88)	133000 (131,000–135000)
	Hispanic	13.26 (13.08–13.45)	227000(224000–230000)
Adults	Non-Hispanic white	6.36 (6.29–6.42)	1,104,000(1 094000–1115000)
	Non-Hispanic black	5.63 (5.56–5.69)	155000 (153000–156000)
	Hispanic	5.58(5.52–5.65)	186000 (184000–188000)

Children are those aged 0 to 17 years and adults older than or equal to 18 years.
From Gilboa SM, Devine OJ, Kucik JE, Oster ME, Riehle-Colarusso T, Nembhard WN, Xu P, Correa A, Jenkins K and Marelli AJ. Congenital Heart Defects in the United States: Estimating the Magnitude of the Affected Population in 2010. Circulation. 2016;134:101-9.

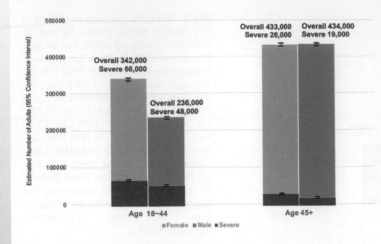

Fig. 2. The distribution of CHDs by sex showing a predominance of women of reproductive age compared with men in the United States in 2010. Corresponding prevalence rates per 1000 (CI). Women: 18~44 overall: 6.10(5.92–6.29), 18~44 severe 1.19(1.10–1.27), 45+ overall 6.70(6.58–6.81), 45+ severe 0.41(0.38–0.44). Men: 18~44 overall: 4.24 (4.08–4.40), 18~44 severe 0.88(0.81–0.96), 45+ overall: 7.59(7.46–7.72), 45+ severe: 0.33(0.30–0.36). (*Data from* Gilboa SM, Devine OJ, Kucik JE, et al. Congenital Heart Defects in the United States: Estimating the Magnitude of the Affected Population in 2010. Circulation. 2016;134:101-9.)

Shifting Mortality—Can We Do Better?

Advances in surgical and clinical management of CHD have allowed more than 90% of children to survive to adulthood, but this development has led not only to a shift but also to a swelling in mortality into adulthood.[16] Consistent with these findings, in Belgium, an analysis of survival trends by cohort and defect type was performed using administrative and clinical records. This showed that overall survival to 18 years of age for children born between 1990 and 1992 was nearly 90%,

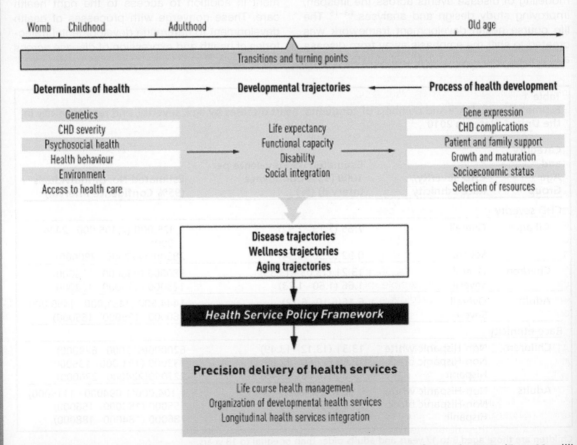

Fig. 3. Life course epidemiology framework illustrating the developmental time frames for CHD. (*From* Marellli AJ. Trajectories of Care in Congenital Heart Disease- The Long Arm of Disease in the Womb. Journal of Internal Medicine. 2020; in press.)

showing significant improvement compared with previous decades.[17] Notwithstanding this progress the question remains: is the glass half empty or half full, and what can we do about it?[18] Despite major progress in CHD mortality due to surgical interventions in children and demonstration that specialized ACHD care can improve mortality where universal health insurance optimizes access,[19] cohorts of patients with ACHD did not show the same degree of benefit as children with CHD between 1973 and 1993.[18,20] Why is this? There are likely a multitude of reasons that are summarized in **Fig. 3**. However, in order to do better there is a need for the growing work force to have access to the specialized health services that will optimize health management as disease becomes increasingly multisystemic in the aging patients with ACHD. This is underscored by the observation that in geriatric CHD populations, it has been shown that the predictors of death relate to cancer, dementia, and kidney disease, with a decreasing emphasis on heart disease itself and with an amplification of acquired cardiovascular complications.[4]

In summary, as demonstrated with population data in Canada, the United States, and Europe, there is no longer any question that CHD is a lifespan condition, with adults comprising the fastest growing segment of this population. The observation that there is a predominance of women of reproductive age compared with men compels us to consider the need for specialized obstetric care as reproductive fitness in women with CHD evolves. This life stage is one of several that patients with ACHD will experience as longevity continues to increase underscoring the need for a novel life course epidemiology construct that accounts for determinants and processes of health more comprehensively. As we seek not just to improve mortality but change outcomes with the goal of improving quality of life, there is an opportunity to address the multisystemic nature of ACHD, seeking to implement interdisciplinary care to tackle potentially reversible multisystemic cardiovascular and noncardiovascular disease complications.

ADULT CONGENITAL HEART DISEASE—A MULTISYSTEM CONDITION
Why Is the Paradigm Shifting?

ACHD is a multisystem disease. Both cardiac and noncardiovascular complications have contributed to this multisystem disease and will require lifelong surveillance (**Box 1**).[21] In a single center trial of 6969 adult patients with CHD who were followed-up between 1991 and 2013, 524

Box 1
Cardiovascular and noncardiovascular complications

Cardiovascular Complications
  Heart failure
  Arrhythmia
  Residual valvular or shunt abnormalities
  Prosthetic materials
Noncardiovascular Complications
  Endocrine
    Bone health
    Calcium hemostasis
    Diabetes
    Dyslipidemia
    Metabolic syndrome
    Obesity
    Thyroid
  Hematology
    Anemia
    Hyperuricemia
    Iron deficiency
    Secondary erythrocytosis
    Thromboembolism
  Immunology/Infectious Disease
    Brain abscess
    Endocarditis
    Pneumonia
    Protein-losing enteropathy
  Liver
    Cardiac cirrhosis
    Congestive hepatopathy
    Fontan-associated liver disease
  Lung
    Plastic bronchitis
    Pulmonary hemorrhage
    Pulmonary hypertension
    Restrictive lung disease
  Oncology
    Age-appropriate cancer screening
    Low-dose ionizing radiation and malignancy
    Hepatocellular carcinoma
  Brain
    Neurocognitive deficits

◀ Depression

　Anxiety

Renal

　Cardiorenal syndrome

　Chronic kidney disease

Vascular

　Aortopathy

　Cerebrovascular disease

　Endothelial dysfunction

　Hypertension

　Peripheral venous/arterial disease

patients died over a median follow-up of 9.1 years.[22] The leading cardiac causes of death were heart failure (42%) and sudden death (7%), whereas noncardiovascular causes were just as important, including pneumonia (10%) and cancer (6%).[22] Acquired cardiovascular risk factors such as diabetes, hypertension, and obesity will also factor into the outcome of older patients with CHD.[23] This section focuses on the multisystem disease that adults with CHD develop over the long term.

Cardiovascular Complications

Residual hemodynamic and electrophysiologic abnormalities play an important role in the cardiovascular outcome of adults with CHD. Nearly 25% of adults with CHD will develop heart failure at the age of 30 years.[24] A multitude of factors can lead to heart failure, including residual ventricular dysfunction, valvular disease, shunts, and arrhythmias. Heart failure with reduced ejection fraction is commonly seen in patients with a morphologic systemic right ventricle or a single ventricle after Fontan palliation, which is predisposed to cardiac dysfunction. Less attention has been paid to heart failure with preserved ejection fraction (HFpEF) in adults with CHD. Although more than 50% of general adult cardiology patients may be affected, HFpEF may be as prevalent in the ACHD population.[25] Fontan failure with preserved ejection fraction remains one of the most challenging types of heart failure to treat and is a marker for worse outcomes with transplantation.[26] There are opportunities to mitigate these cardiac complications through follow-up at ACHD centers, which has been shown to improve survival in this population.[19] It will be important to monitor for repeat intervention on residual hemodynamic lesions;

approximately 20% of patients with CHD will require surgery after they turn adults.[27] The most common indication for reoperation is pulmonary valve replacement in the setting of tetralogy of Fallot (TOF). These operations are often being performed earlier before the onset of symptoms in order to prevent right heart failure and arrhythmia later in adulthood.

Arrhythmia is one of the most frequent indications for hospitalization and cause of death in adults with CHD.[28] More than 50% of adults with CHD are estimated to develop an atrial tachyarrhythmia during their lifetime.[28] There is a 2% to 5% incidence per decade of sudden cardiac death (SCD) in individuals with TOF and transposition of the great arteries after atrial switch.[28,29] Monitoring for arrhythmias and the use of invasive electrophysiologic procedures can be important in risk stratifying individuals with CHD who may be at risk for SCD. Although moderate and complex defects are more likely to suffer from cardiovascular complications, simple defects are not immune. The risk of endocarditis persists lifelong for all defects,[30] with even small unoperated ventricular septal defects having a risk of infective endocarditis (IE) that is 20 to 30 times that of the general population.[31] Guideline-based antibiotic prophylaxis remains important in the reduction of IE risk over a lifetime as well as a low threshold to obtain blood cultures in individuals with CHD before antibiotic treatment in the setting of fever of unknown origin. The importance of routine dental care and updated vaccinations are important preventative strategies.

Noncardiovascular Complications

Noncardiovascular complications are increasingly prevalent in adults with CHD with nearly all organ systems affected (**Fig. 4**). More than 40% to 50% of adults with CHD are noted to have abnormal renal and pulmonary function tests.[32,33] These noncardiac conditions have more than doubled in patients with CHD who have been hospitalized between 1998 and 2010.[34] Renal dysfunction, restrictive lung disease, anemia, and liver cirrhosis have all been associated with reduced survival in patients with CHD.[21] Both cardiac and noncardiac surgery can be affected by these noncardiac comorbidities with an increased likelihood of developing acute renal failure, pneumonia, and respiratory failure postoperatively.[35] Unique endocrine and immunologic complications are seen in individuals with CHD with genetic syndromes.[36] Patients with CHD with residual cyanosis are the most vulnerable to noncardiovascular complications affecting nearly all organ systems including unique complications from

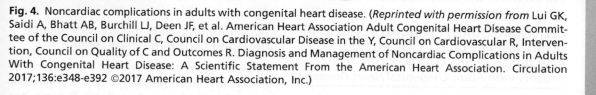

Fig. 4. Noncardiac complications in adults with congenital heart disease. (*Reprinted with permission from* Lui GK, Saidi A, Bhatt AB, Burchill LJ, Deen JF, et al. American Heart Association Adult Congenital Heart Disease Committee of the Council on Clinical C, Council on Cardiovascular Disease in the Y, Council on Cardiovascular R, Intervention, Council on Quality of C and Outcomes R. Diagnosis and Management of Noncardiac Complications in Adults With Congenital Heart Disease: A Scientific Statement From the American Heart Association. Circulation 2017;136:e348-e392 ©2017 American Heart Association, Inc.)

secondary erythrocytosis.[21] Cancer is the second leading cause of noncardiovascular death in adults with CHD.[22] The prevalence of cancer in adults with CHD in Québec is 1.6 to 2 times higher than that of the general population.[37] Risk factors likely include prior radiation exposure, genetic factors, and even unique CHD repairs such as the Fontan palliation, which has been associated with hepatocellular carcinoma.[21] Neurodevelopmental deficits increase in frequency and severity with CHD complexity. There is significant research on the

prevalence and types of neurodevelopmental disabilities in children and young adolescents and a growing body of evidence on the impact of CHD on the brain of patients with ACHD.[38,39] Not only is there an increased incidence of stroke in patients with ACHD,[40] but recent evidence suggests the possibility of an accrued risk of dementia[41] potentially mitigated by the cumulative burden of vascular complications in the brain of patients with CHD.[38] In addition, more than one-third of adults with CHD have reported a mood or anxiety disorder.[42] Both cognitive challenges and psychosocial distress can have profound effects on health care, education, employment, and overall quality of life of patients with CHD. Finally, as the number of adults with CHD older than 65 years increases, acquired cardiovascular diseases will have a significant impact; more than 80% of adults with CHD have more than one atherosclerotic cardiovascular risk factor.[43] Adult comorbidities such as diabetes, coronary artery disease, and hypertension will begin to shift how practitioners who once only focused on the late cardiac sequelae of CHD to managing a multisystem disease including both cardiovascular and noncardiovascular complications of adults with CHD.

In summary, the key to management of extracardiac complications is early detection, which requires an interdisciplinary team with expertise in disciplines such as hepatology, immunology, pulmonology, and nephrology as well as familiarity with complex CHD. The integration of mental health providers into ACHD care teams provide an opportunity for early identification and management of psychosocial distress. In order to improve the long-term outcome of this vulnerable patient population, understanding and managing noncardiovascular complications becomes as important as knowing their cardiac history. As these individuals grow in numbers and age, we need to identify preventative strategies with intervention at an earlier age to mitigate the development of later cardiovascular and noncardiovascular complications. Thus, processes of care become key drivers of the quality of the care that we can plan to deliver. This is especially important as we implement quality improvement (QI) initiatives in partnership with the growing number of care givers that the ACHD workforce mandates.

DELIVERING QUALITY IN ADULT CONGENITAL HEART DISEASE CARE—CAN WE DO IT?
How Do We Define Quality of Care for Patients with Adult Congenital Heart Disease?

Quality of care was defined by the Institute of Medicine (IOM) as "the degree to which health services for individuals and populations increase the likelihood of desired health outcomes and are consistent with current professional knowledge."[44] The basic tenets of delivering quality care from the IOM include that care should be safe, effective, patient centered, timely, efficient, and equitable.[45] Because these tenets were developed in the early 1990s, health care systems and providers have adapted practices to ensure these goals come to fruition. In earlier decades, quality care for CHD used to mean survival. However, with survival to adulthood approaching 90%, the focus of care has turned to addressing morbidity and long-term outcomes, patient experience, and quality of life. Thus, the focus of quality of care has also shifted to include these aspects of care beyond survival.

The foundational aspects of quality of care assessment are based in the models of Donabedian[46] and, more recently, Porter.[47] The Donabedian model frames quality of care into 3 specific areas: structure, process, and outcome. Structure involves the physical context of the health care system including who is seeing patient, in what types of locations, and with what equipment. Process includes the technical aspects of health care delivery including timing and types of testing, procedures and medications, and how patients flow through the system. Outcome includes both that of the patient and the health care system, including aspects such as mortality, clinical outcomes, costs, and efficiency. The Porter model adds on value-based health care and the idea that health care should be centered on outcomes that matter to patients and the costs to achieve those outcomes.

One way to bring these quality assessments into practice is to break them down to 3 components: quality measurement, quality reporting, and QI. Quality measurement is a retrospective approach to assess the quality of care delivered, which may include the proportion of women receiving recommended screening mammography or proportion of people offered flu shots each year. Quality reporting is the transparent approach to sharing quality measurement data to inform future efforts. QI is a prospective approach to improving care to individual patients and health care systems, which might include implementation of decision support tools for mammogram or flu shot reminders.

Importance of Quality of Care for Patients with Adult Congenital Heart Disease

In ACHD, developing consistent mechanisms to measure and improve quality of care is particularly important but also complicated. ACHD comprises patients not only with a great variety of underlying congenital heart conditions but also a variety of treatment strategies. Even for the same underlying conditions, treatment strategies may vary based on the era of birth and the available surgical intervention at that time or in that geographic area. For example, a patient born in 1990 with d-loop transposition of the great arteries may have undergone 1 of 2 surgeries depending on the surgical services available to them at the time. Similarly, a patient with tetralogy of Fallot born in the 1950s would likely have undergone a Blalock-Taussig shunt in infancy or childhood followed by eventual intracardiac repair where a patient born in the 2000s would have had a single intracardiac repair in infancy.

Also contributing to the complexity of devising and delivering quality care to patients with ACHD is the large proportion of patients who have gaps in care or are lost to follow-up and the different types of providers who care for patients with ACHD in adulthood. More than 40% of patients with CHD have gaps in congenital cardiac care of greater than 3 years[48] and these lapses in care start as early as childhood.[49] These lapses in care can change the trajectory of the condition, as those with gaps are more likely to require urgent interventions on return to congenital heart care.[50] Furthermore, as patients with CHD transition to adulthood, many are unable or unaware of the need to find a cardiologist specializing in congenital heart care. Many patients end up in general cardiology care, primary care, or no medical care at all, and the specific needs for the patient with ACHD may not be recognized or met. This is most evident in the care of patients with ACHD with underlying complex CHD where maintaining specialized ACHD care has a documented survival benefit.[19]

The tremendous underlying variation in disease, treatment, and care provision, providing a foundational way to measure and improve quality in this population, is of great importance. Specific quality measures and reporting can also provide consistency in data collection for process and outcomes that are critical for further research and data acquisition. This information can be used to design studies and refine care processes for improvement in ACHD care as well as provide feedback to improve care in pediatrics.

Quality Initiatives in Adult Congenital Heart Disease Care

With the recognition of the need and importance for quality assessment in ACHD care, there have been multiple initiatives to measure and improve quality of care over the past few decades. A key feature of quality of care planning is that information must be easy to spread to many different types of providers across the community. These efforts started with the development of guidelines for care for the patients with ACHD published in Canada[51] and Europe[52] that are being updated. They have been updated in 2018 in the United States to include information about clinical management for the different CHD conditions as well as different types of repairs.[1] Some of the guidelines also include components related to specialized ACHD program design and support.

Additional papers have been published evaluating guideline adherence in different countries. Although guidelines do not substitute for quality measures, they do provide a foundation for consistency of care and for the design of quality measures and QI activities. The observation that adherence to clinical practice guidelines is highly variable for patients with ACHD underscores the heterogeneity of the patient population and the need for more individualized approaches to care as data continue to evolve.[53,54]

Based on the available guidelines at the time, ambulatory quality measures for 6 ACHD conditions were developed in 2013.[55] The conditions included atrial septal defect, coarctation of the aorta, d-loop transposition of the great arteries, tetralogy of Fallot, Fontan procedure, and Eisenmenger syndrome. These measures were developed using the RAND-modified Delphi method[56] and resulted in 55 total measures for ambulatory care across the 6 conditions. Subsequent to this, additional studies have been performed evaluating electronic data collection of measures and implementation of care processes across populations. The measures can also serve as a foundation to design and implement QI projects.

In addition to the quality assessment for processes and outcomes of clinical care described, there have been efforts in ACHD to ensure consistency of training and resources across ACHD providers and programs. Until 2012, there were no criteria for specialized adult congenital heart disease training for health care providers; fellowships existed but were not standardized across programs for content, duration, or competencies. After significant effort by ACHD providers, the American Board of Medical Specialties approved adult congenital heart disease as separate board-certified medical specialty in 2012 and the first board examination was administered in 2015.[57] This has resulted in hundreds of board-certified ACHD specialists across the country and multiple consistent fellowship training programs. In addition to specialty certification for individuals, the Adult Congenital Heart Association, the largest ACHD patient advocacy organization in the United States, worked with its medical advisory board to develop accreditation criteria for ACHD programs across the United States to improve quality and consistency of care across programs and across the country.[58] There are currently 35 accredited programs across 23 states.

In summary, quality assessment has many components including measurement, reporting, and improvement. Efforts in multiple types of quality of care have been developed in ACHD, resulting in quality measures to use for assessment and improvement initiatives as well as building consistency in training and resources across providers and programs. These efforts provide a foundation but will need to go further to improve processes and outcomes in all aspects of care including inpatient, outpatient, and procedures.

SUMMARY AND FUTURE DIRECTIONS

The demographic shifts in the ACHD population are rapidly changing in the United States, with a predominance of adults compared with children (see **Fig. 1**; see **Table 1**). This mandates the need for more adult cardiology care providers with expertise in CHD, a condition considered largely in the prevue of pediatric cardiologist just more than 30 years ago. There is predominance of women (see **Fig. 2**) where sex and gender determinants of outcomes will need to be accounted for in addition to the growing expertise that will be needed in specialized obstetric care. It is becoming increasingly evident that ACHD is a multisystem condition with a myriad of cardiovascular complications but also a growing body of evidence that support the clinical observations of complications distal to the heart including, metabolic complications, liver and kidney disease, vascular health, complications along the heart-brain axis, and cancer (see **Fig. 4**; see **Box 1**). Without a doubt managing multisystem disease will require the close collaboration of interdisciplinary teams where there is ongoing communication not only between pediatric and adult providers but also between adult subspecialties in cardiovascular and other medical subspecialties. Cost containment for populations with chronic, lifelong morbidity challenges our ability to sustain delivery of high-quality care underscoring the need for process-related measures of care quality such as that have been developed for ACHD outpatient management. Surveillance that is patient centered and sufficiently standardized to ensure that care is delivered commensurate with guideline recommendations is critical to prevention of complications but also challenging for a group of patients who are largely active and mobile. This requires organization of care at a systems level in a way that is well aligned with country-specific health insurance models.

As the body of evidence grows that CHD is a dynamic life-long complex series of pathophysiological disturbances, so too the need for shift in conceptual models that will underpin future research directions. As illustrated in **Fig. 3**, the life stages that a patient with CHD lives through

require numerous transitions and turning points in their health management journey. Determinants of health are complex as are the processes of health development for this patient population. Ultimately, the goals of the workforce are to improve life-expectancy and functional capacity, reduce disability, and promote social integration of people with CHD. Increasingly, our interest is not only in improving disease trajectories but also in maximizing wellness trajectories and minimizing biological aging trajectories. This serves as a health services policy framework that moves toward the precision delivery of health services to provide cost-effective life course health management, organized around developmental time frames that will promote the longitudinal integration of health services across the lifespan.[59]

DISCLOSURE

The authors declare no conflict of interest.

REFERENCES

1. Stout KK, Daniels CJ, Aboulhosn JA, et al. 2018 AHA/ACCguideline for the management of adults with congenital heart disease: executive summary: a report of the American College of Cardiology/American Heart Association Task Force on clinical practice guidelines. Circulation 2019;139:e637–97.
2. Marelli AJ, Mackie AS, Ionescu-Ittu R, et al. Congenital heart disease in the general population: changing prevalence and age distribution. Circulation 2007;115:163–72.
3. Marelli AJ, Ionescu-Ittu R, Mackie AS, et al. Lifetime prevalence of congenital heart disease in the general population from 2000 to 2010. Circulation 2014;130:749–56.
4. Afilalo J, Therrien J, Pilote L, et al. Geriatric congenital heart disease: burden of disease and predictors of mortality. J Am CollCardiol 2011;58:1509–15.
5. Gilboa SM, Devine OJ, Kucik JE, et al. Congenital Heart Defects in the United States: estimating the magnitude of the affected population in 2010. Circulation 2016;134:101–9.
6. Raskind-Hood C, Hogue C, Overwyk KJ, et al. Estimates of adolescent and adult congenital heart defect prevalence in metropolitan Atlanta, 2010, using capture-recapture applied to administrative records. Ann Epidemiol 2019;32:72–77 e2.
7. Glidewell J, Book W, Raskind-Hood C, et al. Population-based surveillance of congenital heart defects among adolescents and adults: surveillance methodology. BirthDefects Res 2018;110:1395–403.
8. Akkaya-Hocagil T, Hsu WH, Sommerhalter K, et al. Utility of capture-recapture methodology to estimate prevalence of congenital heart defects among

adolescents in 11 New York State Counties: 2008 to 2010. BirthDefects Res 2017;109:1423–9.

9. Raskind-Hood C, Saraf A, Riehle-Colarusso T, et al. Assessing pregnancy, gestational complications, and co-morbidities in women with congenital heart defects (data from ICD-9-CM Codes in 3 US surveillance sites). Am J Cardiol 2020;125:812–9.

10. Marelli A, Gauvreau K, Landzberg M, et al. Sex differences in mortality in children undergoing congenital heart disease surgery: a United States population-based study. Circulation 2010;122: S234–40.

11. Zomer AC, Ionescu-Ittu R, Vaartjes I, et al. Sex differences in hospital mortality in adults with congenital heart disease: the impact of reproductive health. J Am CollCardiol 2013;62:58–67.

12. Pelletier R, Khan NA, Cox J, et al. Sex versus gender-related characteristics: which predicts outcome after acute coronary syndrome in the young? J Am CollCardiol 2016;67:127–35.

13. Marellli AJ.Trajectories of Care in Congenital Heart Disease- The Long Arm of Disease in the Womb. Journal of Internal Medicine 2020. https://doi.org/10.1111/joim.13048.

14. Halfon N, Hochstein M. Life course health development: an integrated framework for developing health, policy, and research. Milbank Q 2002;80: 433–79, iii.

15. Kuh D, Ben-Shlomo Y, Lynch J, et al. Life course epidemiology. J EpidemiolCommunityHealth 2003; 57:778–83.

16. Khairy P, Ionescu-Ittu R, Mackie AS, et al. Changing mortality in congenital heart disease. J Am CollCardiol 2010;56:1149–57.

17. Moons P, Bovijn L, Budts W, et al. Temporal trends in survival to adulthood among patients born with congenital heart disease from 1970 to 1992 in Belgium. Circulation 2010;122:2264–72.

18. Cohen S, Marelli A. Increasing survival in patients with congenital heart disease-a glass half full or half empty? JAMA Intern Med 2017;177:1690–1.

19. Mylotte D, Pilote L, Ionescu-Ittu R, et al. Specialized adult congenital heart disease care: the impact of policy on mortality. Circulation 2014; 129:1804–12.

20. Mandalenakis Z, Rosengren A, Skoglund K, et al. Survivorship in Children and young adults with congenital heart disease in Sweden. JAMA Intern Med 2017;177:224–30.

21. Lui GK, Saidi A, Bhatt AB, et al, American Heart Association Adult Congenital Heart Disease Committee of the Council on Clinical Cardiology and Council on Cardiovascular Disease in the Young; Council on Cardiovascular Radiology and Intervention; and Council on Quality of Care and Outcomes Research. Diagnosis and management of noncardiac complications in adults with congenital heart disease: a scientific statement from the American Heart Association. Circulation 2017;136:e348–92.

22. Diller GP, Kempny A, Alonso-Gonzalez R, et al. Survival prospects and circumstances of death in contemporary adult congenital heart disease patients under follow-up at a large tertiary centre. Circulation 2015;132:2118–25.

23. Lui GK, Fernandes S, McElhinney DB. Management of cardiovascular risk factors in adults with congenital heart disease. J Am Heart Assoc 2014;3: e001076.

24. Norozi K, Wessel A, Alpers V, et al. Incidence and risk distribution of heart failure in adolescents and adults with congenital heart disease after cardiac surgery. Am J Cardiol 2006;97:1238–43.

25. Vaikunth SS, Lui GK. Heart failure with reduced and preserved ejection fraction in adult congenital heart disease. Heart Fail Rev 2019. https://doi.org/10.1007/s10741-019-09904-z.

26. Griffiths ER, Kaza AK, Wyler von Ballmoos MC, et al. Evaluating failing Fontans for heart transplantation: predictors of death. Ann Thorac Surg 2009;88: 558–63 [discussion: 563–4].

27. Zomer AC, Verheugt CL, Vaartjes I, et al. Surgery in adults with congenital heart disease. Circulation 2011;124:2195–201.

28. Khairy P, Van Hare GF, Balaji S, et al. PACES/HRS expert Consensus statement on the recognition and management of arrhythmias in adult congenital heart disease: developed in partnership between the pediatric and congenital Electrophysiology Society (PACES) and the heart Rhythm Society (HRS). Endorsed by the governing bodies of PACES, HRS, the American College of Cardiology (ACC), the American Heart Association (AHA), the European Heart Rhythm Association (EHRA), the Canadian Heart Rhythm Society (CHRS), and the International Society for Adult Congenital Heart Disease (ISACHD). Heart Rhythm 2014;11:e102–65.

29. Silka MJ, Bar-Cohen Y. A contemporary assessment of the risk for sudden cardiac death in patients with congenital heart disease. PediatrCardiol 2012;33:452–60.

30. Verheugt CL, Uiterwaal CS, van der Velde ET, et al. Mortality in adult congenital heart disease. Eur Heart J 2010;31:1220–9.

31. Berglund E, Johansson B, Dellborg M, et al. High incidence of infective endocarditis in adults with congenital ventricular septal defect. Heart 2016; 102(22):1835–9.

32. Dimopoulos K, Diller GP, Koltsida E, et al. Prevalence, predictors, and prognostic value of renal dysfunction in adults with congenital heart disease. Circulation 2008;117:2320–8.

33. Alonso-Gonzalez R, Borgia F, Diller GP, et al. Abnormal lung function in adults with congenital heart disease: prevalence, relation to cardiac

anatomy, and association with survival. Circulation 2013;127:882–90.

34. O'Leary JM, Siddiqi OK, de Ferranti S, et al. The changing demographics of congenital heart disease hospitalizations in the United States, 1998 through 2010. JAMA 2013;309:984–6.

35. Maxwell BG, Wong JK, Kin C, et al. Perioperative outcomes of major noncardiac surgery in adults with congenital heart disease. Anesthesiology 2013;119:762–9.

36. Fort P, Lifshitz F, Bellisario R, et al. Abnormalities of thyroid function in infants with Down syndrome. J Pediatr 1984;104:545–9.

37. Gurvitz M, Ionescu-Ittu R, Guo L, et al. Prevalence of cancer in adults with congenital heart disease compared with the general population. Am J Cardiol 2016;118(11):1742–50.

38. Marelli A, Miller SP, Marino BS, et al. Brain in congenital heart disease across the lifespan: the cumulative burden of injury. Circulation 2016;133:1951–62.

39. Keir M, Ebert P, Kovacs AH, et al. Neurocognition in adult congenital heart disease: how to monitor and prevent progressive decline. Can J Cardiol 2019; 35:1675–85.

40. Lanz J, Brophy JM, Therrien J, et al. Stroke in adults with congenital heart disease: incidence, cumulative risk, and predictors. Circulation 2015;132:2385–94.

41. Bagge CN, Henderson VW, Laursen HB, et al. Risk of dementia in adults with congenital heart disease: population-based cohort study. Circulation 2018; 137:1912–20.

42. Kovacs AH, Saidi AS, Kuhl EA, et al. Depression and anxiety in adult congenital heart disease: predictors and prevalence. Int J Cardiol 2009;137:158–64.

43. Moons P, Van Deyk K, Dedroog D, et al. Prevalence of cardiovascular risk factors in adults with congenital heart disease. Eur J CardiovascPrevRehabil 2006;13:612–6.

44. Blumenthal D. Part 1: quality of care–what is it? N Engl J Med 1996;335:891–4.

45. Institute of Medicine (U.S.).Committee on Quality of Health Care in America. Crossing the quality chasm : a new health system for the 21st century. Washington, D.C.: National Academy Press; 2001.

46. Donabedian A. The quality of care.howcan it be assessed? JAMA 1988;260:1743–8.

47. Porter ME. What is value in health care? N Engl J Med 2010;363:2477–81.

48. Gurvitz M, Valente AM, Broberg C, et al. Prevalence and predictors of gaps in care among adult congenital heart disease patients: HEART-ACHD (The Health, Education, and Access Research Trial). J Am CollCardiol 2013;61:2180–4.

49. Mackie AS, Ionescu-Ittu R, Therrien J, et al. Children and adults with congenital heart disease lost to follow-up: who and when? Circulation 2009;120: 302–9.

50. Yeung E, Kay J, Roosevelt GE, et al. Lapse of care as a predictor for morbidity in adults with congenital heart disease. Int J Cardiol 2008;125:62–5.

51. Silversides CK, Marelli A, Beauchesne L, et al. Canadian Cardiovascular Society 2009 Consensus Conference on the management of adults with congenital heart disease: executive summary. Can J Cardiol 2010;26:143–50.

52. Baumgartner H, Bonhoeffer P, De Groot NM, et al. ESC Guidelines for the management of grown-up congenital heart disease (new version 2010). Eur Heart J 2010;31:2915–57.

53. Gerardin JF, Menk JS, Pyles LA, et al. Compliance with adult congenital heart disease guidelines: are we following the recommendations? CongenitHeart Dis 2016;11:245–53.

54. Engelfriet P, Tijssen J, Kaemmerer H, et al. Adherence to guidelines in the clinical care for adults with congenital heart disease: the Euro Heart Survey on adult congenital heart disease. Eur Heart J 2006; 27(6):737–45.

55. Gurvitz M, Marelli A, Mangione-Smith R, et al. Building quality indicators to improve care for adults with congenital heart disease. J Am CollCardiol 2013;62: 2244–53.

56. Brook RH, McGlynn EA, Cleary PD. Quality of health care. Part 2: measuring quality of care. N Engl J Med 1996;335:966–70.

57. SpecialtiesABoM.2018-2019 ABMS Board Certification Report. 2012;2020. Available at: https:// www.abms.org/board-certification/abms-board-certification-report/.

58. Association ACH. ACHA Launches National Accreditation Program. 2017;2020. Available at: https://www. achaheart.org/provider-support/accreditation-program/.

59. Marelli A. The future of adult congenital heart disease research: precision health services delivery for the next decade. Can J Cardiol 2019;35: 1609–19.

Access and Delivery of Adult Congenital Heart Disease Care in the United States: Quality-Driven Team-Based Care

Susan M. Fernandes, LPD, PA-C[a],*, Ariane Marelli, MD, MPH[b],
Danielle M. Hile, BS[c], Curt J. Daniels, MD[d]

KEYWORDS

- Adult congenital heart disease • Access and delivery of care • Care models

KEY POINTS

- The adult congenital heart disease (ACHD) population has surpassed current abilities to provide high-quality care.
- To improve access and delivery of high-quality care requires developing and growing ACHD centers in areas of greatest need.
- The ACHD centers of excellence (accredited centers) are grounded in a team-based approach to deliver care.

As described by Marelli and colleagues,[1] the number of adult congenital heart disease (ACHD) patients are growing at a rate faster than those with pediatric congenial heart disease (CHD). These ACHD patients are highly complex, suffer from multi organ disease and require great cardiovascular (CV) care and ACHD expertise. The ability to provide high-quality ACHD care in many areas of the United States is challenging due to a limited number of providers and numerous access to care issues. ACHD as a subspecialty in the United States produced fewer than 100 ACHD cardiologists over 2 decades and fell behind the rising ACHD patient population. More recently, with board certification and certified training pathways, the quality of ACHD care is improving, but access to this care remains well behind patient demand.

Meeting the demands for access to high-quality ACHD care will require not only a focus on increasing the numbers of ACHD cardiologists but also expanding the use of team-based care (TBC). This article defines ACHD TBC, discusses the various team specialists and their responsibilities, demonstrates current gaps in care, and describes areas of need for the future.

TEAM APPROACH TO CARE IN ADULT CONGENITAL HEART DISEASE

The care of adults with CHD, in particular those with more complex disease, requires a capable team that can work together to provide high-quality patient-centered care. TBC, the "provision of health services to individuals, families, and

---

[a] Adult Congenital Heart Program Stanford, Stanford Health Care, Lucile Packard Children's Hospital Stanford, Stanford University, School of Medicine, 150 Governor's Lane, Stanford, CA 94305, USA; [b] McGill Adult Unit for Congenital Heart Disease Excellence (MAUDE Unit), Division of Cardiology, McGill University, RVH/Glen Site, D055108, 1001 Decarie Boulevard, Montreal, Quebec H4A3J1, Canada; [c] Adult Congenital Heart Association, 280 North Providence Road, Suite 6, Media, PA 19063, USA; [d] Columbus Ohio Adult Congenital Heart Disease Program, Department of Internal Medicine and Pediatrics, The Ohio State University, Nationwide Children's Hospital, 451 West 10th Avenue, Columbus, OH 43210, USA
* Corresponding author.
E-mail address: sfernandes@stanford.edu

Cardiol Clin 38 (2020) 295–304
https://doi.org/10.1016/j.ccl.2020.04.012

communities by at least two health providers who work collaboratively with patients and their caregivers to accomplish shared goals and achieve coordinated, high-quality care," has been shown to improve patient care and efficiency while decreasing costs.[2] In CV medicine, TBC has been associated with improvements in medication compliance, care outcomes, and quality of life and with decreased health care costs.[3,4]

TBC has not been studied specifically in the ACHD population but has been accepted as best practice. One of the main goals of the International Society for Adult Congenital Heart Disease is "to promote a holistic team-based approach to the care of the adult with congenital heart disease that is, comprehensive, patient-centered, and interdisciplinary."[5] The Adult Congenital Heart Association (ACHA) ACHD Accreditation Program (www.achaheart.org) also highlights the importance of the TBC, requiring more than 10 different types of providers to meet criteria for program accreditation.

The CHD patient experience with the health system spans pediatric and adult hospitals and takes place in ambulatory, inpatient, and critical care units; operating rooms; advanced imaging suites; and cardiac catheterization, electrophysiology, and exercise testing laboratories. In these settings, they interact with a wide range of providers, including but not limited to surgeons, anesthesiologists, physician assistants (PAs), nurse practitioners (NPs), nurses, pharmacists, technicians, a wide range of congenital and internal medicine cardiologists, and numerous internal medicine subspecialty providers. With the complexity of providing ACHD care, it would be easy for patients to interact with these environments and providers in isolation, but high-performing programs put the ACHD patient in the center of care, with the team members communicating with the patient and each other. Anchoring the model of TBC in ACHD is the core ACHD team (**Table 1**), which typically includes ACHD cardiologists, NPs or PAs, nurses, psychologists, social workers, and administrative support. This front-line team provides patients 24/7 access, coordinates care, and ensures that all physical and emotional needs are addressed. The ACHD cardiologist typically is the leader of this team, providing oversight for the medical care provided by team members, guiding members to function at the top of their skill set, and providing feedback and space for ongoing professional development. Each member of the team, however, should be seen as a potential leader. When a patient care scenario arises for which another member of the team has the best-suited training and expertise to guide the team, that member should be encouraged to step forward into that role. A well-functioning team has shared purpose or goals, effective leadership, communication, cohesion, and mutual respect. They are open to the professional contributions of each team member while recognizing and respecting their unique skills.[6]

ADULT CONGENITAL HEART DISEASE ADMINISTRATIVE SUPPORT

Each member of the ACHD team plays an integral role. Although administrative positions are not required for ACHA ACHD program accreditation, 89% of programs reported having at least 1 person dedicated to an administrative role. This administrative support person often is the first person an ACHD patient interacts with and can set the tone for future interactions with the team. How programs utilize administrative support is highly variable, although frequently this person is in charge of complex scheduling, data gathering, processing paperwork for insurance authorizations and disability approval, and calendar tracking of patient admissions, surgeries, and other procedures. They can guide other schedulers (such as surgical schedulers) in balancing activities for the ACHD team so that adequate resources are available for ACHD consultation. In addition, the administrative support person typically manages the team calendar (team meetings, on-call and on-service times, vacations, and so forth), identifies and books meeting rooms, orders office supplies, and provides additional administrative support services as requested. The title of this administrative role within the ACHD team varies from program to program, with administrative coordinator, patient care coordinator, operations specialist, and administrative associate a few of the common titles.

Over the past few years, there has been an increasing number of programs hiring an administrative program director or manager. Currently, 66% of accredited ACHD programs report having someone in this role. Typically, this person has managerial, financial, and business strategy experience. In partnership with the ACHD medical director, this administrative leadership person can manage program performance tracking (volume and finances), provide justification for additional resources, and identify and support opportunities for growth. They can provide leadership for process improvement projects to optimize efficiency and patient satisfaction. Their direct reporting to hospital administration provides an opportunity for the ACHD team to have visibility at the hospital leadership level and a voice at the decision-making table. This is true particularly when the

Table 1
Team-based care in adult congenital heart disease core team roles

Role	
Administrative support • Administrative coordinator • Patient care coordinator • Operations specialist • Administrative associate	• Performs basic and complex scheduling • Manages data • Obtains outside medical records, imaging, and testing results • Manages support data (volume tracking and finances) • Processes paperwork (insurance and disability) • Manages calendar (patient and team) • Acts as liaison to procedural schedulers • Performs general administrative tasks
Administrative leadership • Program manager • Program director	• Provides managerial, financial, and business support for the ACHD program • Provides leadership for program vision and strategy initiatives • Manages data and database • Tracks activities to support justification for additional resources • Processes improvement activities • Acts as liaison to institutional administrative leadership • Provides leadership for program accreditation initiation and compliance
Nurse coordinator	• Coordinates care • Tracks testing and ensures patients follow and timely review of test results • Manages active patient list • Triages phone • Provides clinic support • Provides patient education • Provides counselling • Coordinates ACHD research and scholarly output • Provides ACHD community engagement
Mental health professional • Social worker • Psychologist	• Evaluates, diagnoses, and provides treatment of mental and emotional disorders • Assesses intellectual functioning (psychologist) • Provides psychotherapy and counseling • Connects patients to local resources (social worker) • Provides logistical support, such as transportation and accommodations (social worker) • Processes insurance and disability paperwork (social worker and nurse case manager) • Provides support for completing legal documents, such as advanced directive (social worker) • Coordinates ACHD research and scholarly output • Provides ACHD community engagement
APP • NP • PA	• Assesses, diagnoses, and manages ACHD patients across all health care settings • Orders and interprets CV testing • Provides patient education • Coordinates ACHD research and scholarly output • Provides ACHD community engagement

(continued on next page)

Table 1 (continued)
Role
ACHD cardiologist

ACHD cardiologist
- Provides leadership for the ACHD team
- Assesses, diagnoses, and manages ACHD patients across all health care settings
- Performs and interprets invasive and noninvasive cardiovascular testing
- Coordinates ACHD research and scholarly output
- Provides ACHD community engagement
- Provides leadership for program vision and strategy initiatives (medical director)
- Provides leadership for activities to improve care quality (medical director)

role is a director-level position. Likely a driving force behind programs adding this type of role is to support initial ACHD program accreditation and to ensure future compliance. Approximately half of those listed in this administrative leadership role, within accredited programs, have administrative backgrounds. The remaining individuals have clinical backgrounds as well, allowing them to carry out the responsibilities, discussed previously, and to provide oversight of the nonphysician members of the ACHD team. This administrative leader benefits programs because they are acutely aware of program needs and the roles of each team member, allowing them to advocate effectively for additional resources as needed. They also can provide data and advocate to keep members from being pulled to other programs or service lines.

NURSE COORDINATOR

In acknowledgment of the vital role that nurses play in the care of the ACHD patients, accreditation requirements mandate that all programs have a full-time dedicated ACHD nurse. In most programs, this role is best described as a nurse coordinator. A 2017 article by Sillman and colleagues,[7] which includes input from nurses representing 10 ACHD programs from 8 countries, provides a comprehensive overview of the essential skills provided by the ACHD nurse coordinator. The nurse coordinator works in tandem with other members of the ACHD team, with the main focus of their activities centered around care coordination, phone triage, patient education, and counseling. There frequently is some overlap between the nurse coordinator and the advanced practice provider (APP) (NP or PA) role in ACHD programs. When nurse coordinators are utilized to their full level of expertise and practice scope, however,

that allows an NP or PA to focus on increasing access to care. Given the shortage of ACHD providers, optimization of each member's role is crucial.

The care coordination provided by the nurse coordinator is supported by the administrative team as the nurse coordinates complex assessments that may require multiple specialists and procedures. They place orders for cosignatures, ensure that patients follow through on recommendations, and ensure that testing results are reviewed promptly by the ACHD providers. Typically, the nurse coordinator is responsible for keeping the active patient list and preparing the list for team meetings while providing updates at these team meetings as needed. The nurse coordinator typically spends large portions of the day triaging patient calls, typically filtered by the administrative team so that only clinical calls move to the nursing team. The calls frequently are related to ongoing symptoms, questions about medications, and psychosocial concerns. The ACHD nurse coordinator must have the skills to guide patients regarding these concerns. In the outpatient clinic, the nurse coordinator can take the lead on providing patient education regarding medication management, heart failure, pregnancy and contraception, self-care management and self-advocacy, preprocedural and postprocedural guidance, endocarditis prevention, and prevention and lifestyle choices. The nurse coordinator also plays a key role in ensuring all patients have an advanced directive on file and typically helps lead the patient-centered discussion regarding care goals and end of life care.

MENTAL HEALTH PROFESSIONAL

Psychosocial challenges are common in the ACHD patient population. Depression, anxiety, and posttraumatic stress disorders are seen more frequently than in the general population.[8–11] Participation in high-risk behaviors also is noted along with challenges regarding relationships, education, and employment attainment, which can have an impact on quality of life for ACHD patients.[12–15] The need for mental health support in ACHD patients is recognized and is a core component of the ACHA ACHD accreditation criteria. A social worker or clinical psychologist plays an integral role in supporting patients through these mental health challenges. The psychologist evaluates and diagnoses mental and emotional disorders and intellectual functioning and provides psychotherapy. Social workers typically provide psychosocial evaluations and counseling; they frequently are able to provide crisis intervention while awaiting an appointment with a psychologist or psychiatrist and can connect the ACHD patient to other local resources and support groups. In some instances, the social worker (or in some programs the ACHD nurse case manager) is involved with supporting activities to obtain disability benefits and insurance access, supporting patients in developing advanced directive plans and providing more logistical support, such as helping to secure financial support for transportation and accommodations to appointments and procedures.

Although there is an overlap in some aspects of training between the mental health professional and the ACHD cardiologist, NP, and PA colleagues, they typically have a greater depth and breadth of training in mental health. Given this, when mental health concerns are the dominating patient issue, the social worker or psychologist should be allowed to step in the ACHD team leadership role to guide the team in how to provide the best care to the patient. When the ACHD provider identifies issues that are having an impact on a patient's emotional well-being, such as a poor prognosis, the mental health professional can play an integral role working with the ACHD team and the patient to ensure a holistic approach to care. This social worker and/or psychologist participating in the care of the ACHD patient also can allow the ACHD providers to focus on CHD issues, ensuring efficiency and effectiveness of patient care while increasing access.

ADVANCED PRACTICE PROVIDER

APPs, such as PAs and NPs, are the fasting growing health care careers in the United States, and the demand for such providers is expected to grow 30% over the next 10 years (U.S. Bureau of Labor Statistics. Occupational Outlook Handbook: Fastest Growing Occupations; https://

www.bls.gov/ooh/fastest-growing.htm). Driving this demand in the United States is an increased number of patients entering the health care system, a shortage of physician providers, and a reduction in trainee work hours (https://www. aamc.org/system/files/c/2/31-2019_update_-_ the_complexities_of_physician_supply_and_ demand_-_projections_from_2017-2032.pdf).

Although there are significant training differences between NPs, who train in an advanced nursing model, and PAs, who train in the medical model, their roles within health care frequently are indistinguishable. As a group, under the umbrella term APP, they have proved themselves high-quality providers who deliver excellent care and increase access to care, while decreasing overall health care costs.[16–19] Based on this evidence, academic medical centers across the United States have embraced APPs as a way to increase access to care, with a median utilization of 1 APP to every 5 physicians.[20]

The American College of Cardiology (ACC) 2020 clinical competencies for cardiovascular NPs and PAs outlines the expected medical knowledge and skills for all CV PAs and NPs and the aspiring knowledge and skills for those with a focused practice area, such as ACHD.[21] This document can inform ACHD cardiologists, administrative leaders, and others involved in building ACHD teams in how to optimize the utilization of APPs. The transition from a general CV APP to a highly specialized ACHD APP requires supportive training and mentoring by an ACHD cardiologist and an active pursuit of professional development by the APP. Over time, the ACHD APP can exhibit, often with significant autonomy, the medical knowledge and clinical skills of a highly competent ACHD provider, providing near similar care to a collaborating ACHD cardiologist.

Given the number of patients, the current shortage of ACHD cardiologists is unlikely to be resolved in the near future. The long training pathway to becoming an ACHD cardiologists also is likely to be a barrier to increasing the number of cardiologists wanting to specialize in ACHD. Expanding the reach of the ACHD cardiologist with the training and utilization of APPs is warranted. A study by Green and colleagues[22] showed that the shortage of primary care providers could be effectively eliminated by shifting care to APPs for 23% of patients. A similar approach in ACHD, with shifting the care of less complex cases to the ACHD APP, could be as effective. There may be a temptation, especially in centers with limited resources, to utilize APPs to do work that can be done by a nurse coordinator, case manager, or social worker. Given the shortage of ACHD cardiologists and that only physicians and APPs can assess, diagnose, manage, and prescribe medications to ACHD patients, APPs must be solely utilized in their advanced practice capacity to increase access to care for ACHD patients.

CARDIOLOGIST

Training for ACHD cardiology was formalized in 2013 with Accreditation Council for Graduate Medical Education (ACGME) approval for a 2-year curriculum after either pediatric or internal medicine cardiology. Prior to formalized training, most cardiologists interested in ACHD completed non-ACGME training, which took the form of either variable time-related training—6 months to 2 years with a mentor or mentors—or completing a full combined internal medicine and pediatric cardiology fellowship over 5 years or 6 years. Over the span of 20 years from 1997 to 2011, only 67 cardiology fellows trained in some capacity at 11 institutions in the United States. The mentorship and nonformalized training provided the early stages of ACHD as a subspecialty in the United States and led to the petition to formalize training through ACGME. This also led to ACHD expertise to submit the petition for ACHD board certification and the development of ACHD clinics and programs around the country. Current ACGME ACHD programs can be found at https://www.acgme.org/Residents-and-Fellows/The-ACGME-for-Residents-and-Fellows.

In 2012, the American Board of Internal Medicine, American Board of Pediatrics, and American Board of Medical Specialties approved the petition for ACHD as a CV subspecialty. Unique and critical to this process was the approval by the American Board of Pediatrics for ACHD as a subspecialty with a pathway through pediatric cardiology. In 2020, there are 455 board-certified ACHD cardiologists in the United States. The distribution of ACHD cardiologists in the United States shows geographic diversity but leaves many areas of the country underrepresented (**Fig. 1**).

Ideally, each patient should have access to a board-certified ACHD cardiologist, but there are insufficient numbers to provide care to the more than 1.5 million ACHD patients in the United States. For the foreseeable future, there will be insufficient number of ACHD cardiologists to match the size and trajectory of patients in the United States. Expanding the reach of the ACHD cardiologist through TBC is warranted.

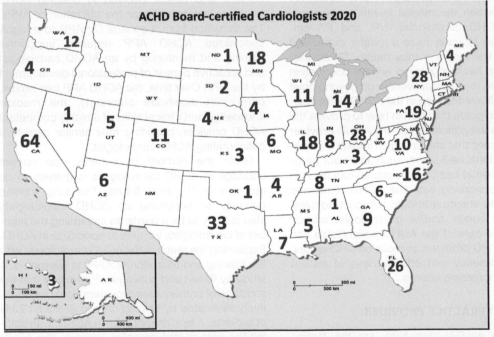

Fig. 1. US map with number of ACHD board-certified (BC) cardiologists per state. There are 455 ACHD American Board of Internal Medicine/American Board of Pediatrics BC cardiologists in the United States. Utilizing estimates from Marelli and colleagues,[33] the number of ACHD patients per state ranges from 158,000 in California to 2200 in Wyoming. Several states and territories have no ACHD BC cardiologists. In states with ACHD BC cardiologists, the ratio of ACHD BC cardiologist to ACHD patients ranges from 1/1254 in Minnesota, to states with large deficits, such as Alabama at 1/19,438; Oklahoma at 1/15,661; and Nevada at 1/12,433.

The ACHD cardiologist is an important and critical piece of the process to deliver high-quality ACHD care; however, the cardiologist is only a part of a larger team approach with multiple service and specialties necessary to deliver care. Attempting to estimate resources to match access and delivery of high-quality ACHD care is challenging.

PROGRAMMATIC RESOURCES

Determining the number of ACHD cardiologists and the number of other providers and support staff necessary for an ACHD program can be challenging. As well, determining the number of ACHD programs per population is equally challenging.

Although ACHA ACHD accreditation standards dictate the minimum number of programmatic resources, identifying program needs beyond accreditation standards need to take into account a program's spectrum of disease complexity, outpatient volume including locations of sites, and surgical and other procedural volumes, with consideration of the ACHD team role in inpatient care (consulting vs primary care team).

If it is assumed that most ACHD programs have an equal number of patients with CHD of simple, moderate, and great complexity,[23] the programmatic resources required for this population are likely to be similar or even more intense than for those cared for in primary care. In primary care, 1 in 4 patients have a chronic disease[18] and 37% of patients 65 years of age and older have a disability.[24] In this setting, it is estimated that it takes 21.7 hours per day to care for a 2500-patient panel.[25] It could be argued that there are few patients in ACHD that can be seen in the typical primary care appointment slot that runs 15 minutes or 20 minutes for a follow-up and 30 minutes for a new patient. Based on this assumption, a combined total of at least 3.0 full-time equivalents of ACHD providers (ACHD cardiologist and APP) would be required to manage an outpatient panel of 2500 patients. Shifting the less complex patients to the APP visit panel would allow an ACHD cardiologist the time to focus on the most complex of patients. Engaging a nurse coordinator and mental health professional to support the ACHD cardiologist and APP also is essential for success. ACHD programs that have a more complex patient panel mix, provide care at off-site clinics, and provide inpatient care, would require additional ACHD providers.

ADULT CONGENITAL HEART DISEASE CENTERS

Recognizing the challenges in providing appropriate care to ACHD patients, the ACC/American Heart Association (AHA) "2008 Guidelines for the Management of Adults with Congenital Heart Disease" were developed to emphasize the recommendation that "health care for ACHD patients should be coordinated by regional ACHD centers of excellence."[23] The concept would prove challenging until 2012 approval of an ACHD CV subspecialty certification.

Even without a formal recognition of CV subspecialty expertise in ACHD, the concept of regional centers began to develop organically after the 2000 Bethesda Conference.[26] In 2010, there were approximately 100 US ACHD centers; however, these centers were self-described centers of excellence.[27] The centers represented a broad spectrum of expertise, resources, and clinical volume, making the ability to demonstrate that these types of specialized centers improved patient outcomes.

In Canada, a federal mandate to shift ACHD care to a few specialized ACHD centers was associated with improved outcomes and survival.[28] Based on these recommendations, the "2018 AHA/ACC Guideline for the Management Adult with Congenital Heart Disease" continued to call for the development of centers of expertise and outline key personnel and recourses that should be part of the new programs.[29,30] Meanwhile, ACHA (a patient advocacy organization) was advocating for and exploring the possibility of a more formalized set of criteria for program's recognized as a regional ACHD centers. The Cystic Fibrosis Foundation had spearheaded efforts through program accreditation with improved outcomes.[31] Given this information, the ACHA began to take actions to move away from self-identified ACHD programs. In 2013, the ACHA had already put together a steering committee of ACHD experts and stakeholders to develop standards for ACHD program accreditation. The working group presented the final criteria for accreditation in 2014, which ultimately were endorsed by the ACC and the AHA.[32] In summary, the criteria for ACHA ACHD program accreditation requires each program to be committed to providing patient-centered care. They must have an adequate number of ACHD cardiologists, APPs, nurses, and social workers. They must have the ability to perform any surgery or procedure an ACHD patient might need at any given time, and they must be able to provide care 24/7.

Five centers participated in the ACHA ACHD accreditation pilot program in 2016 and in 2017 the program was open to all other US ACHD programs. At the time of this publication, 35 centers had completed the rigorous accreditation process (5 were in the process), which included developing more than 100 policy documents, advocating for program resources, and passing a comprehensive site visit.

To date, the ACHA has not announced their goal for a total number of accredited ACHD centers, but data from Marelli and colleagues[33] can provide guidance. **Fig. 2** illustrates the deficit in ACHD centers across the 52 US states and territories. The deficit was calculated by subtracting the actual number of centers per state from the estimated needs. The estimated needs were calculated using the following principles: geographic access to care and/or a minimum of 1 center for a population of 2 million, with the assumption that every ACHD patient should be seen at least once in an ACHD center.[33] Based on these criteria, a minimum of 100 accredited centers is required. Currently only 2 states have the required number of programs (Mississippi and Nebraska), whereas 6 additional states are close with the need for only 1 additional program (Oregon, Utah, New Mexico, Kansas, Wisconsin, and Connecticut). Four states (New York, Florida, Texas, and California) have the highest deficit, requiring at least 6 additional centers.

Fig. 3 captures both the current number and the deficit of ACHD centers. The distribution of current ACHD centers shows that 85% of the

states in the United States have 0 to 1 center, with a gaussian distribution skewed toward the left. These states have either no deficit or a small deficit of 1 to 3 centers. It, therefore, is reasonable to predict that, were there to be the addition of only 1 to 2 additional ACHD centers in these states, distribution across the country would be substantially improved, shifting the gaussian distribution rightward, reflecting a higher quality of care across the United States. The greatest deficits in ACHD centers (deficit of ≥6 centers) are in states where ACHD centers already exist but in insufficient quantities. For these states, comprising approximately 15% of all states in the United States, a different approach to health services delivery of care planning is required.

Currently, there are vast stretches of the United States where ACHD patients do not have access to a specialty ACHD center. Given this, the focus should shift to increase the number of ACHA ACHD–accredited centers in areas that are underserved and develop strategies to support and advance these programs. Once the target areas are identified, ACHD providers and patient advocacy groups should work with state-level policy makers to remove barriers to care access and to support policies that provide incentives to ACHD

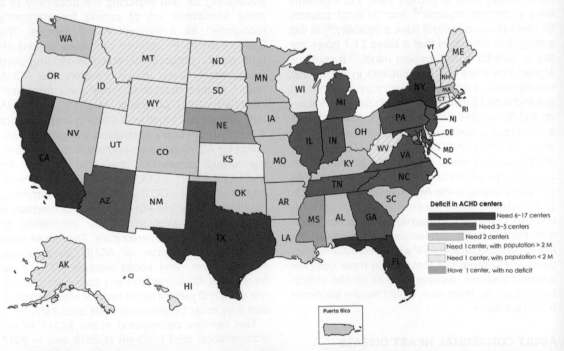

Fig. 2. Map of United States showing the gradient of deficit in ACHD centers per state, from the darkest red, representing a deficit of 6 to 17 centers, to green, showing no deficit with a minimum of 1 center. The states that are textured with diagonal lines are considered in need of an ACHD center for reasons of access rather than a number needed to serve a population of 2 million.

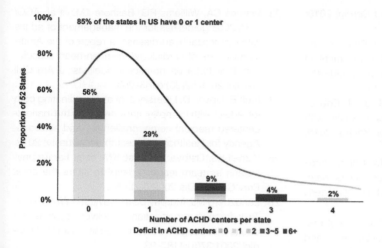

Fig. 3. Distribution of the number of ACHD centers per state and corresponding deficits. The X axis illustrates the current number of ACHD centers per state that vary between 1 center and 4 centers per state. Within each bar, colors indicate the deficit illustrated in **Fig. 1** indexed to the actual number of ACHD centers per state. Notably, 85% of states in the United States currently have either no center or only 1 center, skewing the current gaussian distribution of ACHD centers toward the left.

cardiologists and other members of the ACHD team, to train and work in these underserved target areas. In addition, partnerships between ACHA ACHD–accredited centers and ACHD cardiologists practicing outside these centers need to be established and fostered. Since the Bethesda Conference in 2000,[26] the care of adults with CHD has seen tremendous advances, but there continue to be many ACHD patients without access to such specialty care. Given this, there still is much work to be done.

CONFLICT OF INTEREST

None.

REFERENCES

1. Marelli AJ, Ionescu-Ittu R, Mackie AS, et al. Lifetime prevalence of congenital heart disease in the general population from 2000 to 2010. Circulation 2014;130(9):749–56.
2. United States Department of Health and Human Services. Strategic objective 1.2: expand safe, high-quality healthcare options, and encourage innovation and competition. Strategic goal 1: reform, strengthen and modernize the Nation's Healthcare System Web site. Available at: https://www.hhs.gov/about/strategic-plan/strategic-goal-1/index.html. Accessed January 27, 2020.
3. Arnett DK, Blumenthal RS, Albert MA, et al. 2019 ACC/AHA guideline on the primary prevention of cardiovascular disease: executive summary: a report of the American College of cardiology/American heart association Task force on clinical practice guidelines. J Am Coll Cardiol 2019;74(10):1376–414.
4. Abu-Rish Blakeney E, Lavallee DC, Baik D, et al. Purposeful interprofessional team intervention improves relational coordination among advanced heart failure care teams. J Interprof Care 2019;33(5):481–9.
5. International Society for Adult Congenital Heart Disease. Goals and objectives. Available at: http://www.isachd.org/content/our-mission. Accessed January 27, 2020.
6. Mickan SM, Rodger SA. Effective health care teams: a model of six characteristics developed from shared perceptions. J Interprof Care 2005;19(4):358–70.
7. Sillman C, Morin J, Thomet C, et al. Adult congenital heart disease nurse coordination: essential skills and role in optimizing team-based care a position statement from the International Society for Adult Congenital Heart Disease (ISACHD). Int J Cardiol 2017;229:125–31.
8. Jackson JL, Leslie CE, Hondorp SN. Depressive and anxiety symptoms in adult congenital heart disease: prevalence, health impact and treatment. Prog Cardiovasc Dis 2018;61(3–4):294–9.
9. Gleason LP, Deng LX, Khan AM, et al. Psychological distress in adults with congenital heart disease: focus beyond depression. Cardiol Young 2019;29(2):185–9.
10. Deng LX, Khan AM, Drajpuch D, et al. Prevalence and correlates of post-traumatic stress disorder in adults with congenital heart disease. Am J Cardiol 2016;117(5):853–7.
11. Eslami B. Correlates of posttraumatic stress disorder in adults with congenital heart disease. Congenit Heart Dis 2017;12(3):357–63.
12. Moons P, Luyckx K, Kovacs AH, et al. Prevalence and effects of cigarette smoking, cannabis consumption, and co-use in adults from 15 countries

with congenital heart disease. Can J Cardiol 2019; 35(12):1842–50.

13. Sluman MA, Apers S, Sluiter JK, et al. Education as important predictor for successful employment in adults with congenital heart disease worldwide. Congenit Heart Dis 2019;14(3):362–71.

14. Pfitzer C, Helm PC, Rosenthal LM, et al. Educational level and employment status in adults with congenital heart disease. Cardiol Young 2018; 28(1):32–8.

15. Deng LX, Gleason LP, Awh K, et al. Too little too late? Communication with patients with congenital heart disease about challenges of adult life. Congenit Heart Dis 2019;14(4):534–40.

16. Jiao S, Murimi IB, Stafford RS, et al. Quality of prescribing by physicians, nurse practitioners, and physician assistants in the United States. Pharmacotherapy 2018;38(4):417–27.

17. Yang Y, Long Q, Jackson SL, et al. Nurse practitioners, physician assistants, and physicians are comparable in managing the first five years of diabetes. Am J Med 2018;131(3):276–83.e2.

18. Morgan PA, Smith VA, Berkowitz TSZ, et al. Impact of physicians, nurse practitioners, and physician assistants on utilization and costs for complex patients. Health Aff (Milwood) 2019;38(6):1028–36.

19. Virani SS, Akeroyd JM, Ramsey DJ, et al. Comparative effectiveness of outpatient cardiovascular disease and diabetes care delivery between advanced practice providers and physician providers in primary care: implications for care under the affordable care act. Am Heart J 2016;181:74–82.

20. Moote M, Krsek C, Kleinpell R, et al. Physician assistant and nurse practitioner utilization in academic medical centers. Am J Med Qual 2019;34(5): 465–72.

21. Rodgers GP, Linderbaum JA, Pearson DD, et al. 2020 ACC clinical competencies for nurse practitioners and physician assistants in adult cardiovascular medicine: a report of the ACC competency management committee. J Am Coll Cardiol 2020; 75(19):2483–517.

22. Green LV, Savin S, Lu Y. Primary care physician shortages could be eliminated through use of teams, nonphysicians, and electronic communication. Health Aff (Milwood) 2013;32(1):11–9.

23. Warnes CA, Williams RG, Bashore TM, et al. ACC/AHA 2008 guidelines for the management of adults with congenital heart disease: a report of the American College of cardiology/American heart association Task force on practice guidelines. J Am Coll Cardiol 2008;52(23):e143–263.

24. Rich E, Lipson D, Libersky J, et al. Coordinating care for adults with complex care needs in the patient-centered medical home: challenges and solutions. Agency for Healthcare Research and Quality; 2012.

25. Yarnall KS, Ostbye T, Krause KM, et al. Family physicians as team leaders: "time" to share the care. Prev Chronic Dis 2009;6(2):A59.

26. Landzberg MJ, Murphy DJ Jr, Davidson WR Jr, et al. Task force 4: organization of delivery systems for adults with congenital heart disease. J Am Coll Cardiol 2001;37(5):1187–93.

27. Fernandes SM, Chamberlain LJ, Grady S Jr, et al. Trends in utilization of specialty care centers in California for adults with congenital heart disease. Am J Cardiol 2015;115(9):1298–304.

28. Khairy P, Ionescu-Ittu R, Mackie AS, et al. Changing mortality in congenital heart disease. J Am Coll Cardiol 2010;56(14):1149–57.

29. Stout KK, Daniels CJ, Aboulhosn JA, et al. 2018 AHA/ACC guideline for the management of adults with congenital heart disease: executive summary: a report of the American College of Cardiology/American Heart Association Task Force on Clinical Practice Guidelines. Circulation 2019;139(14): e637–97.

30. Sahay S, Melendres-Groves L, Pawar L, et al. Pulmonary hypertension care center network: improving care and outcomes in pulmonary hypertension. Chest 2017;151(4):749–54.

31. Mogayzel PJ Jr, Dunitz J, Marrow LC, et al. Improving chronic care delivery and outcomes: the impact of the cystic fibrosis Care Center Network. BMJ Qual Saf 2014;23(Suppl 1):i3–8.

32. Association ACH. ACHA ACHD accreditation program. Available at: https://www.achaheart.org/media/2637/achaachdprogramcriteria2020.pdf. Accessed January 27, 2020.

33. Marelli AJ, Therrien J, Mackie AS, et al. Planning the specialized care of ase patients: from numbers to guidelines; an epidemiologic approach. Am Heart J 2009;157(1):1–8.

Psychological Needs, Assessment, and Treatment in the Care of Adults with Congenital Heart Disease

Jamie L. Jackson, PhD[a],*, Kristen R. Fox, PhD[a], Adrienne H. Kovacs, PhD[b]

KEYWORDS

- Congenital heart disease • Emotional distress • Depression • Anxiety • Medical trauma • Treatment

KEY POINTS

- Congenital heart disease survivors are at risk for declining emotional well-being as they age.
- Neurocognitive deficits, physical and emotional repercussions of invasive treatments, and declines in physical functioning over time contribute to emotional distress.
- Brief self-report measures can be used to identify symptoms that warrant further evaluation.
- Psychotherapy, pharmacotherapy, or a combination of both are common treatment options.

Medical advancements have prolonged the lives of congenital heart disease (CHD) survivors as evidenced by more adults currently living with CHD than children.[1] Now that these individuals are living longer, they are also encountering the stressors associated with having a chronic medical condition. This circumstance requires health providers to not only consider the cardiac health of CHD survivors, but also their emotional well-being. For the general population, emotional well-being is an independent risk factor for morbidity and mortality, including the occurrence of cardiac events.[2] Among individuals who have acquired heart disease, the connection between emotional well-being and cardiac health is even more pronounced,[3–5] highlighting the importance of addressing symptoms of emotional distress alongside cardiac follow-up. Emotional well-being represents a continuum that ranges from normative levels of occasional distress experienced by most everyone to symptoms of psychopathology that meet criteria as set forth by the *Diagnostic and Statistical Manual of Mental Disorders* (DSM). Therefore, optimal health care for CHD survivors is achieved when symptoms of emotional distress can be identified and the appropriate referral resources are accessible by the teams caring for these patients.

CHD survivors have several risk factors for declining emotional well-being as they age, and several key ones are shown in **Fig. 1**. These individuals are more likely to experience a cardiac-related event or hospitalization as they age owing to their cardiac lesion or previous interventions.[6,7] Additionally, CHD survivors who have had multiple surgeries and/or have complex disease are at greater risk for neurocognitive deficits.[8,9] Neurocognitive sequalae can contribute to poorer emotional well-being owing to difficulty with executive functions,[9] which are associated with poorer coping[10] and result in an increased risk of developing psychiatric disorders, such as depression and attention deficit hyperactivity disorder.[11] CHD survivors may also

[a] Center for Biobehavioral Health, Abigail Wexner Research Institute, Nationwide Children's Hospital, 700 Children's Drive, NEOB, 3rd Floor, Columbus, OH 43205, USA; [b] Oregon Health and Science University, Knight Cardiovascular Institute, 3181 Southwest Sam Jackson Park Road, UHN-62, Portland, OR 97239, USA
* Corresponding author.
E-mail address: Jamie.jackson2@nationwidechildrens.org

Cardiol Clin 38 (2020) 305–316
https://doi.org/10.1016/j.ccl.2020.04.007
0733-8651/20/© 2020 Elsevier Inc. All rights reserved.

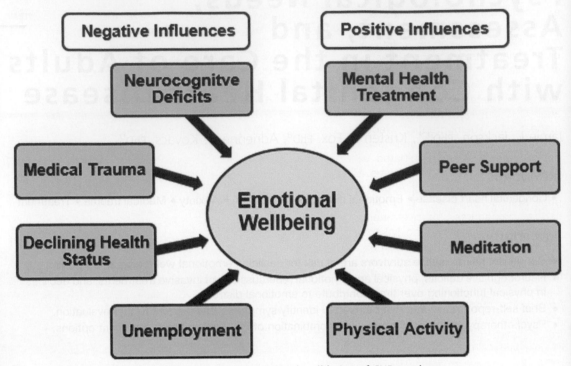

Fig. 1. Negative and positive influences on the emotional well-being of CHD survivors.

experience lasting repercussions from the invasive interventions that are needed to repair or palliate the cardiac lesion. Surgeries can result in significant scarring,[12] recurring chest pain,[13] and the development of arrhythmias.[14] Last, CHD survivors are more likely to experience declining health status at younger ages compared with the general population, and may thus be less capable or perceive themselves as less capable of engaging in peer-appropriate activities.[15,16]

Primary care and cardiology teams may be the first line of defense in recognizing and providing a referral for symptoms of emotional distress. Therefore, the purpose of the current review is to offer health providers information about the psychological needs specific to CHD survivors, identification measures that can be implemented in a clinic setting, and treatment modalities for consideration when developing referral resources.

PSYCHOLOGICAL NEEDS
Stress

Descriptions of disease-related stress for CHD survivors are often reported in anecdotal terms. However, 1 study found that the following items were commonly endorsed as being at least somewhat stressful by adult CHD survivors: the presence of scars from invasive treatments, not being able to engage in activities in which other people

of a similar age engage, and being uncertain about their future health.[17] Within this sample, adolescents (15–18 years of age) reported significantly less disease-related stress than young adults (19–39 years of age). Furthermore, participants with some degree of functional impairment, as denoted by their New York Heart Association (NYHA) functional class (II–IV), endorsed significantly higher levels of disease-related stress compared with participants without functional impairment (NYHA functional class I). The authors concluded that disease-related stress may increase as CHD survivors age and is associated with symptoms of psychopathology and poorer health-related quality of life. Although there is a dearth of longitudinal studies on changes in emotional well-being over time among CHD survivors, one may assume that disease-related stress is a risk factor for the development of symptoms of psychopathology, especially if there is a decline in functional status.

Clinically Significant Emotional Distress

CHD survivors have elevated rates of psychiatric disorders compared with the general population, particularly major depressive disorder (MDD) and anxiety disorders.[18] The diagnosis of a psychiatric disorder negatively impacts quality of life among adult CHD survivors, even when the symptoms are mild.[19] Moreover, depressive and anxiety symptoms, which share cognitive (eg, difficulty concentrating) and somatic (eg, sleep disturbance) elements, often co-occur among adults with CHD.[20]

Numerous demographic, psychosocial, and clinical correlates of emotional distress among adult CHD survivors have been identified. With respect to demographic factors, female sex,[20–22] older age,[20,21] and lower socioeconomic status[20–22] are associated with elevated depressive and anxiety symptoms. Clinical factors, including impaired NYHA functional class,[21] poor exercise capacity,[22] a greater number of cardiac procedures,[23] and greater medical co-morbidity[20] have also been linked with poorer emotional functioning. Lesion complexity (ie, simple vs moderate vs complex), however, has an inconsistent relationship with emotional distress.[24] A meta-analysis found that CHD survivors with moderate lesions reported less emotional distress compared with healthy controls,[25] whereas another study reported that individuals with moderate and complex lesions were more likely to have an anxiety disorder than those with simple lesions.[23] Inconsistencies in the relationship between the traditional lesion complexity classification and emotional distress may be due to the vast heterogeneity in the moderate lesion category. The recently published and more nuanced classification system that incorporates a patient's physiologic stage (eg, NYHA functional class, hemodynamic sequelae, and presence of arrhythmias)[26] may better delineate a patients' current disease severity for use in research studies.

Importantly, emotional distress has been identified as a predictor of health care use and adverse medical outcomes. Individuals with depression and/or an anxiety disorder have a greater number of primary care, cardiology, and emergency department visits, in addition to more hospitalizations.[20] Adolescent and adult CHD survivors with increased depressive symptoms have shorter event-free survival, as well as double the risk of experiencing a major adverse cardiovascular event during a 5-year observation period.[27] Furthermore, a diagnosis of depression and/or anxiety was associated with higher mortality risk among adult CHD patients.[20]

Symptoms of Medical Trauma

CHD survivors are exposed to various stressful medical events that have the potential to precipitate traumatic stress responses. The results of 1 study suggest that more than one-half of CHD survivors report experiencing a medically traumatic event, including cardiac surgery, and one-third of CHD survivors who have undergone cardiac surgery identify the experience as traumatic.[28] This perception of medically traumatic events suggests that CHD survivors may be at risk for posttraumatic stress disorder (PTSD). PTSD is characterized by intrusion, avoidance, and hyperarousal symptoms, as well as alterations in mood and cognition that arise in response to a traumatic stressor.[29] For CHD survivors, posttraumatic stress may present as nightmares about distressing aspects of treatment (intrusion), noncompliance with medical treatment (avoidance), and heightened monitoring and catastrophic interpretation of physical symptoms (arousal).[30]

PTSD among adult CHD survivors is understudied, with a small number of investigations reporting the prevalence and correlates of PTSD in this population. Rates of PTSD among CHD survivors range widely from 3% to 52%.[18,28,30,31] CHD survivors with a history of cardiac surgery[28,31] and stroke[28] are more likely to meet the criteria for PTSD than other CHD survivors. Moreover, earlier age at cardiac surgery is associated with PTSD,[28] suggesting that cardiac surgery has long-term effects on emotional well-being.

ASSESSMENT OF EMOTIONAL DISTRESS

The gold standard for determining whether symptoms of emotional distress meet the formal criteria for a psychiatric disorder is by conducting a structured clinical interview. Available research versions of structured interviews require extensive training and can vary in length depending on the number of mental disorders being assessed (30–180 minutes). A clinical interview is important in clarifying a diagnosis, although is not necessary for identifying individuals who should be referred for mental health services. Many patients will self-identify as experiencing psychological distress and thus seek mental health referrals. In addition, there are many self-report measures available that can be administered quickly with minimal training in an outpatient clinic setting. The administration of such measures may facilitate the recognition of clinically significant emotional stress and trigger discussion with patients about possible mental health referrals.

The adverse effects of emotional distress on psychosocial and physical functioning among adults with CHD highlight the importance of routine assessment of depressive and anxiety symptoms. Encouragingly, 70% of cardiologists express willingness to implement a self-report measure to identify depression in their patients.[32] Individuals with acquired heart disease tend to follow-up on recommended health care after depression and anxiety screening[33]; therefore, increased implementation of self-report measures that identify emotional distress may enhance care for adults with CHD.

The following are commonly used self-report measures that have cutoff scores to help make determinations about the degree of psychological distress, and thus consideration for mental health services. Many of these measures have been administered in studies investigating psychological outcomes in CHD. See **Table 1** for additional details about the self-report measures described elsewhere in this article. All instruments are brief and take approximately 5 minutes or less to complete.

Symptoms of Emotional Distress

Beck Anxiety Inventory
The Beck Anxiety Inventory[34] has been used infrequently to measure anxiety in CHD survivors, but the Beck Anxiety Inventory is quick to administer and can be easily scored.

Beck Depression Inventory – Second Edition (BDI – II)
Westhoff-Bleck and colleagues[19] found that the Beck Depression Inventory – Second Edition,[35] detected MDD with a sensitivity of 75% and a specificity of 90%. Although the Beck Depression Inventory – Second Edition has multiple strengths, because it contains a question about suicidal ideation it might require prompt review to determine whether urgent further assessment by a mental health professional is indicated.

Center for Epidemiologic Studies Scale - Depression
The Center for Epidemiologic Studies Scale - Depression[36] was found by Moon and colleagues[37] to detect the presence of depressive and anxiety disorders among adults with CHD, with sensitivity ranging from 73% to 87% and specificity ranging from 60% to 80%. The Center for Epidemiologic Studies Scale - Depression may be readily implemented in a clinic setting.

Generalized Anxiety Disorder Questionnaire – 7
The Generalized Anxiety Disorder Questionnaire – 7[38] has a sensitivity and specificity of 89% and 82%, respectively, among primary care patients.[38] Tablet-based administration of the Generalized Anxiety Disorder Questionnaire – 7 is acceptable

to patients presenting to a variety of outpatient clinics.[39]

Hospital Depression and Anxiety Scale
The Hospital Depression and Anxiety Scale[40] contains depression (HADS-D) and anxiety (HADS-A) subscales. For adults with CHD, the HADS-D has a sensitivity of 76% and a specificity of 92% for identifying MDD. Strengths of the HADS are that it measures more than 1 component of emotional distress with a relatively small number of items and was developed specifically for medical populations.

Patient Health Questionnaire – 9
The Patient Health Questionnaire – 9 (PHQ-9)[41] functions as an indicator of both probable depression diagnosis and symptom severity, although the severity classification system has greater sensitivity as compared with the diagnostic algorithm.[42] Among primary care patients, the PHQ-9 has a sensitivity of 88% and a specificity of 88% for identifying MDD.[41] Of note, 2.2% of adult CHD survivors endorsed the suicidal ideation and self-harm item,[39] indicating that the PHQ-9 may be best implemented in clinic settings with access to a mental health professional. Tablet-based administration of the PHQ-9 has proven acceptable to medical outpatients.[39] Another benefit of the PHQ-9 is the availability of proposed treatment actions that correspond to severity scores, which may assist with decisions regarding referral (ie, score of 5–9 suggests watching, waiting, and reassessment; and a score of ≥10 suggests that treatment is needed).[43]

Symptoms of Medical Trauma

Because there is no available measure of posttraumatic stress specific to medical trauma, self-report measures commonly used in other trauma-exposed populations have been used to assess PTSD in CHD survivors. Of note, the observed prevalence of PTSD seems to vary as a function of the selected screening instrument, though this trend also affects assessment of PTSD in healthy populations. For example, two studies have compared rates of PTSD among adult CHD survivors and healthy adults, and neither study found a difference in prevalence between the two populations (2.7% vs 2.4% and 52.3% vs 48.4% for CHD survivors and healthy adults, respectively).[18,31] PTSD measures are included in **Table 1** and are described elsewhere in this article with an emphasis on their usefulness to assess PTSD diagnostic criteria according to fifth edition of the DSM (DSM-5).[29]

Table 1
Commonly used measures of emotional distress

Assessment Tool	Description	No. of Items	General Population: Clinical Cutoff/Severity Classification	CHD-Specific Clinical Cutoff (Mean ± SD)	Fee for Use?
Depression specific					
Beck Depression Inventory – Second Edition (BDI-II)	Severity of affective, cognitive, and somatic depressive symptoms over the past 2 wks	21	≥16 = presence of MDD	>11 = MDD 7.7±8.7[19]	Yes
Center for Epidemiologic Studies Scale – Depression (CES-D)	Frequency of affective, cognitive, and somatic depressive symptoms over the past week	20	≥16 = presence of MDD	≥18 = depressive/ anxiety disorder[37] 18.4±5.9[37]	No
Patient Health Questionnaire – 9 (PHQ-9)	Frequency of affective, cognitive, and somatic depressive symptoms over the last 2 wks	9	≥10 = presence of MDD ≤4 = minimal 5–9 = mild 10–14 = moderate 15–19 = moderately severe ≥20 = severe	6.6% had probable MDD based on diagnostic algorithm[39] 5.5% score ≥10[39]	No
Anxiety specific					
Beck Anxiety Inventory (BAI)	Severity of affective and somatic anxiety symptoms over the past week	21	≥7 = minimal 8–15 = mild 16–25 = moderate ≥ 26 = severe	19% score ≥16[70]	Yes
Generalized Anxiety Disorder Questionnaire – 7 (GAD-7)	Frequency of generalized anxiety symptoms over the past 2 wks and degree of impairment	7	≥10 = presence of GAD	17% score ≥10[39]	No
Anxiety and depressive symptoms					

(continued on next page)

Table 1
(continued)

Assessment Tool	Description	No. of Items	General Population: Clinical Cutoff/Severity Classification	CHD-Specific Clinical Cutoff (Mean ± SD)	Fee for Use?
Hospital Anxiety and Depression Scale (HADS)	Frequency and severity of depressive and anxiety symptoms over past week	14	8–10 = mild 11–14 = moderate 15–21 = severe	HADS-D: >5 = MDD[19] HADS-A: 9.2±4.4[71]	Yes
PTSD symptoms					
Impact of Events Scale – Revised (IES-R)	Severity of intrusion, avoidance, and hyperarousal symptoms over the past 7 days	22	≥33 = presence of PTSD	11% score ≥33[28]	No
Posttraumatic Diagnostic Scale (PTDS)	Frequency of intrusion, avoidance, and hyperarousal symptoms over past month	17	≤10 = mild 11–20 = moderate 21–35 = moderate to severe ≥36 = severe	52% had probable PTSD based on diagnostic algorithm[31] 14.2 ± 11.1[31]	Yes
PTSD Civilian Checklist Version (PCL-C)	Severity of intrusion, avoidance, hyperarousal, cognitive, and affective symptoms during the past month	17	≥44 = presence of PTSD	21% score ≥44[28]	No

Abbreviations: GAD, generalized anxiety disorder; SD, standard deviation.

Impact of Events Scale – Revised

The Impact of Events Scale – Revised (IES-R)[44] has a sensitivity of 91% and a specificity of 82% for diagnosing PTSD. One advantage of the IES-R is that clinicians and researchers are able to specify the traumatic stressor, making the IES-R a good candidate for the assessment of cardiac-specific trauma. Moreover, despite changes in PTSD diagnostic criteria by the DSM-5, the IES-R continues to be considered a useful measure of posttraumatic stress.[45]

Posttraumatic Diagnostic Scale

According to its diagnostic algorithm, the Post-traumatic Diagnostic Scale (PTDS)[46] provides a sensitivity of 89% and a specificity of 75%. A symptom severity score may also be derived. The PTDS has been revised to reflect DSM-5 changes in the diagnostic criteria for PTSD,[47] but this measure has not yet been used to examine posttraumatic stress among CHD survivors. Compared with other self-report measures, the PTDS is more complicated to score. However, it assesses impairment related to posttraumatic stress, a consideration that is omitted by other brief screening instruments.

PTSD Checklist Civilian Version

The PTSD Checklist Civilian Version (PCL-C)[48] has a sensitivity of 94% and a specificity of 86% for diagnosing PTSD. The PCL-C has been revised to reflect the PTSD criteria outlined in the DSM-5 (PCL-5).[49] The scores on the PCL-5 and PCL-C are strongly correlated,[49] but the PCL-5 has yet to be used among CHD survivors.

TREATMENT OF EMOTIONAL DISTRESS

Several options are available to address symptoms of emotional distress, some of which are shown in **Fig. 1**. The most common options include psychotherapy, which is also known as "talk therapy," and pharmacotherapy, including antidepressant and anxiolytic medications. This review also briefly summarizes additional treatment modalities that can be considered. It is important to note that there is a paucity of research on these interventions among adult CHD survivors. However, many of these treatments have been studied with adults with acquired heart disease, who may share some similarities as those with complex CHD in functional limitations and uncertainty about the progression of their condition.

In 2009, Kovacs and colleagues[50] surveyed 155 adult CHD survivors about their history and interest in mental health treatment. Approximately 51% of respondents reported interest in receiving psychological treatment for at least 1 area (eg, stress management, coping with a cardiac condition, mood/anxiety management). Furthermore, 41% expressed interest in receiving psychotherapy alone, 9% preferred pharmacotherapy alone, 34% reported that either option would be acceptable, and 16% were uninterested in either option. Therefore, a majority of adult CHD survivors are amenable to receiving treatment and are amenable to either psychotherapy or pharmacotherapy.

Psychotherapy

Psychotherapy (talk therapy) is an effective form of treatment for symptoms of emotional distress in the general population. For those with acquired heart disease, psychotherapy often includes a combination of education, cognitive restructuring (ie, examining and challenging dysfunctional thoughts), relaxation training, and/or improving stress management skills. Richards and colleagues[51] conducted a systematic review of psychological interventions for individuals with acquired heart disease, which reported small to moderate improvements in depressive and anxiety symptoms, as well as a positive effect on cardiac mortality. Another systematic review and meta-analysis found that psychological interventions resulted in improved depressive symptoms and social support, though did not decrease anxiety symptoms.[52] The interventions included in these reviews varied widely in treatment length, type of personnel delivering the intervention, and current level of depression and anxiety symptoms.

Research on the effectiveness of psychotherapy interventions for adult CHD survivors is scarce. Promising preliminary results from a pilot randomized clinical trial examining the efficacy of a cognitive–behavioral protocol for treating depressive and anxiety symptoms among adults with CHD indicated decreases in depressive and anxiety symptoms.[53] The intervention incorporated psychoeducation on living with CHD and cognitive–behavioral techniques including relaxation training, cognitive restructuring, and self-awareness training. Ferguson and Kovacs[54] also presented findings on integrating psychology service as part of an adult CHD outpatient clinic using a general cognitive-behavioral framework, and reported that 88% of the patients who received psychological treatment after referral by their cardiologist reported reduced or no emotional distress after treatment. Although these studies have shown promise for psychotherapy among adult CHD survivors, additional research is needed to determine the impact of psychotherapy on

Table 2
Benefits (+) and drawbacks (−) of psychotherapy and pharmacotherapy

	Psychotherapy	Pharmacotherapy
Expense	+ A specified number of outpatient therapy sessions are covered by most insurances. − However, not all therapists accept all forms of insurance and there may still be high copay fees.	+ Antidepressants are typically covered by most insurances. + Medication is typically inexpensive, though total cost depends on the duration of use.
Side effects	+ Although some may experience a temporary exacerbation of emotional distress when beginning therapy, it is typically short lived.	− Medication side effect profiles can interfere with adherence. Initial side effects may subside after a few weeks of adjusting to the medication. − Sudden discontinuation of antidepressants can result in significant side effects. Patients are advised to slowly titrate off of a medication under the supervision of the prescriber.
Ease of access	− Access to individuals providing psychotherapy can be limited in certain communities. Patients should consult their insurance to determine which providers are considered in network. − Providers may have varying degrees of familiarity with the needs of individuals with cardiovascular conditions.	+ Many primary care physicians are willing to prescribe and manage antidepressant medications. − Some mental disorders require significant medication management (eg, bipolar disorder and schizophrenia), and should be monitored by a psychiatrist. Psychiatrists are less available in certain communities and may have long wait lists. − Providers may have varying degrees of familiarity with the needs of individuals with cardiovascular conditions.
Convenience	− Some may need to travel a significant distance to a provider and appointments are traditionally held weekly. − Appointments are 50–60 min and typically occur during normal business hours, which may not be feasible for all patients.	+ Filling and picking up a prescription is convenient for many people.
Treatment duration	+ Duration of psychotherapy is often discussed in the early stages of treatment and is commonly ≥8 sessions.	− Duration of medication varies, but could last ≥1 y.
Treatment effect sustainability	+ Psychotherapy addresses current symptoms of emotional distress and provides tools for recurrence prevention.	− Symptoms of emotional distress may return when medication is discontinued.

(continued on next page)

Table 2
(continued)

	Psychotherapy	Pharmacotherapy
Patient experience	− Improvement in symptoms takes time. + Strategies are learned to reduce the likelihood of symptom recurrence. − Some patients may have negative perceptions about psychotherapy owing to stereotyped portrayals in the media. − Patient–provider relationship is important for participation in psychotherapy, therefore changing providers may disrupt treatment progress. + Patient–provider relationship is a powerful tool alone, irrespective of the type of psychotherapy.	− Improvement in symptoms takes time, with the exception of anxiolytics used to treat physiologic symptoms of panic. − Not uncommonly, multiple medications are sequentially trialed before symptoms are optimally reduced. − Symptoms may return once medication is discontinued. − Patients who are already taking medications for other health needs may be hesitant to add another. + If care must be reestablished (eg, after a move), prescriptions can be easily transferred to another pharmacy, though finding a new prescriber may be more challenging.

symptoms of emotional distress, as well as any special considerations for CHD survivors as compared with the general population or those with acquired heart disease.

Pharmacotherapy

Selective serotonin reuptake inhibitors are commonly used to treat symptoms of mood (eg, MDD) or anxiety disorders (eg, generalized anxiety disorder and obsessive–compulsive disorder). A 2013 review on selective serotonin reuptake inhibitor use in patients with either coronary heart disease or heart failure concluded that they are generally safe and may even decrease first or recurrent cardiovascular events.[55] However, the benefit for those with heart failure was unclear. Diller and colleagues[56] reported that, of the 6162 adult CHD survivors followed, 3.3% were taking an antidepressant, which included selective serotonin reuptake inhibitors or tricyclic antidepressants. Over an 11-year follow-up period, 8.2% of the patients had died. The mortality rate was not directly related to use of antidepressant medication.

Anxiolytic medications, such as benzodiazepines, are also prescribed to treat physical symptoms of anxiety. Benzodiazepines are not considered first-line treatments for anxiety disorders, in large part owing to their adverse effects with long-term and/or high dosage use, including the potential for physical and psychological dependence.[57] The long-term consequences of

anxiolytic use among individuals with acquired heart disease or CHD has not been reported.

In choosing between psychotherapy, pharmacotherapy, or a combination of both, the benefits and drawbacks of each treatment option must be weighed (**Table 2**). The treatment preferences of each patient should be assessed before providing a referral, given that the drawbacks for either psychotherapy or pharmacotherapy may be more prohibitive for some individuals. Once a referral is made, mental health providers will assist the patient in choosing the right treatment option for them while taking into account best practices for addressing the reported symptoms. If both psychotherapy and pharmacotherapy are indicated, there may be multiple providers who will collaborate (eg, a psychologist and psychiatrist).

Other Treatment Modalities for Symptoms of Emotional Distress

In addition to medication and therapy, other intervention modalities may enhance the emotional well-being of adults with CHD. Given that loneliness is related to psychological distress among adults with CHD,[50] it may be hypothesized that peer support interventions could decrease emotional distress. Adult CHD survivors identify peer support as a necessary aspect of positive emotional well-being,[58] and many endorse interest in receiving peer support.[59] Although peer support programs have been highlighted as a complement to psychological services in the care of adults with

CHD,[60] research on peer support is limited. Of note, the Adult Congenital Heart Association (www.achaheart.org) offers Heart to Heart, a program that matches patients with trained peer mentors (ambassadors) for support related to concerns such as adjustment to health status and cardiac procedures.[61]

Mindfulness-based interventions are recognized for having a positive impact on stress, as well as depressive and anxiety symptoms, among adults with cardiovascular disease.[62] Among adults with cardiovascular disease, mindfulness-based stress reduction interventions that include meditation, relaxation, and cognitive restructuring components have been shown to decrease stress, depression, and anxiety[63] and to promote self-efficacy and enhance quality of life.[64] A statement from the American Heart Association highlighted meditation as a low-cost and low-risk adjunctive approach to stress and other cardiovascular risk reduction.[65]

Physical activity has also gained empirical support as a treatment option for depressive symptoms.[66] Being physically active promotes positive mood maintenance[67] and decreases the cardiotoxicity of stress.[68] The emotional benefits of physical activity among children and adults with CHD were emphasized in an American Heart Association Scientific Statement.[69] Given the cardiovascular and emotional benefits of physical activity, health providers should consider having conversations not only about the presence or absence of physical activity restrictions, but also educate patients about the multitude of benefits of engaging in physical activity levels appropriate for that individual and their unique cardiovascular considerations.

SUMMARY

Although the majority of adult CHD survivors are thriving, there is a significant portion who will encounter emotional distress that warrants treatment. Identifying these individuals in an outpatient clinic setting is feasible given the wide variety of available measures. The critical step, however, is ensuring sufficient referral resources for further assessment and treatment. This may necessitate communication with mental health providers in one's institution or in the local community, including psychologists, social workers, and psychiatrists. Establishing these collaborations is vital for ensuring optimal emotional and physical well-being of adult CHD survivors.

CONFLICTS OF INTEREST

None.

REFERENCES

1. Gilboa SM, Devine OJ, Kucik JE, et al. Congenital heart defects in the United States: estimating the magnitude of the affected population in 2010. Circulation 2016;134(2):101–9.
2. Gan Y, Gong Y, Tong X, et al. Depression and the risk of coronary heart disease: a meta-analysis of prospective cohort studies. BMC Psychiatry 2014; 14:371.
3. Meijer A, Conradi HJ, Bos EH, et al. Prognostic association of depression following myocardial infarction with mortality and cardiovascular events: a meta-analysis of 25 years of research. Gen Hosp Psychiatry 2011;33(3):203–16.
4. Park JH, Tahk SJ, Bae SH. Depression and anxiety as predictors of recurrent cardiac events 12 months after percutaneous coronary interventions. J Cardiovasc Nurs 2015;30(4):351–9.
5. Lichtman JH, Froelicher ES, Blumenthal JA, et al. Depression as a risk factor for poor prognosis among patients with acute coronary syndrome: systematic review and recommendations: a scientific statement from the American Heart Association. Circulation 2014;129(12):1350–69.
6. Opotowsky AR, Siddiqi OK, Webb GD. Trends in hospitalizations for adults with congenital heart disease in the U.S. J Am Coll Cardiol 2009;54(5):460–7.
7. Burchill LJ, Gao L, Kovacs AH, et al. Hospitalization trends and health resource use for adult congenital heart disease-related heart failure. J Am Heart Assoc 2018;7(15):e008775.
8. Ilardi D, Ono KE, McCartney R, et al. Neurocognitive functioning in adults with congenital heart disease. Congenit Heart Dis 2017;12(2):166–73.
9. Marelli A, Miller SP, Marino BS, et al. Brain in congenital heart disease across the lifespan: the cumulative burden of injury. Circulation 2016;133(20): 1951–62.
10. Jackson JL, Gerardo GM, Monti JD, et al. Executive function and internalizing symptoms in adolescents and young adults with congenital heart disease: the role of coping. J Pediatr Psychol 2018;43(8): 906–15.
11. Calderon J, Bellinger DC. Executive function deficits in congenital heart disease: why is intervention important? Cardiol Young 2015;25(7):1238–46.
12. Crossland DS, Jackson SP, Lyall R, et al. Patient attitudes to sternotomy and thoracotomy scars. Thorac Cardiovasc Surg 2005;53(2):93–5.
13. Agarwal S, Sud K, Khera S, et al. Trends in the burden of adult congenital heart disease in US emergency departments. Clin Cardiol 2016;39(7):391–8.
14. Lundqvist CB, Potpara TS, Malmborg H. Supraventricular arrhythmias in patients with adult congenital heart disease. Arrhythm Electrophysiol Rev 2017; 6(2):42–9.

15. Amedro P, Dorka R, Moniotte S, et al. Quality of life of children with congenital heart diseases: a multi-center controlled cross-sectional study. Pediatr Cardiol 2015;36(8):1588–601.

16. Bruto VC, Harrison DA, Fedak PW, et al. Determinants of health-related quality of life in adults with congenital heart disease. Congenit Heart Dis 2007; 2(5):301–13.

17. Jackson JL, Gerardo GM, Daniels CJ, et al. Perceptions of disease-related stress: a key to better understanding patient-reported outcomes among survivors of congenital heart disease. J Cardiovasc Nurs 2016;32(6):587–93.

18. Westhoff-Bleck M, Briest J, Fraccarollo D, et al. Mental disorders in adults with congenital heart disease: unmet needs and impact on quality of life. J Affect Disord 2016;204:180–6.

19. Westhoff-Bleck M, Winter L, Aguirre Davila L, et al. Diagnostic evaluation of the hospital depression scale (HADS) and the Beck depression inventory II (BDI-II) in adults with congenital heart disease using a structured clinical interview: impact of depression severity. Eur J Prev Cardiol 2020. https://doi.org/10.1177/2047487319865055.

20. Benderly M, Kalter-Leibovici O, Weitzman D, et al. Depression and anxiety are associated with high health care utilization and mortality among adults with congenital heart disease. Int J Cardiol 2019; 276:81–6.

21. Jackson JL, Leslie CE, Hondorp SN. Depressive and anxiety symptoms in adult congenital heart disease: prevalence, health impact and treatment. Prog Cardiovasc Dis 2018;61(3–4):294–9.

22. Kovacs AH, Moons P. Psychosocial functioning and quality of life in adults with congenital heart disease and heart failure. Heart Fail Clin 2014;10(1):35–42.

23. Khanna AD, Duca LM, Kay JD, et al. Prevalence of mental illness in adolescents and adults with congenital heart disease from the Colorado Congenital Heart Defect Surveillance System. Am J Cardiol 2019;124(4):618–26.

24. Warnes CA, Williams RG, Bashore TM, et al. ACC/AHA 2008 guidelines for the management of adults with congenital heart disease: a report of the American College of Cardiology/American Heart Association Task Force on practice guidelines. J Am Coll Cardiol 2008;52(23):e143–263.

25. Jackson JL, Misiti B, Bridge JA, et al. Emotional functioning of adolescents and adults with congenital heart disease: a meta-analysis. Congenit Heart Dis 2015;10(1):2–12.

26. Deen JF, Krieger EV, Slee AE, et al. Metabolic syndrome in adults with congenital heart disease. J Am Heart Assoc 2016;5(2):e001132.

27. Kourkoveli P, Rammos S, Parissis J, et al. Depressive symptoms in patients with congenital heart disease: incidence and prognostic value of self-rating depression scales. Congenit Heart Dis 2015;10(3): 240–7.

28. Deng LX, Khan AM, Drajpuch D, et al. Prevalence and correlates of post-traumatic stress disorder in adults with congenital heart disease. Am J Cardiol 2016;117(5):853–7.

29. American Psychiatric Association. Diagnostic and statistical manual of mental disorders. 5th edition. Arlington (VA): American Psychiatric Association; 2013.

30. Moreland P, Santacroce SJ. Illness uncertainty and posttraumatic stress in young adults with congenital heart disease. J Cardiovasc Nurs 2018;33(4):356–62.

31. Eslami B. Correlates of posttraumatic stress disorder in adults with congenital heart disease. Congenit Heart Dis 2017;12(3):357–63.

32. Hare DL, Stewart AGO, Driscoll A, et al. Screening, referral and treatment of depression by Australian cardiologists. Heart Lung Circ 2019;29:401–4.

33. Larsen KK, Vestergaard CH, Schougaard LM, et al. Contacts to general practice and antidepressant treatment initiation after screening for anxiety and depression in patients with heart disease. Dan Med J 2016;63(2):A5185.

34. Beck AT, Epstein N, Brown G, et al. An inventory for measuring clinical anxiety: psychometric properties. J Consult Clin Psychol 1988;56(6):893–7.

35. Beck AT, Steer RA, Brown GK. Manual for the Beck Depression Inventory-II. San Antonio (TX): Psychological Corporation; 1996.

36. Radloff LS. The CES-D scale: a self-report depression scale for research in the general population. Appl Psychol Meas 1977;1(3):385–401.

37. Moon JR, Huh J, Song J, et al. The Center for Epidemiologic Studies Depression Scale is an adequate screening instrument for depression and anxiety disorder in adults with congenital heart disease. Health Qual Life Outcomes 2017;15(1):176.

38. Spitzer RL, Kroenke K, Williams JB, et al. A brief measure for assessing generalized anxiety disorder: the GAD-7. Arch Intern Med 2006;166(10): 1092–7.

39. Rayner L, Matcham F, Hutton J, et al. Embedding integrated mental health assessment and management in general hospital settings: feasibility, acceptability and the prevalence of common mental disorder. Gen Hosp Psychiatry 2014;36(3): 318–24.

40. Zigmond AS, Snaith RP. The hospital anxiety and depression scale. Acta Psychiatr Scand 1983; 67(6):361–70.

41. Kroenke K, Spitzer RL, Williams JB. The PHQ-9: validity of a brief depression severity measure. J Gen Intern Med 2001;16(9):606–13.

42. Manea L, Gilbody S, McMillan D. A diagnostic meta-analysis of the Patient Health Questionnaire-9 (PHQ-9) algorithm scoring method as a screen for depression. Gen Hosp Psychiatry 2015;37(1):67–75.

43. Kroenke K, Spitzer RL. The PHQ-9: a new depression diagnostic and severity measure. Psychiatr Ann 2002;32(9):509–15.

44. Creamer M, Bell R, Failla S. Psychometric properties of the impact of event scale - revised. Behav Res Ther 2003;41(12):1489–96.

45. Hosey MM, Bienvenu OJ, Dinglas VD, et al. The IES-R remains a core outcome measure for PTSD in critical illness survivorship research. Crit Care 2019; 23(1):362.

46. Foa EB, Cashman L, Jaycox L, et al. The validation of a self-report measure of post-traumatic stress disorder: the post-traumatic diagnostic scale. Psychol Assess 1997;9(4):445–51.

47. Foa EB, McLean CP, Zang Y, et al. Psychometric properties of the posttraumatic stress disorder symptom scale interview for DSM-5 (PSSI-5). Psychol Assess 2016;28(10):1159–65.

48. Blanchard EB, Jones-Alexander J, Buckley TC, et al. Psychometric properties of the PTSD checklist (PCL). Behav Res Ther 1996;34(8):669–73.

49. Bovin MJ, Marx BP, Weathers FW, et al. Psychometric properties of the PTSD checklist for diagnostic and statistical manual of mental disorders-fifth edition (PCL-5) in veterans. Psychol Assess 2016; 28(11):1379–91.

50. Kovacs AH, Saidi AS, Kuhl EA, et al. Depression and anxiety in adult congenital heart disease: predictors and prevalence. Int J Cardiol 2009;137(2):158–64.

51. Richards SH, Anderson L, Jenkinson CE, et al. Psychological interventions for coronary heart disease. Cochrane Database Syst Rev 2017;(4):CD002902.

52. Ski CF, Jelinek M, Jackson AC, et al. Psychosocial interventions for patients with coronary heart disease and depression: a systematic review and meta-analysis. Eur J Cardiovasc Nurs 2016;15(5):305–16.

53. Kovacs AH, Grace SL, Kentner AC, et al. Feasibility and outcomes in a pilot randomized controlled trial of a psychosocial intervention for adults with congenital heart disease. Can J Cardiol 2018; 34(6):766–73.

54. Ferguson M, Kovacs AH. An integrated adult congenital heart disease psychology service. Congenit Heart Dis 2016;11(5):444–51.

55. Andrade C, Kumar CB, Surya S. Cardiovascular mechanisms of SSRI drugs and their benefits and risks in ischemic heart disease and heart failure. Int Clin Psychopharmacol 2013;28(3):145–55.

56. Diller GP, Bräutigam A, Kempny A, et al. Depression requiring anti-depressant drug therapy in adult congenital heart disease: prevalence, risk factors, and prognostic value. Eur Heart J 2016;37(9): 771–82.

57. Bystritsky A, Khalsa SS, Cameron ME, et al. Current diagnosis and treatment of anxiety disorders. P T 2013;38(1):30–57.

58. Pagé MG, Kovacs AH, Irvine J. How do psychosocial challenges associated with living with congenital heart disease translate into treatment interests and preferences? A qualitative approach. Psychol Health 2012;27(11):1260–70.

59. Kovacs AH, Bendell KL, Colman J, et al. Adults with congenital heart disease: psychological needs and treatment preferences. Congenit Heart Dis 2009; 4(3):139–46.

60. Callus E, Pravettoni G. The role of clinical psychology and peer to peer support in the management of chronic medical conditions - a practical example with adults with congenital heart disease. Front Psychol 2018;9:731.

61. Heart to heart peer mentors. ahcaheart.org. Available at: https://www.achaheart.org/get-involved/community/heart-to-heart/. Accessed February 19, 2020.

62. Scott-Sheldon LAJ, Gathright EC, Donahue ML, et al. Mindfulness-based interventions for adults with cardiovascular disease: a systematic review and meta-analysis. Ann Behav Med 2020;54(1): 67–73.

63. Parswani MJ, Sharma MP, Iyengar S. Mindfulness-based stress reduction program in coronary heart disease: a randomized control trial. Int J Yoga 2013;6(2):111–7.

64. Jalali D, Abdolazimi M, Alaei Z, et al. Effectiveness of mindfulness-based stress reduction program on quality of life in cardiovascular disease patients. Int J Cardiol Heart Vasc 2019;23:100356.

65. Levine GN, Lange RA, Bairey-Merz CN, et al. Meditation and cardiovascular risk reduction: a scientific statement from the American Heart Association. J Am Heart Assoc 2017;6(10):e002218.

66. Blumenthal JA, Smith PJ, Hoffman BM. Is exercise a viable treatment for depression? ACSMs Health Fit J 2012;16(4):14–21.

67. Chan JSY, Liu G, Liang D, et al. A systematic review on the effects of exercise intensity, duration, and modality. J Psychol 2019;153(1):102–25.

68. O'Keefe EL, O'Keefe JH, Lavie CJ. Exercise counteracts the cardiotoxicity of psychosocial stress. Mayo Clin Proc 2019;94(9):1852–64.

69. Longmuir PE, Brothers JA, de Ferranti SD, et al. Promotion of physical activity for children and adults with congenital heart disease: a scientific statement from the American Heart Association. Circulation 2013;127(21):2147–59.

70. Bang JS, Jo S, Kim GB, et al. The mental health and quality of life of adult patients with congenital heart disease. Int J Cardiol 2013;170(1):49–53.

71. Eslami B, Sundin O, Macassa G, et al. Anxiety, depressive and somatic symptoms in adults with congenital heart disease. J Psychosom Res 2013; 74(1):49–56.

Atrial Septal Defect

Elisa A. Bradley, MD[a],*, Ali N. Zaidi, MD[b]

KEYWORDS

- Atrial septal defect • Congenital heart disease • Pulmonary arterial hypertension
- Ostium secundum defect • Ostium primum defect • Sinus venosus defect

KEY POINTS

- Atrial septal defects are among the most common types of congenital heart disease that may go undiagnosed in childhood and may initially be found in adulthood.
- Adults with an atrial septal defect are often asymptomatic, but may present with nonspecific symptoms such as dyspnea on exertion or exercise intolerance.
- Pulmonary arterial hypertension and atrial arrhythmias may develop as a consequence of a long-standing unrepaired atrial septal defect.
- Management of the adult with an atrial septal defect must include consideration of whether or not pulmonary arterial hypertension is present, degree of shunting, and anatomy.
- Therapeutic considerations for an unrepaired atrial septal defect in the adult include pulmonary arterial vasodilator therapy, interatrial septal rim assessment, and candidacy for percutaneous versus surgical repair.

 Video content accompanies this article at http://www.cardiology.theclinics.com.

INTRODUCTION

Atrial septal defects (ASD) are considered one of the most common congenital heart defects (CHD) found in the adult. The estimated prevalence of ASDs in adults is 0.88 per 1000 patients.[1] Frequently, the reason that this lesion is not detected sooner is that many patients are asymptomatic until the second to fourth decades of life, a time after which increased pulmonary blood flow may lead to pulmonary vascular remodeling and ultimately affect shunt direction and end-organ perfusion. Although this lesion is classified as a simple form of CHD, complex physiologic changes related to pulmonary vascular remodeling and shunt direction often complicate the presentation. Therefore, the assessment and treatment options vary widely between patients and require

evaluation by specialized and experienced providers in the field of adult CHD.[2]

The purpose of this review is to describe ASD anatomy and various physiologic presentations in the adult. The goal is to review common clinical presentations and findings on imaging and special testing, and to discuss both practical and advanced management strategies inclusive of medical therapeutic considerations, surgical repair options, and percutaneous closure.

ANATOMY AND PHYSIOLOGY
Anatomy

There are 4 main types of defects that occur in the atrial septum and lead to the formation of an ASD (**Fig. 1**).[2] The most common type of ASD is the ostium secundum defect, which accounts for

[a] Department of Internal Medicine, Division of Cardiovascular Medicine, The Ohio State University, Columbus, OH, USA; [b] Mount Sinai Cardiovascular Institute, The Children's Heart Center, Kravis Children's Hospital, Icahn School of Medicine at Mount Sinai, 1 Gustave L. Levy Place, Box 1030, New York, NY 10029, USA
* Corresponding author. Davis Heart Lung Research Institute, 473 West 12thAvenue, Columbus, OH 43210.
E-mail addresses: Elisa.bradley@osumc.edu; elisa_a_bradley@yahoo.com
Twitter: @drelisabradley (E.A.B.); @AliZaidi MD (A.N.Z.)

Cardiol Clin 38 (2020) 317–324
https://doi.org/10.1016/j.ccl.2020.04.001

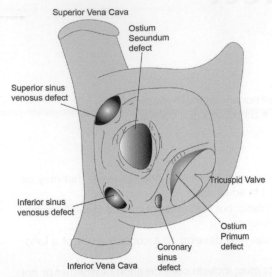

Superior Vena Cava

Ostium
Secundum
defect

Superior sinus
venosus defect

Tricuspid Valve

Inferior sinus
venosus defect

Ostium
Primum
defect

Coronary
sinus
defect

Inferior Vena Cava

Fig. 1. Anatomy of the interatrial septum and septal defects. Anatomy of the interatrial septum demonstrating the location(s) of the 4 main types of ASDs: secundum, primum, sinus venosus, and coronary sinus, as viewed from the RA.

approximately 80% of ASDs. This defect arises owing to a deficiency of tissue at the level of the fossa ovalis. Ostium primum ASDs account for about 10% of septal defects and develop owing to a deficiency in tissue near the atrioventricular valves. Ostium primum ASDs are associated with a cleft in the left-sided atrioventricular valve and are often more aptly referred to by the synonymous term, partial atrioventricular septal defect. Sinus venosus defects occur more commonly in the superior (vs inferior) portion of the embryologic sinus venosus and commonly occur with partial anomalous pulmonary venous return, particularly of the right upper pulmonary vein. Coronary sinus defects, frequently referred to as unroofed coronary sinus, are the least common type of ASD and often are missed on traditional imaging modalities. However, an unroofed coronary sinus may be detected when agitated saline contrast bubbles from the left upper extremity enter the left atrium (LA) first, before the right atrium (RA).

Normal Physiology

When resting cardiopulmonary hemodynamics are normal in the presence of an ASD, blood shunts from the oxygenated LA through the ASD to the deoxygenated blood pool in the RA, creating a step-up in oxygen saturation at the level of the RA. Hemodynamics in the setting of an ASD are governed by Ohm's law as it relates to fluid flow in the pulmonary vascular bed

(ΔPressure = Flow × Resistance, $\Delta P = QR$). So long as flow and resistance are low, the degree of shunting that occurs is based on end-diastolic filling pressures, compliance, and the anatomy and size of the defect. This lesion is generally well-tolerated in children, adolescents, and the young adult, in part owing to low filling pressures in the heart and high compliance in a system with normal pulmonary vascular resistance (PVR). However, in the case of a sizable ASD, over time the increased left-to-right flow across the defect leads to enlargement of the RA and right ventricle. This finding may be the first clue to the presence of an ASD.

Abnormal Physiology

In a minority of patients, the pulmonary overcirculation that results from a septal defect may contribute to abnormal pulmonary vascular remodeling and elevation in PVR, culminating in the development of pulmonary arterial hypertension (PAH). Up to 16% of adults who present with an ASD have concomitant PAH.[3] In most cases, although pulmonary artery pressures are elevated, they remain lower than the systemic blood pressure. However, in a minority of cases, the pulmonary vascular pressures increase to systemic or suprasystemic levels, resulting in reversal of the shunt (right-to-left flow) and peripheral desaturation with cyanosis, a condition called Eisenmenger syndrome. In general, therapeutic options for the patient that has developed frank Eisenmenger syndrome are limited in comparison with the adult with an unrepaired ASD and mild to moderate PAH. Recent studies have shown that those patients with ASD and mild to moderate PAH may respond favorably to PAH-specific medical therapy, and potentially regress PVR to a level at which septal defect repair may be possible, and perhaps impact long-term morbidity and mortality (**Table 1**).

CLINICAL PRESENTATION

Most adults who present with a newly diagnosed unrepaired ASD are asymptomatic, and the finding is incidental. However, in a minority of patients, a careful medical history and clinical examination may suggest the presence of an unrepaired ASD. In these patients, the history often reveals a gradual change in exercise capacity, commonly reported as subtle, and occasionally overt, dyspnea on exertion. Typically, a patient may describe this change occurring over the preceding months to years; however, if PAH is present, this change can occur more abruptly, on the order of weeks to months. Less frequently, palpitations may

Table 1
Studies evaluating delayed ASD closure in moderate to severe PAH

Author, Year	Timeframe	Location	N	Therapy	Outcomes
Cho et al,[17] 2011	2004–2009	Korea	16	PDE5i, ERA, Inh Prost	All closed with fenestration (PVR od 9.8)
Fujino et al,[12] 2015	2013	Japan	5	ERA, Inh Prost	1 patient had preclosure treatment
Bradley et al,[13] 2013	1998–2012	U.S.	15	PDE5i, ERA, Prost	5 (33%) underwent closure PVR of 8.8 (7.2 → 4.6 vs 9.9 → 8.2)
Kijima et al,[14] 2016	2006–2014	Japan	8 (22)	PDE5i, ERA, Inh Prost	All received closure (PVR 9.6 → 4.0)
Song et al,[15] 2016	2001–2012	Korea	7 (17)	PDE5i, ERA, Inh Prost	All closed with fenestration (PVR 9.2 → 6.3)
Bradley et al,[16] 2018	1996–2017	US	69	PDE5i, ERA, PC	19 (28%) underwent closure, closure group: ↑ RV function, ↑ 6MWTD, trend ↑ survival.

Abbreviations: 6MWTD, 6-minute walk test distance; ERA, endothelin receptor antagonist; Inh, inhaled; PC, prostacyclin; PDE5i, phosphodiesterase type 5 inhibitor; RV, right ventricle.

occur, especially in those that have developed an occult atrial arrhythmia, which is more common in the patient who presents at an older age. On physical examination, there may be a soft systolic crescendo–decrescendo outflow tract murmur owing to increased flow across the pulmonary valve, accompanied by a fixed split in the S2 heart sound owing to delayed closure of the pulmonic valve.

INVESTIGATION AND ASSESSMENT

Often the first test that a new patient with dyspnea receives is an electrocardiogram. This test can be helpful if an ASD is suspected, because these patients commonly demonstrate an incomplete right bundle branch block. More specifically, in the presence of a secundum ASD right axis deviation and crochetage (crochet-like hook) of the inferior lead R waves may be seen. In primum ASD, incomplete right bundle branch block is more likely to occur in the presence of left axis deviation. If a chest radiograph is sought, it is often normal. However, if the patient has developed PAH, there may be cardiomegaly and increased pulmonary vascularity.

Ultimately, imaging is required to confirm the diagnosis of an ASD. Frequently, a transthoracic echocardiogram is the preferred initial imaging test. The limitation of the transthoracic echocardiogram is that it may be impacted by poor acoustic windows related to the adult body habitus. However, image quality is often sufficient to

evaluate the size of the RA and right ventricle, which are typically enlarged. This study can also provide information about pulmonary artery pressure, and may be the first clue as to the presence of PAH. In the patient with good transthoracic echocardiogram image quality, the interatrial septum can be visualized and color Doppler interrogation may be used to determine if a defect is present. Agitated saline contrast is often administered to determine if there is a septal defect present and, in the case of an ASD, demonstrates extravasation of saline contrast microbubbles from the RA to the LA at the level of the interatrial septum.

In most cases, a transesophageal echocardiogram (TEE) is required to more closely examine the interatrial septum to determine both the type and size of the ASD. These factors become important when considering therapeutic options with respect to closure and repair of the defect. Typically, the interatrial septum and defect are imaged in at least 3 different TEE planes: 0° and 90° at the mid esophagus, and 30° at the high esophageal level (**Fig. 2**, Videos 1–3). Although these views provide an adequate evaluation of the interatrial septum and rims, the inferior vena caval rim is often not well-visualized on TEE and, if it is suspected to be deficient, may require intravascular echocardiography at the time of hemodynamic evaluation.

Although advanced cardiac imaging such as computed tomography and cardiac MRI are not required to make the diagnosis of an ASD, these

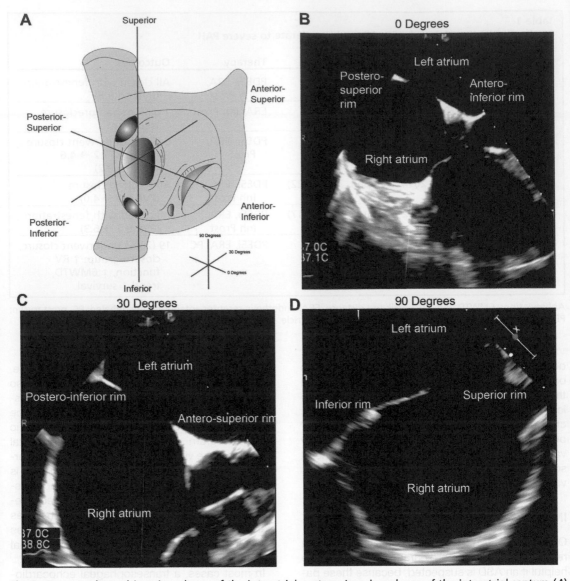

Fig. 2. Transesophageal imaging planes of the interatrial septum. Imaging planes of the interatrial septum (*A*) when evaluated by TEE include mid esophageal views at 0° (*B*) demonstrating the posterosuperior and anteroinferior rims and at 90° show the superior and inferior rims (*D*). High esophageal views at 30° (*C*) are required to demonstrate the posteroinferior and anteroinferior rims.

tests may be completed during the clinical workup. Advanced imaging provides high quality data on chamber size and function and can be helpful in determining whether or not anomalous pulmonary venous return is present, particularly when the pulmonary veins are not fully evaluated on TEE (**Fig. 3**). Additionally, flow quantification on cardiac MRI may be used to evaluate Qp:Qs in the presence of a septal defect.

Invasive hemodynamic right heart catheterization (RHC) is usually one of the last tests to be completed in the presence of an ASD, particularly

when defect repair is being considered. RHC allows for the evaluation of shunt flow and in particular is helpful in quantifying the degree and direction of shunting. Intravascular echocardiography is frequently undertaken during RHC if TEE images are inadequate in evaluation of the defect, and if or when percutaneous closure is being considered. Intravascular echo is often used to provide direct visualization of the interatrial septum and allows for real-time 2-dimensional imaging guidance at the time of percutaneous closure.

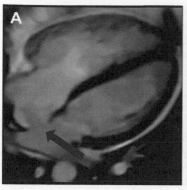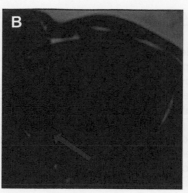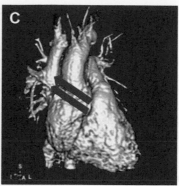

Fig. 3. Cardiac MRI evaluation for ASDs. Routine cardiac MRI sequences used to define the atrial septum on bright blood images (gradient echo sequences) (*A*) and dark blood images (fast spin echo sequences) (*B*). These images allow definition of atrial septal anatomy (*red arrow*, secundum ASD), atrial and ventricular morphology and are used to assess volumetric data and to quantify ventricular function. High spatial resolution MR angiography with 3-dimentional volume rendered imaging is used to define cardiac anatomy and morphology of the great vessels and systemic and/or pulmonary veins (*C*). The *double red arrows* demonstrate anomalous return of right-sided pulmonary veins to the superior vena cava.

Finally, exercise testing may be done before or after RHC in select cases. This testing can be accomplished in the form of a 6-minute walk test or more formal cardiopulmonary exercise testing. The purpose of exercise testing is not only to evaluate objective exercise tolerance, but also to assess oxygenation at rest and with peak exercise. In patients with normal resting hemodynamics (and in the absence of significant lung disease), oxygen saturation is typically normal. However, with exercise, a minority of patients demonstrate significant increases in the PVR. This hemodynamic change can cause a previous left-to-right or minimally bidirectional shunt to become right-to-left with activity, and results in exercise-induced desaturation. In this situation, closure of the defect may be unsafe and often PAH-specific medical therapy may be considered, even when resting pulmonary artery pressures may be normal (see **Table 1**).

MEDICAL DECISION MAKING AND THERAPEUTIC CONSIDERATIONS
Indications for Repair

Small ASDs may spontaneously close in childhood; however, larger defects may contribute to hemodynamic abnormalities and clinical symptoms if left unrepaired. The decision to repair an ASD is based on clinical and anatomic information, including the size and location of the defect, magnitude of hemodynamic impact of the shunt, and the presence and degree of PAH, if present. Patients with decreased functional capacity caused by hemodynamically significant ASD's (moderate or large left-to-right shunts, a Qp:Qs of >1.5 and evidence of right heart volume overload in the absence of significant PAH) typically benefit from surgical or transcatheter closure of the ASD.[4] Asymptomatic patients with a significant left-to-right shunt (Qp:Qs of >1.5) and evidence of right heart enlargement also benefit from closure, because continued overcirculation in an already dilated right heart increases the likelihood of late clinical complications, including decreased functional capacity, atrial arrhythmia, and the development of PAH.[5,6]

Contraindications for Repair

Closure of an ASD is not recommended in patients with a clinically significant right-to-left shunt and those with severe PAH (PVR of >8 Wood units or irreversible pulmonary vascular occlusive disease, desaturated at rest). There are emerging data that support that patients with a pulmonary artery pressure of less than two-thirds of the systemic arterial pressure, a PVR of less than two-thirds of the systemic resistance, or a positive response to pulmonary vasodilator testing may be considered for ASD closure.[6] A fenestrated device is often considered in these cases to ensure that an adequate "popoff" is present so that if RA pressure rises above the LA pressure, cardiac output is conserved. Relative contraindications to closure typically are regarded for percutaneous cases and include: defects larger than 36 mm, inadequate margins and rims to safely anchor the device, and/or interference of the device with the atrioventricular valves or venous drainage.[7]

Surgical Repair Options and Outcomes

Cardiothoracic surgery is the gold standard approach for ASD repair and implies direct visualization of the defect using an open sternotomy approach with cardiopulmonary bypass. Surgical repair is typically achieved by the use of autologous pericardial or synthetic patches made of polyester polymer (Dacron) or polytetrafluoroethylene. In an ostium primum defect, surgical repair may be more complicated because the patch has to be attached at the crux of the ventricular septum and atrioventricular valves. Mitral valve repair, including closure of the cleft mitral leaflet with possible annuloplasty, may be necessary. In rare cases, mitral valve replacement may be required. In the case of a sinus venosus defect, partial anomalous pulmonary venous return is typical, with 1 or more of the pulmonary veins draining into the RA. The ASD must be patch closed, allowing for anomalous pulmonary venous drainage to be diverted into the LA. Surgical repair before 25 years of age results in a 30-year survival rate comparable to that of age- and sex-matched control subjects; however, with repair between the ages of 25 and 40 years, surgical survival is attenuated, although not significantly if pulmonary artery pressures are normal.[8] Although surgical repair of an ASD in adulthood is associated with a significant reduction in mortality, there is no beneficial impact on the risk of current or future atrial arrhythmias.

Overall mortality with ASD repair is low; however, morbidities such as atrial arrhythmia, bleeding, pneumothorax, and pericardial or pleural effusions may occur.[7]

Percutaneous Repair Options and Outcomes

Transcatheter closure has become an accepted alternative for surgical repair in adults with a secundum ASD and adequate tissue rims.[9] Although many devices have been studied, only the following ASD closure devices have become routinely available in the United States: Amplatzer Septal Occluder, the Gore Helex septal occluder, and the Gore Cardioform Septal Occluder (Table 2). The Amplatzer Septal Occluder is currently the most widely used device in the United States because it is easy to implant and is manufactured in sizes that permit safe closure of relatively large defects. Percutaneous transcatheter ASD closure has a postprocedural complication risk of 7.2% compared with a postoperative complication risk of 24%.[9] Complications associated with percutaneous closure include arrhythmias, atrioventricular block, device erosion, and thromboembolism. Device embolization and malpositioning typically occur as a result of inadequate sizing or device placement, with an incidence of less than 1%. When ASDs are closed percutaneously, patients require antiplatelet therapy typically for 6 months, although this requirement varies based on operator and center expertise.

Table 2
Percutaneous ASD devices in the United States

Device	Description	Maximum Size of the Defect
Amplatzer Septal Occluder	Self-expanding, recapturable prosthesis made of nitinol wire mesh, 2 round discs with a polyester patch inside, and a connecting short waist.	36 mm
Gore Helex Septal Occluder	Corkscrew-type nitinol wire frame covered by expanded polytetrafluoroethylene to reduce friction with the cardiac adjacent structures; thereby reducing the risk of erosion; size varies from 15 to 30 mm, but is not recommended for defects >18 mm	18 mm
Gore Cardioform Septal Occluder	Flexible, retrievable, double-disc device with a petal design made of a nitinol frame covered by expanded polytetrafluoroethylene to facilitate rapid endothelialization	17 mm
Gore Cardioform ASD Occluder	Implantable occluder and a delivery system to treat a range of defects from 8 to 35 mm with unique conformability to adapt to secundum ASD	35 mm

SPECIAL CASES: SHUNT-RELATED PULMONARY ARTERIAL HYPERTENSION

Improvements in the diagnosis and management of CHD has contributed to an increasing number of adult CHD survivors, including those with PAH and either repaired or unrepaired CHD. This cohort includes patients with unrepaired ASDs with PAH who are evaluated and then classified into 1 of 4 categories of shunt-related PAH.[10] The most well-known of these clinical categories is Eisenmenger's syndrome, which occurs when the PVR increases to systemic levels and the intracardiac shunt reverses, such that there is pulmonary-to-systemic shunting at rest and manifest cyanosis. It is clear that this group of patients would be unsafe to consider defect repair, because cardiac output depends on the shunt in the presence of severely elevated PVR. However, it is less clear that this is the case in the second clinical category, namely, PAH associated with prevalent systemic-to-pulmonary shunt. In this group, the defect is typically moderate to large in size and the PVR is elevated, yet still substantially lower than the systemic vascular resistance, characterized predominantly by systemic-to-pulmonary shunting. Although resting cyanosis is not present in this group, PVR may increase, particularly with exercise, and this may manifest as cyanosis with exercise, implying that physical activity may change hemodynamics such that the Qp:Qs approaches 1.0 (bidirectional shunting). Defect repair in this setting, particularly with significantly elevated PVR and after PAH-specific medical therapy, is controversial. However, several studies have implied that there may be a subset of patients in whom repair may be achieved safely and impact long-term outcome favorably.[11–16] This area requires further study, and to date these decisions are made on an individual basis with careful consideration and coordination of an experienced adult CHD and pulmonary hypertension team. The final 2 categories of CHD with PAH include those patients with PAH and small/coincidental defect and those with PAH after defect correction. In both cases, PAH develops in the absence of a current hemodynamically significant shunt, highlighting that likely more than a single mechanism is responsible for PAH in this CHD patient. As such, ASD repair in these last 2 categories is not typically a therapeutic consideration.

SUMMARY

Although an ASD is considered a type of simple CHD, you can see here that it is not always a simple condition to manage. There is variability in the anatomy of the defect, resultant physiology, and late hemodynamic and arrhythmia-driven comorbidities. These factors ultimately impact therapeutic management and repair strategies. For the straightforward adult patient with a sizable secundum ASD and normal physiology, transcatheter repair is a safe and acceptable option. For an adult with any other type of ASD and abnormal physiology, the management algorithm changes and is impacted commonly by anatomic considerations of the defect(s), arrhythmia, heart failure, and/or PAH. For these reasons, it is important that adult patients with an ASD be referred for specialized and expert care by a team with experience in adult CHD.

DISCLOSURE

The authors have nothing to disclose.

SUPPLEMENTARY DATA

Supplementary data related to this article can be found online at https://doi.org/10.1016/j.ccl.2020.04.001.

REFERENCES

1. Marelli AJ, Ionescu-Ittu R, Mackie AS, et al. Lifetime prevalence of congenital heart disease in the general population from 2000 to 2010. Circulation 2014;130:749–56.
2. Stout KK, Daniels CJ, Aboulhosn JA, et al. 2018 AHA/ACC guideline for the management of adults with congenital heart disease: executive summary: a report of the American College of Cardiology/American Heart Association Task Force on clinical practice guidelines. Circulation 2019;139:e637–97.
3. Gabriels C, De Meester P, Pasquet A, et al. A different view on predictors of pulmonary hypertension in secundum atrial septal defect. Int J Cardiol 2014;176:833–40.
4. Stout KK, Daniels CJ, Aboulhosn JA, et al. 2018 AHA/ACC guideline for the management of adults with congenital heart disease: a report of the American College of Cardiology/American Heart Association Task Force on clinical practice guidelines. Circulation 2019;139:e698–800.
5. Stout KK, Daniels CJ, Aboulhosn JA, et al. 2018 AHA/ACC guideline for the management of adults with congenital heart disease: a report of the American College of Cardiology/American Heart Association Task Force on clinical practice guidelines. J Am Coll Cardiol 2019;73:e81–192.
6. Fraisse A, Latchman M, Sharma SR, et al. Atrial septal defect closure: indications and contra-indications. J Thorac Dis 2018;10:S2874–81.

7. Geva T, Martins JD, Wald RM. Atrial septal defects. Lancet 2014;383:1921–32.

8. Murphy JG, Gersh BJ, McGoon MD, et al. Long-term outcome after surgical repair of isolated atrial septal defect. Follow-up at 27 to 32 years. N Engl J Med 1990;323:1645–50.

9. Yang MC, Wu JR. Recent review of transcatheter closure of atrial septal defect. Kaohsiung J Med Sci 2018;34:363–9.

10. Galie N, Hoeper MM, Humbert M, et al. Guidelines for the diagnosis and treatment of pulmonary hypertension: the Task Force for the diagnosis and treatment of pulmonary hypertension of the European Society of Cardiology (ESC) and the European Respiratory Society (ERS), endorsed by the International Society of Heart and Lung Transplantation (ISHLT). Eur Heart J 2009;30:2493–537.

11. Cho YH, Jun TG, Yang JH, et al. Surgical strategy in patients with atrial septal defect and severe pulmonary hypertension. Heart Surg Forum 2012;15: E111–5.

12. Fujino T, Yao A, Hatano M, et al. Targeted therapy is required for management of pulmonary arterial hypertension after defect closure in adult patients with atrial septal defect and associated pulmonary arterial hypertension. Int Heart J 2015;56:86–93.

13. Bradley EA, Chakinala M, Billadello JJ. Usefulness of medical therapy for pulmonary hypertension and delayed atrial septal defect closure. Am J Cardiol 2013;112:1471–6.

14. Kijima Y, Akagi T, Takaya Y, et al. Treat and repair strategy in patients with atrial septal defect and significant pulmonary arterial hypertension. Circulation 2016;80:227–34.

15. Song J, Huh J, Lee SY, et al. Hemodynamic follow-up in adult patients with pulmonary hypertension associated with atrial septal defect after partial closure. Yonsei Med J 2016;57:306–12.

16. Bradley EA, Ammash N, Martinez SC, et al. "Treat-to-close": non-repairable ASD-PAH in the adult: results from the North American ASD-PAH (NAAP) Multi-center Registry. Int J Cardiol 2019;291:127–33.

17. Cho MJ, Song J, Kim SJ, et al. Transcatheter closure of multiple atrial septal defects with the Amplatzer device. Korean Circ J 2011;41:549–51.

Aortopathy in Congenital Heart Disease

Timothy B. Cotts, MD[a],*, Katherine B. Salciccioli, MD[b], Sara K. Swanson, MD, PhD[c], Anji T. Yetman, MD[d,e]

KEYWORDS

• Aortopathy • Congenital heart disease • Aortic dissection • Bicuspid aortic valve

KEY POINTS

• Normal values for aortic dimensions may vary by age and body size prompting the need to consult nomograms when evaluating individual patients.
• High-risk patients include those with the "aortic root phenotype" and those with syndromic or familial aortopathies including Marfan syndrome, Loeys-Dietz syndrome, and Turner syndrome.
• The most significant functional alteration in aortopathy is increased wall stiffness, which is seen in patients with Marfan syndrome and bicuspid aortic valves and patients with other familial thoracic aortic aneurysms and dissections.
• Aortic dilatation is common in patients with conotruncal congenital heart defects, and rarely results in aortic dissection.

Over the last few decades, an accumulating body of medical literature has documented the presence of aortic dilation in patients with congenital heart defects (CHD) and explored the clinical importance of this common radiographic finding.[1–9] The impetus of a clinical review published a decade ago was to alert cardiologists to the potential for progressive, clinically significant aortic dilation in patients with CHD, a disease entity that had previously received little attention.[1] As often is the case in clinical medicine, the pendulum swung toward intervention, perhaps too far, and only more recently has begun to right itself.[4–6] Although progressive aortic dilation is seen commonly in adults with congenital heart disease, aortic dissection is rare.[9] Progressive aortic dilation is seen most commonly in bicuspid aortic valve

(BAV) and conotruncal defects, both of which are discussed in this article.[7,8,10]

THE NORMAL AORTA

The thoracic ascending aorta (TAA) is considered dilated or ectatic when its size measures more than 1.1 to 1.5 times normal and aneurysmal if greater.[6,11,12] The normal aorta is larger in older individuals and patients with greater body surface area and/or height, with an average increase of 1.2 mm for each decade in age and 1 mm for each 0.23 m² in body surface area.[8,11] In a large American population-based study of more than 5000 participants age 45 to 84 years, the upper limit of normal for the TAA luminal diameter for white women was 35.8 mm (22 mm/m²) and 40.3 mm (20 mm/m²) for white men as determined

---

[a] Internal Medicine and Pediatrics, University of Michigan, Michigan Congenital Heart Center, 1540 East Hospital Drive, Ann Arbor, MI 48109-4204, USA; [b] University of Michigan, Michigan Congenital Heart Center, 1540 East Hospital Drive, Ann Arbor, MI 48109-4204, USA; [c] Pediatrics, University of Nebraska Medical Center, Children's Hospital & Medical Center, and Nebraska Medicine, 8200 Dodge Street, Omaha, NE 68114, USA; [d] Pediatrics, Aortopathy Program, University of Nebraska Medical Center, Children's Hospital & Medical Center, and Nebraska Medicine, 8200 Dodge Street, Omaha, NE 68114, USA; [e] Medicine, Aortopathy Program, University of Nebraska Medical Center, Children's Hospital & Medical Center, and Nebraska Medicine, 8200 Dodge Street, Omaha, NE 68114, USA

* Corresponding author.
E-mail address: cottstim@med.umich.edu

Cardiol Clin 38 (2020) 325–336
https://doi.org/10.1016/j.ccl.2020.04.002
0733-8651/20/© 2020 Elsevier Inc. All rights reserved.

by MRI.[11] Aortic diameters were greater in Chinese Americans, smaller in African Americans, and not significantly different in Hispanic individuals.[11] Within the general population, gender is thought to have a significant impact on aortic size and the risk for, and outcome of, aortic dissection. Female gender has been associated with greater rates of TAA growth, higher rates of TAA dissection, and lower 5-year event-free survival.[13] In light of the normal variations in aortic size described previously, use of gender-specific nomograms that index aortic size for body size and age are recommended and readily available.[14–17] Gone are the days when an aortic diameter less than 4 cm is considered normal.

STRUCTURAL AND FUNCTIONAL ALTERATIONS OF THE DILATED AORTA
Structural Alterations

The same picture of maladaptive remodeling of the aortic media seen in Marfan syndrome is also noted in patients with BAV and conotruncal defects.[18–22] In contrast to degenerative ascending aortic aneurysms, there is extracellular matrix degradation associated with noninflammatory loss of vascular smooth muscle cells.[8] The vascular smooth muscle cell apoptosis is thought to occur secondary to excessive activity of a group of degradative enzymes known as matrix metalloproteinases (MMPs). The increase in MMP activity may arise because of an imbalance of these enzymes and their tissue inhibitors (TIMPs).[8] As with Marfan syndrome, the transforming growth factor-β superfamily of cytokines has also been implicated in aneurysm formation in patients with CHD.[20,22] The underlying impetus that triggers the maladaptive remodeling process in all of these disorders remains poorly understood. Either because of a fibrillin deficiency as documented in BAV, an altered fibrillin product as is the case in Marfan syndrome, or a hemodynamic stressor the MMP cascade is triggered resulting in the common pathologic appearance.[8,21] Despite the similarities in the pathophysiology, the frequency of aortic dilation, and more importantly, the risk of aortic dissection, differs considerably among the aortopathies of Marfan syndrome, BAV, and conotruncal defects.[3,6] In light of these differences, the criteria for surgical intervention differ.[1,4–6,23]

Functional Alterations

The most significant functional alteration in aortopathy is increased wall stiffness, which is seen in patients with Marfan syndrome and BAV and patients with other familial thoracic aortic aneurysms and

dissections.[24–28] This increased stiffness is also seen with increasing age and with diabetes.[29,30] Stiffness is measured in many different ways depending on the modality used (ie, echo vs MRI), but in general is a measure of the relative change in vessel dimension compared with changes in pressure between systole and diastole.[24,25,31,32]

There has been historical debate as to whether increased stiffness leads to dilation or aneurysm formation. Stiffness is believed to predict more significant aortic dilation in patients with Marfan syndrome and BAV, even in the absence of significant valvular dysfunction.[24,32–35] More recent studies, however, have shown stiffness to be a consequence of the previously discussed cellular remodeling rather than a stimulus for said remodeling.[24,26] Two smaller recent studies have shown increased aortic stiffness to be associated with slowed arterial dilation and aneurysm formation, suggesting stiffness may be protective.[24,26] However, more work is needed to refine the understanding of the causal relationship between stiffness and dilation and to determine whether prospective monitoring of aortic stiffness by echocardiography or MRI can be used to predict change in aortic size or, more importantly, to provide useful input into medical and surgical decision-making.

BICUSPID AORTIC VALVE AORTOPATHY

BAV is the most common congenital cardiac defect with a prevalence of 1% to 2% of the general population, with males comprising approximately 70% of all BAV cases.[6,36] Although stenosis and insufficiency are the most common complications of BAV, aortic aneurysms occur in 40% to 50% of patients.[1–6] Aortic dilation often begins in early childhood and is progressive, increasing at a more rapid rate than age-matched healthy control subjects.[2] BAV aortopathy-related mortality estimates vary widely, which likely relates to the fact that BAV aortopathy is a heterogeneous disorder. In 1978, before the advent of modern-day echo, Edwards and colleagues[37] noted at 6.14% lifetime risk of aortic dissection in all-comers with BAV. With modern echo techniques and routine thoracic screening performed for a multitude of noncardiac disorders, many more patients with a normally functioning BAV are diagnosed. As the denominator has increased with inclusion of much milder forms of the disease, estimates of dissection risk have decreased. The incidence of aortic dissection was 0.1% per patient year of follow-up in a Toronto study involving more than 600 patients with a BAV.[9] Similarly, Michelena and colleagues[38] documented no increase in mortality or dissection over age-matched control subjects over a period of 20 years in a young adult cohort with a normal functioning BAV receiving routine cardiac care. Despite the low mortality rate in this cohort, morbidity remained high with combined cardiovascular medical or surgical events (heart failure, stroke, endocarditis, valve or aortic surgery) occurring in 42% at 20 years after diagnosis.

Although the risk of aortic dissection has been shown to be lower than once thought, BAV aortopathy remains a common indication for surgical intervention with studies demonstrating significant regional variations in surgical practice and practice patterns that are not guideline-driven.[39] Efforts are being made to distinguish between high- and low-risk patients to provide timely surgery to only those at higher risk of dissection. Aortic size alone has been shown to be insufficient in predicting the risk of ascending aortic dissection because most patients experiencing dissection do so at less than the current surgical criteria of 5.5 cm.[40] Although this has been an impetus for some to operate at smaller diameters, the vast denominator of those with smaller aortas who do not dissect suggests the pitfall in relying in aortic size alone.[41] Substantial efforts are currently being made to improve risk prediction of aortic catastrophes in BAV patients. Circulating levels of MMPs, TIMPs, transforming growth factor-β1 levels, specific microRNA signatures, and levels of sRAGE, an immunoglobulin superfamily of surface molecules that bind proinflammatory mediators, have all shown promise correlating with the degree of aortic disease in different at-risk BAV populations.[42–45] Although none of these circulating biomarkers are yet ready for routine introduction into clinical practice, the hope is that serologic testing may soon offer complementary information to radiographic imaging. Additionally, imaging measurements of aortic stiffness may become more clinically useful in the future.

Genetics of Bicuspid Aortic Valve and Bicuspid Aortic Valve Aortopathy

The role of a genetic versus hemodynamic alteration as the source of BAV aortopathy remains controversial.[3,8] There are ample data to support a role for both and the weight of either may vary from patient to patient. Familial studies suggest an autosomal-dominant mode of inheritance with incomplete penetrance.[46,47] Loscalzo and colleagues[48] noted an increased incidence of aortic dilation and aortic dissection in family members of patients with BAV even in the absence of a BAV suggesting the aortopathy and valve abnormality were two different manifestations of a common developmental anomaly. Familial studies have documented a 9% to 20% chance of identifying BAV in first-degree relatives of an affected proband and form the basis for the guidelines recommending echocardiographic screening in all first-degree relatives.[3–6,8,31,46,49] Despite high heritability, only a few genes to date have been linked to isolated familial nonsyndromic BAV aortopathy, including *NOTCH-1*, *SMAD6*, and *MAT2A*.[47,50,51] Within patients with Turner syndrome, *TIMP3* and *TIMP1* (genes for the TIMPs) have been implicated in BAV aortopathy.[52]

Hemodynamic Perturbations and Bicuspid Aortic Valve Aortopathy

The hemodynamics of BAV aortopathy are relevant in that the altered flow patterns caused by the abnormal valve are related to aortic morphology.[53–57] Additionally, valve morphology, independent of valve function, correlates with the type of aortic dilation present, suggesting that there are predictable patterns of flow that lead to specific aortopathy patterns.[55,57] Different patterns of leaflet fusion (eg, right-left coronary cusp fusion vs right-noncoronary cusp fusion) lead to predictably different flow acceleration through and beyond the valve. These altered flows lead to focal increases in wall shear stress in characteristic locations in the ascending aorta, with right-left cusp fusion leading to an anteriorly directed jet and right-nonfusion leading to a more posteriorly directed jet.[58] The phenotypic patterns of dilation seen in these two different populations of patients correspond with their respective characteristic areas of maximum wall shear stress.[53–56,58] These flow patterns have been extensively studied using MRI, but to date this information has not been translated into routine clinical application.

Surveillance of Patients with Bicuspid Aortic Valve

The rationale for periodic visits for patients with BAV is not only to monitor the status of valve function but to monitor the rate of progression of aortic dilation, monitor and treat elevated blood pressure, reassess whether the patient falls into a high-risk category, use such information to determine the appropriate timing of surgery (**Table 1**), and provide and reinforce lifestyle recommendations aimed at mitigating disease progression.

Medical Therapy for Bicuspid Aortic Valve and Bicuspid Aortic Valve Aortopathy

There have been no randomized trials demonstrating improved outcomes for BAV aortopathy, either dilation or dissection, with the use of any

Table 1
Syndrome and nonsyndromic aortopathies with increased prevalence of bicuspid aortic valve

Gene	Disorder	History	Incidence of BAV	Examination Findings	Timing of Aortic Replacement
FBN-1	Marfan syndrome	Positive family history in 75%	5%	www.marfan.org/dx/score	<5.0 cm
TGFBRI/TGFBRII	Loeys-Dietz syndrome	Skin fragility, wide scars	6%	Bifid uvula, pectus, translucent skin, wide-set eyes, Marfan features, aortic tortuosity	4.0–4.5 cm
ELN	Autosomal-dominant cutis laxa	Hypermobility	25%	Pendulous cheeks, loose skin folds	5.0 cm
SMAD3	Osteoarthritis aortopathy syndrome	Early onset arthritis, disk degeneration, easy bruising	5%	Marfan features, wide-set eyes, dolichocephaly, MVP, aortic tortuosity	4.0–4.5 cm
ACTA2	Smooth muscle dysfunction syndrome	Bowel obstructions, peripartum dissections	4%	Fixed dilated pupils, livedo reticularis, moyamoya, vessel occlusive disease	4.5–5.0 cm
X chromosome	Turner syndrome	Short stature, delayed puberty, infertility	40%	Short stature, webbed neck, ↑ carrying angle	Aorta/BSA >2.5 cm/m^2

Abbreviations: BSA, body surface area; MVP, mitral valve prolapse.
Data from Refs. 5,13,66–71

specific medications. As a result, no specific medical therapy is recommended in the 2014 American College of Cardiology (ACC)/American Heart Association (AHA) guideline for management of patients with valvular heart disease or the 2018 guidelines on bicuspid aortopathy.[6,49] Blood pressure control and general cardiovascular risk reduction are recommended, as in nonheritable thoracic aortopathy.[59,60] Beta-blockers and renin-angiotensin system inhibitors are often used based on extrapolation from data in patients with Marfan syndrome, but there is no evidence that these classes of antihypertensives are superior.[61–63] Additionally, there is no evidence that blood pressure targets lower than the general population are indicated.[60]

THE HIGH-RISK BICUSPID AORTIC VALVE PATIENT

Patients with BAV at higher risk for aortic dissection have been identified and include those with (1) an aortic root phenotype, (2) a familial syndromic or nonsyndromic thoracic aortic aneurysm syndrome, and (3) Turner syndrome.[3,5,8,31,46,64]

Root Phenotype

Several classification schemes for BAV aortopathy have been proposed, but in general terms, two phenotypes exist: one where the aortic root is primarily involved, and one where the primary site of dilation is the ascending or tubular portion of the aorta.[3,5] The aortic root phenotype is the rarest and is associated with a younger age at diagnosis, male gender, and aortic insufficiency; more recent four-dimensional flow MRI has also shown an association with fusion of the right-coronary and noncoronary cusps.[3,7,58] This pattern is thought to carry a higher rate of aortic dilation and dissection, which may be explained by the fact that this pattern of BAV aortopathy is seen in association with several different systemic syndromic and nonsyndromic disorders.[65–71]

Syndromic or Nonsyndromic Aortopathy

One of the great clinical dilemmas when evaluating the patient with a nonstenotic BAV is determining whether the valve abnormality is an isolated problem or whether it is a feature of an underlying systemic disorder that carries significant risk of aortic dissection. Personal medical history, family history, and clinical examination should all be directed toward assessing for features that may suggest the presence of a syndrome associated with a higher risk of rapid aortic dilation and dissection. BAV has been documented to occur with increased frequency in several conditions independently associated with aortic dissection, such as Marfan syndrome, Loeys-Dietz syndrome, smooth muscle dysfunction syndrome, aortopathy-osteoarthritis syndrome, and in patients with autosomal-dominant cutis laxa depending on the exon involved.[66–71] Although the yield of routine genetic testing in patients with BAV is low, the presence of suggestive clinical signs or symptoms should trigger genetic testing for the suspected underlying disorder.[72] Timing of surgical intervention is dictated by the underlying genetic mutation in these cases (see **Table 1**).

Turner Syndrome

BAV is present either alone, or in combination with aortic coarctation in approximately 40% of patients with Turner syndrome.[73] The risk of aortic dissection is higher than that of the general population and often occurs at smaller aortic diameters even when accounting for the short stature of most patients; as such, surgical criteria differ (see **Table 1**). Given the strong male predilection of BAV, a diagnosis of Turner syndrome should be considered in a female without a family history of BAV disease.

Method of Surveillance

Although various imaging modalities are used to evaluate BAV disease, per AHA/ACC guidelines, transthoracic echocardiography (TTE) is the standard diagnostic tool.[5,49,74] The frequency of imaging depends on the degree of valvar dysfunction, the degree of aortic dilation, and the presence or absence of associated syndromic or nonsyndromic systemic aortopathies.[5,6,49] TTE provides a comprehensive evaluation of the aortic valve including identification of valve morphology and assessment of valve function, and the aorta. Valve morphology is determined based on visual assessment of the number of valve leaflets, leaflet motion, thickness, and presence of calcification. Identification of the valve morphology and pattern of dilation is important for reasons mentioned previously. The severity of aortic stenosis is evaluated with Doppler velocity and pressure measurements and quantitative measures, such as aortic valve area determined by the continuity equation. Assessment of aortic regurgitation focuses on color and Doppler parameters and measures of the left ventricle. Left ventricular volumes and systolic function, and in certain populations, global longitudinal strain measurements, can aid in prognosis and timing of an intervention.[75] Limitations of echocardiography mainly relate to poor acoustic windows, which can lead to inadequate visualization or incomplete evaluation of cardiac structures. Evaluation for ascending aortic dilation is more difficult, but techniques are used to adequately image the mid or distal ascending aorta.[73] If, despite use of high parasternal and right parasternal imaging, TTE provides inadequate imaging, other modalities, such as transesophageal echocardiography, cardiac MRI (CMR), and computed tomography (CT), can complement and provide further assessment. **Fig. 1** demonstrates diffuse aortic involvement in a patient with BAV and familial aortopathy.

The 2018 guidelines on bicuspid aortopathy recommend repeat TTE every 3 to 5 years if the initial aortic measurements are normal.[6] If any segment of the aorta measures 40 to 49 mm, confirmation should be obtained using CT or CMR, with repeat imaging in 12 months to determine rate of change.[6] If measurements are stable, repeat imaging every 2 to 3 years using the same modality (echo or cross-sectional imaging, depending on echo

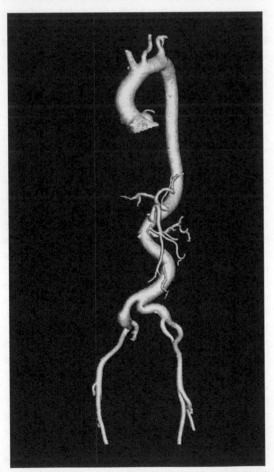

Fig. 1. Aortic CT scan of patient with bicuspid aortic valve and familial aortopathy. There is involvement of the proximal thoracic aorta and aortic tortuosity and iliac artery aneurysm.

images) is appropriate.[6] These recommendations differ slightly from the 2014 ACC/AHA Guidelines for Management of Patients with Valvular Heart Disease, which state that repeat examination frequency is at the discretion of the clinician based on the previous rate of change of diameter and family history until the aorta measures greater than 4.5 cm, at which point annual cross-sectional imaging should be performed.[49]

CMR provides a comprehensive assessment of BAV disease and is used as a valuable adjunctive imaging modality to assess aortic disease specifically when TTE is inadequate.[76] Cine images of the aortic root depict aortic valve morphology and allow for measurement of its dimensions. Phase-contrast flow measurements accurately quantify the regurgitation fraction of the aortic valve. Left ventricular volumes, mass, and function are determined from short-axis cine images. Delayed enhancement imaging identifies regions of myocardial fibrosis, which may be present in a subset of patients. Contrast-enhanced magnetic resonance angiography provides a comprehensive evaluation of the thoracic aorta, demonstrating any evidence of dilation or aneurysm. Thoracic aorta diameters are accurately measured using multiplanar reconstruction in double-oblique cross-sectional planes. Currently, research with CMR using four-dimensional flow sequences and analysis of aortic wall stress in individuals with BAV aortopathy have demonstrated how different valve morphologies impact flow patterns, dilation, and wall stress in the aorta and contribute or cause aortopathy.[57,58,77] Limitations of CMR include availability, cost, and the need for patients to tolerate lying flat for longer examination times.

Cardiac CT provides high spatial resolution images of the thoracic aorta and is useful for the morphologic assessment of the bicuspid valve and evaluation of calcification. A CT of a patient with BAV and familial aortopathy is shown in **Fig. 1**. Additionally, if needed, coronary artery anatomy can be concurrently evaluated. Aortic measurements are obtained using multiplanar reconstruction in double-oblique cross-sectional planes. If candidacy for transcatheter aortic valve replacement is being considered, CT has a role for preoperative assessment, aiding in accurate annular dimensions for valve sizing. Limitations of CT include radiation dose, need for iodinated contrast, and a lack of functional information regarding severity of valve disease.

In addition to risk stratification, clinical visits should cover the following topics where appropriate:

1. Pregnancy: Female patients require timely counseling regarding the potential risks of pregnancy.

Such counseling should commence before the onset of sexual activity and be reinforced at regular intervals during the childbearing years. Pregnancy has been documented to have an effect on aortic size in healthy patients, with greater aortic size associated with greater parity.[78] Pregnancy in itself is recognized as an independent risk factor for aortic dissection.[79] However, provided that a woman does not have BAV as a feature of an underlying genetic aortopathy, the risk of aortic dissection associated with BAV in a woman with an aortic diameter greater than 5 cm is exceedingly small; the data do not substantiate a risk greater than that of the general peripartum population.[79] Most published peripartum aortic dissections have involved women with a trileaflet aortic valve.[80] Despite claims to the contrary, a higher risk of aortic dissection in the general population of woman with BAV and an aortic diameter less than 5 cm is not born out by the numbers, and there is no basis for recommendations to consider replacement of the aorta at a smaller size if a woman desires pregnancy.[81,82] Because the denominator of patients experiencing pregnancy with a normal-functioning BAV is exceedingly large, the overall risk quite small.

2. Avoidance of fluoroquinolones: There are accumulating data documenting the risk of aortic aneurysm ± dissection in patients using fluoroquinolones.[83–85] A propensity-matched study of patients receiving amoxicillin or a fluoroquinolone by Pasternak and colleagues[83] demonstrated a 66% increased risk of an aortic dissection in patients receiving the fluoroquinolone, with increased incidence most pronounced within the first 10 days of treatment. Other observational studies have documented a similar association.[84,85] Furthermore, administration of ciprofloxacin to an aneurysm-prone mouse model significantly increased the incidence of aortic dissection.[86] The mechanism of action has been purported to be increased activity of MMPs.[83–85] In December of 2018, the Food and Drug Administration issued a drug safety announcement advising that fluoroquinolones can increase the risk of aortic dissection. It is recommended that this class of antibiotics not be used in patients at risk for aortic aneurysm including those with aortic dilation, hypertension, genetic disorders associated with aneurysm, and the elderly.[87]

3. Athletics: More than a decade ago, Elefteriades[88] reported on the association of ascending aortic dissection and high-intensity weight lifting. These data, in combination with studies of healthy volunteers documenting

blood pressures in excess of 300 to 400 mm Hg with weight lifting, form the basis of exercise recommendations for patients with BAV aortopathy.[89] Patients with moderate (45 mm) or greater aortic dilation should avoid heavy weight lifting and extreme sports.[3] Aerobic/endurance exercise, however, is recommended if concomitant valve disease does not preclude such.[3] The blood pressure lowering effect of routine aerobic exercise is thought to be beneficial.[5]

The recommendations of the ACC/AHA that follow are for patients with BAV and associated aortic root enlargement[49]:

1. Patients with BAV with no aortic root dilatation (less than 40 mm or the equivalent according to body surface area in children and adolescents) and no significant aortic stenosis or aortic regurgitation may participate in all competitive sports.

2. Patients with BAV and dilated aortic roots between 40 and 45 mm may participate in low and moderate static or low and moderate dynamic competitive sports (classes IA, IB, IIA, and IIB), but should avoid any sports in these categories that involve the potential for bodily collision or trauma.

3. Patients with BAV and dilated aortic root greater than 45 mm can participate only in low-intensity competitive sports (class IA).

If such patients also have significant valvar stenosis, insufficiency, or Marfan syndrome these recommendations should be considered in concert with those discussed in the document related to these valvular and connective tissue diseases.

Conotruncal Defects and Aortopathy

Although there is clear evidence of increased risk of dissection caused by BAV aortopathy, this is not the case for other types of complex congenital heart disease. Conotruncal defects including truncus arteriosus, transposition of the great arteries (TGA), tetralogy of Fallot, and double outlet right ventricle are frequently associated with thoracic aortic dilation.[19,90–96] A representative magnetic resonance angiography of an adult with tetralogy of Fallot and aortic dilatation is shown in **Fig. 2**. The mechanism of this dilation is thought to be related to hemodynamically significant right-to-left shunting before repair, because increased volume loading of the aorta has consistently been shown to be associated with increased diameter.[19,97] Additionally, histologic studies have shown cystic medial necrosis in the aortic wall in patients with tetralogy of Fallot, suggesting there

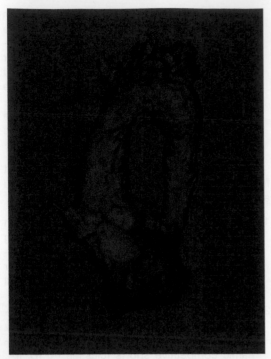

Fig. 2. Three-dimensional steady-state free precession MRI in a 39-year-old man with tetralogy of Fallot. Sagittal projection with the right heart removed demonstrates dilatation of the aortic root and ascending aorta, and focal dilatation of the proximal descending aorta. The maximal sinus-to-sinus measurement is 58 mm. (*Courtesy of* Jimmy Lu, MD, Ann Arbor, MI.)

is an additional cellular-level cause of decreased elasticity.[18,19,90,98]

Despite frequent dilation, dissection is rare. In a study of children and young adults with aortic dissection, patients with CHD were more likely than the general population to have aortic dissection, but the incidence of aortic dissection in children, with and without CHD, was extremely low and, unsurprisingly, well lower than that of the general adult population.[99] The discussion of this study postulated that some of these dissections were procedure-related because the diagnosis was not present on admission.

There is a single reported case of dissection in D-TGA occurring following Mustard procedure at maximum diameter of 70 mm. Aortic dilation is much more commonly seen following arterial switch operation compared with Mustard procedure and no case reports of dissection following arterial switch have been published, although two cases of dissection following unspecified D-TGA repair were included in a recent database study.[10,100] The same database study, examining dissection in all inpatients in the state of Texas, documented a single case of dissection in a patient with truncus arteriosus, but no other cases have been reported.[10] There have been no documented cases of dissection in patients with double outlet right ventricle.

The few existing case reports of dissection in patients with tetralogy of Fallot occurred in individuals with massive aortic dilation or older age: three cases in patients 30 years or younger had maximum aortic dimensions of 70 mm, 70 mm, and 93 mm, respectively.[101–103] An additional report described a dissection in a 60-year-old patient had maximum aortic dimension of 53 mm.[104] A recent review of thoracic aortic dissection in patients with tetralogy of Fallot was performed by Egbe and colleagues[105] using the National Inpatient Sample looking at all hospitalizations nationally over a 15-year period. They identified 11 total dissections in more than 18,000 admissions for patients with tetralogy of Fallot corresponding to 6 dissections per 10,000 admissions (0.06%), a number that is certainly even lower for the total tetralogy of Fallot population including nonhospitalized patients. When compared with the frequency of thoracic aortic aneurysm in patients with tetralogy of Fallot, with different studies suggesting prevalence of 28% to 69%, the rate of dissection is vanishingly small.[19,31,90,91,95–97,102,105,106]

Given limited data, neither the 2018 ACC/AHA Guideline for the Management of Adults with Congenital Heart Disease nor the 2010 European Society of Cardiology make specific recommendations regarding intervention for patients with conotruncal defects and aortic dilatation. The 2018 ACC/AHA guideline describes the identification of adults at risk for aortic dissection as a knowledge gap meriting further investigation. Dearani and colleagues[23] recommended surgery for aortic aneurysm in conotruncal congenital heart disease based on criteria similar to the general population (>55 mm) with consideration for earlier intervention if the patient was planning for cardiac surgery for another lesion. Based on the previously mentioned data about the low incidence of dissection despite larger aortic dimensions, more conservative management, particularly in those without additional risk factors (age, hypertension, genetic disorder), is likely warranted in conotruncal congenital heart disease. More data are needed, however, to determine the dimensions at which intervention is warranted.

DISCLOSURE

None of the authors have any disclosures to report.

REFERENCES

1. Yetman AT, Graham T. The dilated aorta in patients with congenital cardiac defects. J Am Coll Cardiol 2009;53(6):461–7.

2. Beroukhim RS, Kruzick TL, Taylor AL, et al. Progression of aortic dilation in children with a functionally normal bicuspid aortic valve. Am J Cardiol 2006;98(6):828–30.

3. Verma S, Siu SC. Aortic dilatation in patients with bicuspid aortic valve. N Engl J Med 2014; 370(20):1920–9.

4. Hiratzka LF, Creager MA, Isselbacher EM, et al. Surgery for aortic dilatation in patients with bicuspid aortic valves: a statement of clarification from the American College of Cardiology/American Heart Association Task Force on clinical practice guidelines. J Am Coll Cardiol 2016;67(6):724–31.

5. Hiratzka LF, Bakris GL, Beckman JA, et al. 2010 ACCF/AHA/AATS/ACR/ASA/SCA/SCAI/SIR/STS/ SVM guidelines for the diagnosis and management of patients with thoracic aortic disease. A report of the American College of Cardiology Foundation/ American Heart Association Task Force on Practice Guidelines, American Association for Thoracic Surgery, American College of Radiology, American Stroke Association, Society of Cardiovascular Anesthesiologists, Society for Cardiovascular Angiography and Interventions, Society of Interventional Radiology, Society of Thoracic Surgeons, and Society for Vascular Medicine. J Am Coll Cardiol 2010; 55(14):e27–129.

6. Borger MA, Fedak PWM, Stephens EH, et al. The American Association for Thoracic Surgery consensus guidelines on bicuspid aortic valve-related aortopathy: full online-only version. J Thorac Cardiovasc Surg 2018;156(2):e41–74.

7. Rutz T, Max F, Wahl A, et al. Distensibility and diameter of ascending aorta assessed by cardiac magnetic resonance imaging in adults with tetralogy of Fallot or complete transposition. Am J Cardiol 2012;110(1):103–8.

8. Tadros TM, Klein MD, Shapira OM. Ascending aortic dilatation associated with bicuspid aortic valve: pathophysiology, molecular biology, and clinical implications. Circulation 2009;119(6):880–90.

9. Tzemos N, Therrien J, Yip J, et al. Outcomes in adults with bicuspid aortic valves. JAMA 2008; 300(11):1317–25.

10. Frischhertz BP, Shamszad P, Pedroza C, et al. Thoracic aortic dissection and rupture in conotruncal cardiac defects: a population-based study. Int J Cardiol 2015;184:521–7.

11. Turkbey EB, Jain A, Johnson C, et al. Determinants and normal values of ascending aortic diameter by age, gender, and race/ethnicity in the Multi-Ethnic Study of Atherosclerosis (MESA). J Magn Reson Imaging 2014;39(2):360–8.

12. Fixler DE, Nembhard WN, Xu P, et al. Effect of acculturation and distance from cardiac center on congenital heart disease mortality. Pediatrics 2012;129(6):1118–24.

13. Saeyeldin AA, Velasquez CA, Mahmood SUB, et al. Thoracic aortic aneurysm: unlocking the "silent killer" secrets. Gen Thorac Cardiovasc Surg 2019; 67(1):1–11.

14. Devereux RB, de Simone G, Arnett DK, et al. Normal limits in relation to age, body size and gender of two-dimensional echocardiographic aortic root dimensions in persons >/=15 years of age. Am J Cardiol 2012;110(8):1189–94.

15. Vriz O, Aboyans V, D'Andrea A, et al. Normal values of aortic root dimensions in healthy adults. Am J Cardiol 2014;114(6):921–7.

16. Campens L, Demulier L, De Groote K, et al. Reference values for echocardiographic assessment of the diameter of the aortic root and ascending aorta spanning all age categories. Am J Cardiol 2014; 114(6):914–20.

17. Wolak A, Gransar H, Thomson LE, et al. Aortic size assessment by noncontrast cardiac computed tomography: normal limits by age, gender, and body surface area. JACC Cardiovasc Imaging 2008;1(2):200–9.

18. Niwa K, Perloff JK, Bhuta SM, et al. Structural abnormalities of great arterial walls in congenital heart disease: light and electron microscopic analyses. Circulation 2001;103(3):393–400.

19. Niwa K. Aortic root dilatation in tetralogy of Fallot long-term after repair–histology of the aorta in tetralogy of Fallot: evidence of intrinsic aortopathy. Int J Cardiol 2005;103(2):117–9.

20. Sophocleous F, Milano EG, Pontecorboli G, et al. Enlightening the association between bicuspid aortic valve and aortopathy. J Cardiovasc Dev Dis 2018;5(2) [pii:E21].

21. Fedak PW, de Sa MP, Verma S, et al. Vascular matrix remodeling in patients with bicuspid aortic valve malformations: implications for aortic dilatation. J Thorac Cardiovasc Surg 2003;126(3):797–806.

22. Cheung YF, Chow PC, So EK, et al. Circulating transforming growth factor-beta and aortic dilation in patients with repaired congenital heart disease. Sci Rep 2019;9(1):162.

23. Dearani JA, Burkhart HM, Stulak JM, et al. Management of the aortic root in adult patients with conotruncal anomalies. Semin Thorac Cardiovasc Surg Pediatr Card Surg Annu 2009;122–9. https://doi. org/10.1053/j.pcsu.2009.01.013.

24. de Wit A, Vis K, Jeremy RW. Aortic stiffness in heritable aortopathies: relationship to aneurysm growth rate. Heart Lung Circ 2013;22(1):3–11.

25. Rooprai J, Boodhwani M, Beauchesne L, et al. Thoracic aortic aneurysm growth in bicuspid aortic valve patients: role of aortic stiffness and pulsatile hemodynamics. J Am Heart Assoc 2019;8(8): e010885.

26. Boonyasirinant T, Rajiah P, Flamm SD. Abnormal aortic stiffness in patients with bicuspid aortic

valve: phenotypic variation determined by magnetic resonance imaging. Int J Cardiovasc Imaging 2019;35(1):133–41.

27. Nistri S, Grande-Allen J, Noale M, et al. Aortic elasticity and size in bicuspid aortic valve syndrome. Eur Heart J 2008;29(4):472–9.

28. Nistri S, Sorbo MD, Basso C, et al. Bicuspid aortic valve: abnormal aortic elastic properties. J Heart Valve Dis 2002;11(3):369–73 [discussion: 73–4].

29. van der Meer RW, Diamant M, Westenberg JJ, et al. Magnetic resonance assessment of aortic pulse wave velocity, aortic distensibility, and cardiac function in uncomplicated type 2 diabetes mellitus. J Cardiovasc Magn Reson 2007;9(4):645–51.

30. Lakatta EG, Levy D. Arterial and cardiac aging: major shareholders in cardiovascular disease enterprises: Part I: aging arteries: a "set up" for vascular disease. Circulation 2003;107(1):139–46.

31. Christensen JT, Lu JC, Donohue J, et al. Relation of aortic stiffness and strain by cardiovascular magnetic resonance imaging to age in repaired tetralogy of fallot. Am J Cardiol 2014;113(6):1031–5.

32. Nollen GJ, Groenink M, Tijssen JG, et al. Aortic stiffness and diameter predict progressive aortic dilatation in patients with Marfan syndrome. Eur Heart J 2004;25(13):1146–52.

33. Cecconi M, Manfrin M, Moraca A, et al. Aortic dimensions in patients with bicuspid aortic valve without significant valve dysfunction. Am J Cardiol 2005;95(2):292–4.

34. Keane MG, Wiegers SE, Plappert T, et al. Bicuspid aortic valves are associated with aortic dilatation out of proportion to coexistent valvular lesions. Circulation 2000;102(19 Suppl 3). III35–I39.

35. Ferencik M, Pape LA. Changes in size of ascending aorta and aortic valve function with time in patients with congenitally bicuspid aortic valves. Am J Cardiol 2003;92(1):43–6.

36. Wang L, Ming Wang L, Chen W, et al. Bicuspid aortic valve: a review of its genetics and clinical significance. J Heart Valve Dis 2016;25(5):568–73.

37. Edwards WD, Leaf DS, Edwards JE. Dissecting aortic aneurysm associated with congenital bicuspid aortic valve. Circulation 1978;57(5):1022–5.

38. Michelena HI, Desjardins VA, Avierinos JF, et al. Natural history of asymptomatic patients with normally functioning or minimally dysfunctional bicuspid aortic valve in the community. Circulation 2008;117(21):2776–84.

39. Verma S, Yanagawa B, Kalra S, et al. Knowledge, attitudes, and practice patterns in surgical management of bicuspid aortopathy: a survey of 100 cardiac surgeons. J Thorac Cardiovasc Surg 2013;146(5):1033–40.e4.

40. Parish LM, Gorman JH 3rd, Kahn S, et al. Aortic size in acute type A dissection: implications for preventive ascending aortic replacement. Eur J Cardiothorac Surg 2009;35(6):941–5.]discussion: 5–6].

41. Paruchuri V, Salhab KF, Kuzmik G, et al. Aortic size distribution in the general population: explaining the size paradox in aortic dissection. Cardiology 2015;131(4):265–72.

42. Wang Y, Wu B, Dong L, et al. Circulating matrix metalloproteinase patterns in association with aortic dilatation in bicuspid aortic valve patients with isolated severe aortic stenosis. Heart Vessels 2016;31(2):189–97.

43. Forte A, Bancone C, Cobellis G, et al. A possible early biomarker for bicuspid aortopathy: circulating transforming growth factor beta-1 to soluble endoglin ratio. Circ Res 2017;120(11):1800–11.

44. Branchetti E, Bavaria JE, Grau JB, et al. Circulating soluble receptor for advanced glycation end product identifies patients with bicuspid aortic valve and associated aortopathies. Arterioscler Thromb Vasc Biol 2014;34(10):2349–57.

45. Gallo A, Agnese V, Coronnello C, et al. On the prospect of serum exosomal miRNA profiling and protein biomarkers for the diagnosis of ascending aortic dilatation in patients with bicuspid and tricuspid aortic valve. Int J Cardiol 2018;273:230–6.

46. Andreassi MG, Della Corte A. Genetics of bicuspid aortic valve aortopathy. Curr Opin Cardiol 2016;31(6):585–92.

47. Pileggi S, De Chiara B, Magnoli M, et al. Sequencing of NOTCH1 gene in an Italian population with bicuspid aortic valve: preliminary results from the GISSI OUTLIERS VAR study. Gene 2019;715:143970.

48. Loscalzo ML, Goh DL, Loeys B, et al. Familial thoracic aortic dilation and bicommissural aortic valve: a prospective analysis of natural history and inheritance. Am J Med Genet A 2007;143A(17):1960–7.

49. Nishimura RA, Otto CM, Bonow RO, et al. 2014 AHA/ACC guideline for the management of patients with valvular heart disease: a report of the American College of Cardiology/American Heart Association Task Force on practice guidelines. J Thorac Cardiovasc Surg 2014;148(1):e1–132.

50. Gillis E, Kumar AA, Luyckx I, et al. Candidate gene resequencing in a large bicuspid aortic valve-associated thoracic aortic aneurysm cohort: SMAD6 as an important contributor. Front Physiol 2017;8:400.

51. Guo DC, Gong L, Regalado ES, et al. MAT2A mutations predispose individuals to thoracic aortic aneurysms. Am J Hum Genet 2015;96(1):170–7.

52. Corbitt H, Morris SA, Gravholt CH, et al. TIMP3 and TIMP1 are risk genes for bicuspid aortic valve and aortopathy in Turner syndrome. PLoS Genet 2018;14(10):e1007692.

53. Lorenz R, Bock J, Barker AJ, et al. 4D flow magnetic resonance imaging in bicuspid aortic valve disease demonstrates altered distribution of aortic blood flow helicity. Magn Reson Med 2014;71(4):1542–53.

54. Bissell MM, Loudon M, Hess AT, et al. Differential flow improvements after valve replacements in bicuspid aortic valve disease: a cardiovascular magnetic resonance assessment. J Cardiovasc Magn Reson 2018;20(1):10.

55. Bissell MM, Hess AT, Biasiolli L, et al. Aortic dilation in bicuspid aortic valve disease: flow pattern is a major contributor and differs with valve fusion type. Circ Cardiovasc Imaging 2013;6(4):499–507.

56. Bissell MM, Dall'Armellina E, Choudhury RP. Flow vortices in the aortic root: in vivo 4D-MRI confirms predictions of Leonardo da Vinci. Eur Heart J 2014;35(20):1344.

57. Mahadevia R, Barker AJ, Schnell S, et al. Bicuspid aortic cusp fusion morphology alters aortic three-dimensional outflow patterns, wall shear stress, and expression of aortopathy. Circulation 2014;129(6):673–82.

58. Rodriguez-Palomares JF, Dux-Santoy L, Guala A, et al. Aortic flow patterns and wall shear stress maps by 4D-flow cardiovascular magnetic resonance in the assessment of aortic dilatation in bicuspid aortic valve disease. J Cardiovasc Magn Reson 2018;20(1):28.

59. Hiratzka LF, Bakris GL, Beckman JA, et al. 2010 ACCF/AHA/AATS/ACR/ASA/SCA/SCAI/SIR/STS/SVM guidelines for the diagnosis and management of patients with thoracic aortic disease: executive summary. A report of the American College of Cardiology Foundation/American Heart Association Task Force on Practice Guidelines, American Association for Thoracic Surgery, American College of Radiology, American Stroke Association, Society of Cardiovascular Anesthesiologists, Society for Cardiovascular Angiography and Interventions, Society of Interventional Radiology, Society of Thoracic Surgeons, and Society for Vascular Medicine. Catheter Cardiovasc Interv 2010;76(2):E43–86.

60. Borger MA, Fedak PWM, Stephens EH, et al. The American Association for Thoracic Surgery consensus guidelines on bicuspid aortic valve-related aortopathy: executive summary. J Thorac Cardiovasc Surg 2018;156(2):473–80.

61. Ahimastos AA, Aggarwal A, D'Orsa KM, et al. Effect of perindopril on large artery stiffness and aortic root diameter in patients with Marfan syndrome: a randomized controlled trial. JAMA 2007;298(13):1539–47.

62. Bin Mahmood SU, Velasquez CA, Zafar MA, et al. Medical management of aortic disease in Marfan syndrome. Ann Cardiothorac Surg 2017;6(6):654–61.

63. Danyi P, Elefteriades JA, Jovin IS. Medical therapy of thoracic aortic aneurysms: are we there yet? Circulation 2011;124(13):1469–76.

64. Gravholt CH, Andersen NH, Conway GS, et al. Clinical practice guidelines for the care of girls and women with Turner syndrome: proceedings from the 2016 Cincinnati International Turner Syndrome Meeting. Eur J Endocrinol 2017;177(3):G1–70.

65. Girdauskas E, Geist L, Disha K, et al. Genetic abnormalities in bicuspid aortic valve root phenotype: preliminary results. Eur J Cardiothorac Surg 2017;52(1):156–62.

66. Nistri S, Porciani MC, Attanasio M, et al. Association of Marfan syndrome and bicuspid aortic valve: frequency and outcome. Int J Cardiol 2012;155(2):324–5.

67. Patel ND, Crawford T, Magruder JT, et al. Cardiovascular operations for Loeys-Dietz syndrome: Intermediate-term results. J Thorac Cardiovasc Surg 2017;153(2):406–12.

68. van de Laar I, Arbustini E, Loeys B, et al. European reference network for rare vascular diseases (VASCERN) consensus statement for the screening and management of patients with pathogenic ACTA2 variants. Orphanet J Rare Dis 2019;14(1):264.

69. Hostetler EM, Regalado ES, Guo DC, et al. SMAD3 pathogenic variants: risk for thoracic aortic disease and associated complications from the Montalcino Aortic Consortium. J Med Genet 2019;56(4):252–60.

70. Callewaert B, Renard M, Hucthagowder V, et al. New insights into the pathogenesis of autosomal-dominant cutis laxa with report of five ELN mutations. Hum Mutat 2011;32(4):445–55.

71. Hadj-Rabia S, Callewaert BL, Bourrat E, et al. Twenty patients including 7 probands with autosomal dominant cutis laxa confirm clinical and molecular homogeneity. Orphanet J Rare Dis 2013;8:36.

72. Arrington CB, Sower CT, Chuckwuk N, et al. Absence of TGFBR1 and TGFBR2 mutations in patients with bicuspid aortic valve and aortic dilation. Am J Cardiol 2008;102(5):629–31.

73. Yetman AT, Starr L, Sanmann J, et al. Clinical and echocardiographic prevalence and detection of congenital and acquired cardiac abnormalities in girls and women with the turner syndrome. Am J Cardiol 2018;122(2):327–30.

74. Stout KK, Daniels CJ, Aboulhosn JA, et al. 2018 AHA/ACC guideline for the management of adults with congenital heart disease: a report of the American College of Cardiology/American Heart Association Task Force on clinical practice guidelines. J Am Coll Cardiol 2019;73(12):e81–192.

75. Kong WKF, Vollema EM, Prevedello F, et al. Prognostic implications of left ventricular global longitudinal strain in patients with bicuspid aortic valve

disease and preserved left ventricular ejection fraction. Eur Heart J Cardiovasc Imaging 2019. https://doi.org/10.1093/ehjci/jez252.

76. Tsai SF, Trivedi M, Daniels CJ. Comparing imaging modalities for screening aortic complications in patients with bicuspid aortic valve. Congenit Heart Dis 2012;7(4):372–7.

77. Toufan Tabrizi M, Rahimi Asl R, Nazarnia S, et al. Evaluation of relationship between bicuspid aortic valve phenotype with valve dysfunction and associated aortopathy. J Cardiovasc Thorac Res 2018;10(4):236–42.

78. Gutin LS, Merz AE, Bakalov VK, et al. Parity and aortic dimensions in healthy women. Int J Cardiol 2013;165(2):383–4.

79. Kamel H, Roman MJ, Pitcher A, et al. Pregnancy and the risk of aortic dissection or rupture: a cohort-crossover analysis. Circulation 2016;134(7):527–33.

80. Yuan SM. Postpartum aortic dissection. Taiwan J Obstet Gynecol 2013;52(3):318–22.

81. De Martino A, Morganti R, Falcetta G, et al. Acute aortic dissection and pregnancy: review and meta-analysis of incidence, presentation, and pathologic substrates. J Card Surg 2019;34(12):1591–7.

82. Immer FF, Bansi AG, Immer-Bansi AS, et al. Aortic dissection in pregnancy: analysis of risk factors and outcome. Ann Thorac Surg 2003;76(1):309–14.

83. Pasternak B, Inghammar M, Svanstrom H. Fluoroquinolone use and risk of aortic aneurysm and dissection: nationwide cohort study. BMJ 2018;360:k678.

84. Lee CC, Lee MT, Chen YS, et al. Risk of aortic dissection and aortic aneurysm in patients taking oral fluoroquinolone. JAMA Intern Med 2015;175(11):1839–47.

85. Lee CC, Lee MG, Hsieh R, et al. Oral fluoroquinolone and the risk of aortic dissection. J Am Coll Cardiol 2018;72(12):1369–78.

86. LeMaire SA, Zhang L, Luo W, et al. Effect of ciprofloxacin on susceptibility to aortic dissection and rupture in mice. JAMA Surg 2018;153(9):e181804.

87. FDA Drug Safety Communication: FDA updates warnings for oral and injectable fluoroquinolone antibiotics due to disabling side effects 2016. Available at: https://www.fda.gov/drugs/drug-safety-and-availability/fda-drug-safety-communication-fda-updates-warnings-oral-and-injectable-fluoroquinolone-antibiotics. Accessed January 9, 2020.

88. Elefteriades JA. Thoracic aortic aneurysm: reading the enemy's playbook. Curr Probl Cardiol 2008;33(5):203–77.

89. MacDougall JD, Tuxen D, Sale DG, et al. Arterial blood pressure response to heavy resistance exercise. J Appl Physiol (1985) 1985;58(3):785–90.

90. Niwa K. Aortic dilatation in complex congenital heart disease. Cardiovasc Diagn Ther 2018;8(6):725–38.

91. Tan JL, Gatzoulis MA, Ho SY. Aortic root disease in tetralogy of Fallot. Curr Opin Cardiol 2006;21(6):569–72.

92. Warnes CA. The adult with congenital heart disease: born to be bad? J Am Coll Cardiol 2005;46(1):1–8.

93. Kay WA. Molecular and genetic insights into thoracic aortic dilation in conotruncal heart defects. Front Cardiovasc Med 2016;3:18.

94. Nagy CD, Alejo DE, Corretti MC, et al. Tetralogy of Fallot and aortic root dilation: a long-term outlook. Pediatr Cardiol 2013;34(4):809–16.

95. Rieker RP, Berman MA, Stansel HC. Postoperative studies in patients with tetralogy of Fallot. Ann Thorac Surg 1975;19(1):17–26.

96. Egbe AC, Miranda WR, Ammash NM, et al. Aortic disease and interventions in adults with tetralogy of Fallot. Heart 2019;105(12):926–31.

97. Seki M, Kuwata S, Kurishima C, et al. Mechanism of aortic root dilation and cardiovascular function in tetralogy of Fallot. Pediatr Int 2016;58(5):323–30.

98. Tan JL, Davlouros PA, McCarthy KP, et al. Intrinsic histological abnormalities of aortic root and ascending aorta in tetralogy of Fallot: evidence of causative mechanism for aortic dilatation and aortopathy. Circulation 2005;112(7):961–8.

99. Shamszad P, Barnes JN, Morris SA. Aortic dissection in hospitalized children and young adults: a multiinstitutional study. Congenit Heart Dis 2014;9(1):54–62.

100. Nowitz A. Acute ascending aortic dissection 41 years after mustard procedure. J Cardiothorac Vasc Anesth 2013;27(4):735–9.

101. Kim WH, Seo JW, Kim SJ, et al. Aortic dissection late after repair of tetralogy of Fallot. Int J Cardiol 2005;101(3):515–6.

102. Konstantinov IE, Fricke TA, d'Udekem Y, et al. Aortic dissection and rupture in adolescents after tetralogy of Fallot repair. J Thorac Cardiovasc Surg 2010;140(5):e71–3.

103. Rathi VK, Doyle M, Williams RB, et al. Massive aortic aneurysm and dissection in repaired tetralogy of Fallot; diagnosis by cardiovascular magnetic resonance imaging. Int J Cardiol 2005;101(1):169–70.

104. Wijesekera VA, Kiess MC, Grewal J, et al. Aortic dissection in a patient with a dilated aortic root following tetralogy of Fallot repair. Int J Cardiol 2014;174(3):833–4.

105. Egbe AC, Crestanello J, Miranda WR, et al. Thoracic aortic dissection in tetralogy of fallot: a review of the national inpatient sample database. J Am Heart Assoc 2019;8(6):e011943.

106. Grotenhuis HB, Dallaire F, Verpalen IM, et al. Aortic root dilatation and aortic-related complications in children after tetralogy of Fallot repair. Circ Cardiovasc Imaging 2018;11(12):e007611.

Aortic Coarctation

Yuli Y. Kim, MD[a,*], Lauren Andrade, MD[a], Stephen C. Cook, MD[b]

KEYWORDS

- Aortic coarctation • Congenital heart disease • Aorta • Aortopathy • Stent therapy

KEY POINTS

- Aortic coarctation is a discrete narrowing of the thoracic aorta and often associated with other forms of congenital heart disease.
- Invasive gradients greater than 20 mm Hg or mean gradient greater than 20 mm Hg by Doppler constitute indication for repair.
- Multimodality imaging is a major component of diagnosis and surveillance.
- Hypertension remains a significant morbidity even in the setting of successful repair.
- Lifelong surveillance by specialists in congenital heart disease is indicated to identify potential long-term complications.

INTRODUCTION

Aortic coarctation accounts for 6% to 8% of all congenital heart disease[1] and occurs with an incidence of 3 to 4 cases out of 10,000 live births with a male predominance of 2:1.[2] It is defined as a narrowing of the thoracic aorta, typically located at the insertion of the ductus arteriosus just distal to the left subclavian artery but can be located distant to the ductus as well. Aortic coarctation is often a discrete stenosis but can be long-segment and/or tortuous. Discrete coarctation can occur in isolation but is often associated with other congenital heart defects, including bicuspid aortic valve (60%), aortic arch hypoplasia and other arch anomalies (18%), ventricular septal defect (13%), mitral valve abnormalities (8%), subaortic stenosis (6%), among others.[3] Shone syndrome is a constellation of left-sided obstructive defects, including supramitral ring, parachute mitral valve, subaortic stenosis, along with aortic coarctation, which suggests a common developmental origin.[4]

The underlying cause of aortic coarctation is not fully elucidated but a genetic underpinning has been implicated. Several candidate genes have been identified, including NOTCH1,[5,6] MCTP2,[7] and FOXC1.[8] For example, NOTCH1 mutations have been identified in patients with other left-sided lesions, including bicuspid aortic valve and hypoplastic left heart syndrome. The high prevalence of aortic coarctation in Turner syndrome as well as PHACE, DiGeorge, and Noonan syndromes also support a genetic component to this condition.[9]

Aortic Coarctation: An Aortopathy

Morphologically, aortic coarctation is characterized by infolding of ductal tissue posteriorly composed of an intimal and medial component that can extend around the entire circumference of the aorta.[10] Under electron microscopy, the intimal component is laminated, staining for fibrin, with progressive thickening over time[11] and with alterations in smooth muscle cell phenotype.[12] Histologically, there is evidence of cystic medial necrosis and elastic fiber formation, which may form the basis of aortic dilation, aneurysm formation, and dissection in aortic coarctation.[13,14]

[a] Philadelphia Adult Congenital Heart Center, Perelman School of Medicine at the University of Pennsylvania, Penn Medicine and Children's Hospital of Philadelphia, Perelman Center for Advanced Medicine, 3400 Civic Center Boulevard, Philadelphia, PA 19104, USA; [b] Adult Congenital Heart Disease Program, Congenital Heart Center, Helen DeVos Children's Hospital, Frederik Meijer Heart & Vascular Institute, Pediatrics and Human Development, Michigan State University, 25 Michigan Street NE Suite 4200, Grand Rapids, MI 49503, USA
* Corresponding author.
E-mail address: Yuli.Kim@pennmedicine.upenn.edu

Cardiol Clin 38 (2020) 337–351
https://doi.org/10.1016/j.ccl.2020.04.003

Aortic coarctation is considered a diffuse aortopathy as demonstrated by abnormal histologic findings, impaired vascular properties, and inflammation. The pathophysiology of the aorta in coarctation is notable for endothelial dysfunction and abnormal elastic properties even after repair.[15–17] Cardiac magnetic resonance (CMR) imaging and vascular ultrasound studies in patients with aortic coarctation demonstrate reduced aortic distensibility, which is associated with higher central systolic blood pressure.[18,19] Circulating levels of proinflammatory molecules involved in atherogenesis are also increased.[17] Positron emission tomography/computed tomography with ^{18}F-fluorodeoxyglucose imaging of normotensive patients with repaired coarctation demonstrated vascular inflammation in the aorta.[20] A small open-label study on 34 young adults with repaired aortic coarctation demonstrated salutary effects of atorvastatin on vascular function and levels of proinflammatory cytokines and molecules.[21]

Natural History

Unrepaired, the natural history of aortic coarctation carries a dismal prognosis. A seminal study by Campbell in 1970 describes autopsy findings of 304 patients who survived beyond the age of 1 year. The mean age of death was 34 years with cause of death ascribed to congestive heart failure (25.5%), aortic rupture (21%), bacterial endocarditis (18%), and intracranial hemorrhage (11.5%).[22] The paper goes on to state "This poor outlook makes an operative mortality in the region of 5% a small price to pay for the greatly increased security afterward" reflecting a risk–benefit ratio highly favoring surgical repair.[22]

However, the prognosis for aortic coarctation after repair is not altogether benign. With evolutions in diagnosis and treatment, including transcatheter options, survival prospects have improved greatly but are still lower than the general population. Patients with aortic coarctation are at continued risk for morbidities delineated by Campbell and others, including heart failure, hypertension, recoarctation, aortic aneurysm/dissection, and sudden death.

CLINICAL PRESENTATION

The clinical presentation of native coarctation in the adult depends on the severity of the lesion. Hemodynamically, the increased afterload due to obstruction of flow from the left ventricle may be accompanied by significant hypertension in the aorta and branch vessels proximal to the coarctation site and may be associated with systemic ventricular dysfunction, vessel aneurysm formation,

and effects of premature atherosclerosis. Distal to the coarctation, there is diminished flow, and collaterals may develop to supplement areas of relative hypoperfusion.

In patients without aortic obstruction, the aortic pulse should be transmitted at equal speed and intensity from the left ventricle to the radial and femoral pulses that are approximately equidistant from the left ventricle. In patients with significant aortic coarctation, pulse wave propagation is both slowed and diminished distal to the coarctation, thereby delaying and diminishing femoral pulse relative to radial pulse. Standard practice dictates that all pulses should be checked at least once in the evaluation of all patients with systemic hypertension to rule out significant aortic coarctation.[23] Four extremity blood pressures should be measured to assess for gradients, but may be misleadingly lower than expected in the setting of significant collateral formation.

Most adult patients are asymptomatic but can present with severe hypertension leading to headaches, epistaxis, heart failure, and/or aortic dissection. Collateral vessel formation around the coarctation when severe, may mitigate the severity of some of these symptoms (**Fig. 1**). **Table 1** summarizes the clinical presentation and physical examination of the adult presenting with aortic coarctation.

DIAGNOSIS AND IMAGING
Transthoracic Echocardiography

Transthoracic echocardiography is often the first-line modality to assess for suspected aortic coarctation due to familiarity and easy accessibility. It can also assess for left ventricular mass, both systolic and diastolic function, and other associated congenital heart lesions. Particular attention should be paid to examining left-sided structures (eg, mitral valve, papillary muscle architecture, left ventricular outflow tract, and aortic valve).

In the suprasternal long-axis, 2D as well as color and spectral Doppler can be used to localize the anatomy of aortic coarctation and estimate the degree of narrowing, but a number of caveats exist. The typical "saw tooth" continuous-wave Doppler appearance of severe coarctation (**Fig. 2**) representing peak systolic acceleration during systole and velocity decay during diastole is affected by aortic compliance. The absence of such may not always indicate mild degrees of coarctation.[24]

The modified Bernoulli equation has been used to calculate the peak instantaneous gradient across the coarcted segment, but many physiologic conditions can affect the accuracy of these estimations. Decompressing collaterals can decrease the peak systolic velocity across the

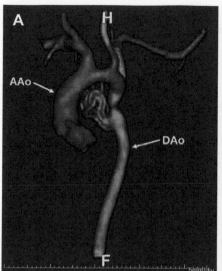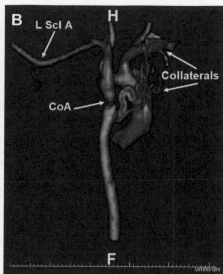

Fig. 1. Volume-rendered 3D reconstruction from a computed tomography of the aorta (*A*, anterior view; *B*, posterior view) in a 43-year-old man who presented to the emergency department with long-standing, poorly controlled hypertension. The study obtained demonstrates severe, native coarctation of the aorta in the presence of marked collateral formation. AAo, ascending aorta; DAo, descending aorta; L Scl A, left subclavian artery.

coarctation leading to underestimation of severity. Increased stiffness proximal to the narrowing increases the degree of proximal velocity acceleration resulting in overestimation of the gradient, even when using the expanded Bernoulli equation.[25] Long-segment stenosis and serial obstructions (ie, associated subaortic obstruction and/or supravalvar aortic stenosis) are also other conditions in which Doppler-derived gradients are less reliable.

Imaging of the aorta by transthoracic echocardiography, however, is often limited by body habitus and technique (**Figs. 3** and **4**). The mainstay of diagnosis and assessment of aortic pathology in the adult is advanced 3D imaging: computed tomographic angiography (CTA) and CMR imaging.

Cardiac Computed Tomographic Angiography

Cardiac CTA provides superior spatial resolution over other modalities, such as CMR and affords advantages in evaluation of vascular anatomy and aortic dimensions, morphology, and evaluation of the coronary arteries. It is the gold standard for imaging aortic dissection—a known complication of adult patients with coarctation, bicuspid aortic valve and especially those with aortic aneurysm.[26] For the adult who has undergone transcatheter intervention, it can also be used to assess luminal patency and is the preferred method to evaluate for long-term complications after stent therapy, including fracture, restenosis, or endoleak (**Fig. 5**). It is also the imaging modality

of choice to evaluate the thoracic aorta in patients with contraindications to CMR, such as a pacemaker or defibrillator. The disadvantages of CTA include the use of ionizing radiation and intravenous dye and associated contrast-induced nephropathy. Fortunately, there have been significant advances in radiation dose reduction strategies, resulting in substantial reductions of total radiation dose for cardiac CTA.[27] This now provides cardiac CTA as a suitable imaging tool for the cardiologist providing care for this population of congenitally affected adults. Still, it is important to balance the risk–benefit ratio of radiation exposure in the young adult with congenital heart disease when considering this imaging modality.

Cardiac Magnetic Resonance Imaging

CMR, which includes MR angiography, is advantageous given its lack of ionizing radiation or risk of contrast-induced nephropathy. It not only affords excellent visualization of aortic anatomy by angiography (**Fig. 6**) but also provides quantitative data on biventricular volumes, mass, and systolic function. In addition, phase contrast flow sequences can be used to quantify velocity acceleration in either discrete coarctation or recoarctation, estimate shunt fraction to evaluate for associated intracardiac shunts, and detect collateral flow in the intercostal arteries.[28,29] The usefulness of CMR in this population has been thoroughly investigated. In a study of adult patients with coarctation referred for routine

Table 1
Clinical presentation and diagnosis of aortic coarctation

Symptoms	Headache
	Epistaxis
	Exertional intolerance
	Dizziness
	Lower extremity claudication
	Abdominal angina
	Intracranial hemorrhage
	Heart failure
Physical examination	Upper extremity hypertension
	Gradient between upper and lower extremity blood pressures
	Weak or absent femoral pulses
	Brachio-femoral delay
	Prominent, nondisplaced apical impulse
	Loud A2
	Systolic ejection click and midsystolic murmur if associated bicuspid aortic valve
	Systolic or continuous murmur radiating to scapula or over thorax from collaterals
Diagnostic testing	CXR
	• Cardiomegaly
	• "E" or "reverse 3" sign from dilated left subclavian artery proximal to and poststenotic dilation distal to coarctation
	• Rib notching from collaterals
	• Dilated ascending aorta if associated bicuspid aortic valve
	ECG
	• Left ventricular hypertrophy
	TTE
	• 2D imaging of ascending aorta, aortic arch, isthmus, and descending aorta
	• Doppler-derived gradient across coarctation
	• Left ventricular size, systolic and diastolic function, hypertrophy
	• Other associated congenital heart defects (eg, bicuspid aortic valve, ventricular septal defect, mitral valve anomalies, subaortic stenosis)

Abbreviations: CXR, chest X-ray; ECG, electrocardiogram; TTE, transthoracic echocardiogram.

surveillance examinations, CMR identified clinically significant recoarctation and/or local aneurysm formation in 27% of the cohort.[30] Finally, CMR has been used to identify predictors of

coarctation severity as assessed by invasive measurements, which include (1) smallest aortic cross-sectional area measured by gadolinium-enhanced 3D magnetic resonance angiography and (2) heart

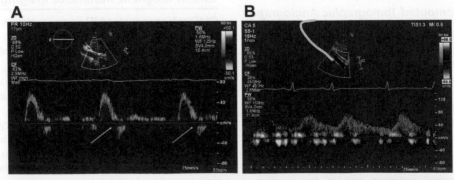

Fig. 2. Normal pulsed-waved Doppler interrogation of the abdominal aorta (*A*) typically demonstrates a brisk upstroke and downstroke followed by early diastolic flow reversal (*arrows*). In contrast, the abdominal Doppler examination in a 21-year-old man (*B*) who underwent previous end-to-end anastomosis demonstrates a dampened, low-velocity signal with continuation throughout diastole suggests significant recoarctation.

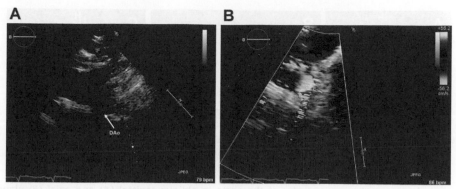

Fig. 3. Suprasternal notch view in an obese 62-year-old man with known bicuspid aortic valve and coarctation of the aorta who underwent previous subclavian flap angioplasty. Images suggest narrowing of the proximal descending aorta (DAo) (*A*). Narrowed appearance supported by color Doppler interrogation (*B*).

rate-corrected mean flow deceleration in the descending aorta measured by phase-velocity cine sequences.[31] CMR provides unrestricted access to the chest and is often regarded as the "gold standard" of imaging in the adult with congenital heart disease. CMR has made valuable contributions to the diagnosis as well as lifelong follow-up evaluation to the adult with CoA.

Cardiac Catheterization

With the advent of advanced 3D imaging techniques, cardiac catheterization is no longer used as a primary diagnostic modality. However, invasive assessment of gradients across the coarctation segment is the gold standard and angiography is essential for assessment of candidacy and planning for transcatheter-based treatment. In older patients with risk factors for coronary artery disease, coronary angiography should be performed as an adjunct diagnostic procedure in preparation for repair.

TREATMENT

Significant coarctation is defined as:

- Resting peak-to-peak gradient greater than 20 mm Hg across the stenosis in the catheterization laboratory or mean Doppler systolic

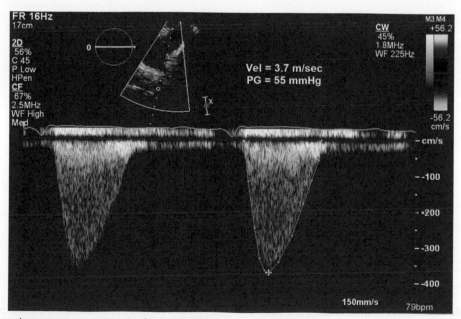

Fig. 4. From the suprasternal view, in the same patient, use of guided Continuous Doppler demonstrates a high-velocity envelope reflective of moderately severe arch obstruction. Advanced imaging is required to further evaluate the arch anatomy.

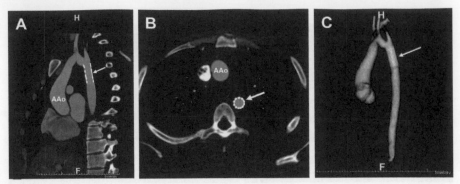

Fig. 5. Computed tomography angiography of the aorta in oblique sagittal (*A*) and axial (*B*) planes demonstrating no evidence of in-stent stenosis (*arrows*) in a 32-year-old patient with coarctation who underwent previous end-to-end anastomosis and later required transcatheter therapy for recoarctation. 3D reconstruction (*C*) displays the luminal contour of the Palmaz stent.

gradient greater than 20 mm Hg by echocardiography OR
- Resting peak-to-peak gradient greater than 10 mm Hg or mean Doppler systolic gradient greater than 10 mm Hg in the presence of decreased left ventricular systolic function, aortic insufficiency, or collateral flow.[32]

However, relatively few data exist to support these cut points historically used to signify risk of sequelae.[33] Several factors need to be considered in selecting the most appropriate method for repair, including age, anatomy of the transverse and descending aorta, history of previous repair, and institutional expertise.

The first surgical repair was performed by Clarence Crafoord in 1944 with resection and end-to-end anastomosis.[34] Since then, many surgical techniques to address coarctation have evolved over time (**Fig. 7**).[35] The patch aortoplasty involves ligating and dividing ductal tissue, creating a longitudinal incision across the coarctation and prosthetic patch enlargement of the region. Although advantageous in that it can be applied to longer regions of aortic narrowing, avoids a circumferential suture line in the end-to-end anastomosis, and less recoarctation, it is marked by a high rate of aneurysm in the long term—between 18% and 47%[36,37] (**Fig. 8**). Subclavian flap aortoplasty is a technique in which the left subclavian artery is

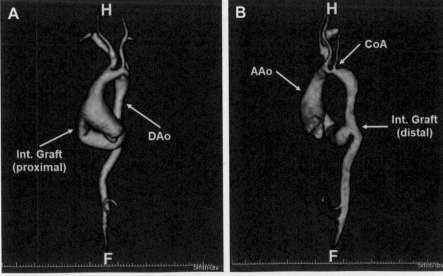

Fig. 6. Volume-rendered 3D reconstructions from a contrast-enhanced MRA examination (*A*, anterior view; *B*, posterior view) in a 57-year-old man with a history of coarctation who underwent surgical repair with an ascending to descending interposition graft (no. 22 mm Hemashield graft). AAo, ascending aorta; CoA, coarctation of the aorta; Dao, descending aorta; Int. Graft, interposition graft.

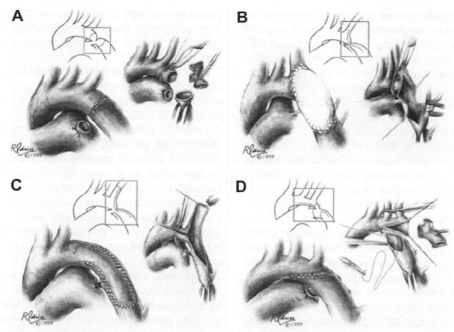

Fig. 7. Surgical techniques of aortic coarctation repair. (*A*) Resection and end-to-end anastomosis. The coarcted segment is resected and a circumferential end-to-end anastomosis is created. (*B*) Patch aortoplasty. Ductal tissue is divided by an incision across the coarctation and patch sutured across the site to enlarge the region. (*C*) Subclavian flap aortoplasty. The left subclavian artery is ligated and divided. A longitudinal incision from the proximal left subclavian artery is made and extended beyond the coarctation. The subclavian flap is turned down and enlarges this area. (*D*) Resection with extended end-to-end anastomosis. The coarcted segment is broadly resected and an oblique anastomosis made between the undersurface of the transverse arch and the proximal descending aorta. (*Adapted from* Dodge-Khatami A, Backer CL, Mavroudis C. Risk factors for recoarctation and results of reoperation: a 40-year review. *J Card Surg.* 2000;15(6):369-377; with permission.)

ligated and divided and turned down onto a longitudinal incision from the proximal left subclavian artery beyond the area of coarctation.[38] Similar to patch aortoplasty in that it avoids circumferential suture lines and can be used for long-segment stenosis, subclavian flap repair can cause retrograde blood flow down the vertebral

artery (subclavian steal) and hypoplasia of the left upper extremity with associated claudication. Some patients have been repaired with coarctectomy and interposition graft but this approach is limited by lack of aortic growth in keeping with somatic size when performed in children. The extended end-to-end anastomosis introduced in

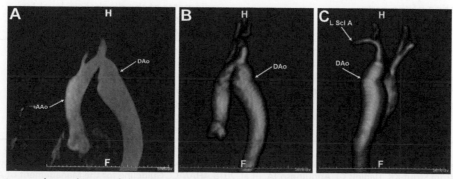

Fig. 8. Contrast-enhanced MRA of the aorta (*A*, oblique sagittal view) and volume-rendered 3D reconstructions (*B*, lateral view; *C*, posterior view) demonstrate an aneurysm in the proximal descending aorta in a 54-year-old man with coarctation of the aorta who underwent patch arterioplasty repair at age 16 years. AAo, ascending aorta; DAo, descending aorta; L Scl A, left subclavian artery.

1977 is a modification of the original technique in which a broad longitudinal incision and anastomosis across the proximal aorta/arch is created.[39]

In 1983, Lock and colleagues[40] described the first use of balloon angioplasty to treat coarctation in infants and children. Although effective in relieving obstruction acutely, balloon angioplasty carries a significant rate of recoarctation in 15%[41] and aneurysm in 24% to 35%.[41,42] Elastic recoil, especially in those of young patients, is believed to be contribute to recoarctation. Intimal and medial tears resulting from balloon angioplasty leading to aortic wall injury may play a role in the long-term development of aortic aneurysm.

Stent implantation became a treatment option in the early 1990s and may be appropriate in adults and adult-size adolescents.[43] Advantages of stent therapy in aortic coarctation include less need for over dilation of the aorta and structural support resulting in lower rates of aortic wall injury and restenosis. In a large observational registry study out of the Congenital Cardiovascular Interventional Study Consortium, outcomes of surgical, stent, balloon and stent angioplasty for native coarctation in 350 patients across 36 institutions were compared. Balloon angioplasty was notable for higher rate of acute and longer-term aortic wall injury.[44]

The Coarctation of the Aorta Stent Trial (COAST) reported short and intermediate outcomes of 105 children and young adults who underwent implantation of a Cheatham-Platinum bare metal stent. At 2 years, 14 patients (13%) required repeat stent dilation but no need for surgical intervention. Twelve of these 14 patients returned for planned reintervention as a result of somatic growth or planned staged therapy. One important outcome was stent fractures that were found in 23, but none were clinically significant. Both acute and late aortic wall injury defined as dissection, aneurysm, or rupture was documented but relatively uncommon.[45]

In general, stent therapy is considered safe and effective in the treatment of native coarctation and is a reasonable option for the adult with simple, discrete native coarctation. Guideline recommendations for therapy and treatment of the adult in aortic coarctation are summarized in **Table 2**.

Table 2
Guideline recommendations for the treatment of the adult with aortic coarctation

AHA/ACC Recommendation	Class/LOE	ESC Recommendation	Class/LOE
Surgical repair or catheter-based stenting is recommended for adults with hypertension and significant native or recurrent coarctation of the aorta.	I/B	All patients with a noninvasive pressure difference >20 mm Hg between upper and lower limbs, regardless of symptoms but with upper limb hypertension (>140/90 mm Hg in adults), pathologic blood pressure response during exercise, or significant LVH should have intervention.	I/C
Guideline-directed management and therapy is recommended for treatment of hypertension in patients with coarctation of the aorta.	I/C	Independent of the pressure gradient, hypertensive patients with ≥50% aortic narrowing relative to the aortic diameter at the diaphragm level (on CMR, CT, or invasive angiography) should be considered for intervention.	IIa/C
Balloon angioplasty for adults with native and recurrent coarctation of the aorta may be considered if stent placement is not feasible and surgical intervention is not an option.	IIb/B	Independent of the pressure gradient and presence of hypertension, patients with ≥50% aortic narrowing relative to the aortic diameter at the diaphragm level (on CMR, CT, or invasion angiography) may be considered for intervention.	IIb/C

Abbreviations: AHA/ACC, American Heart Association/American College of Cardiology; CMR, cardiac magnetic resonance; CT, computed tomography; ESC, European Society of Cardiology; LOE, level of evidence; LVH, left ventricular hypertrophy.
Adapted from Stout KK, Daniels CJ, Aboulhosn JA, et al. 2018 AHA/ACC Guideline for the Management of Adults with Congenital Heart Disease: A Report of the American College of Cardiology/American Heart Association Task Force on Clinical Practice Guidelines. J Am Coll Cardiol. 2019;73:1494-1563; and Baumgartner H, Bonhoeffer P, De Groot NM, et al. ESC Guidelines for the management of grown-up congenital heart disease (new version 2010). Eur Heart J. 2010;31:2915–2957.

OUTCOMES

Long-term survival is lower than that of the general population with an overall incidence of mortality of 5%.[46] A large single-center series described long-term outcome of 819 patients (mean age at repair 17.2 ± 13.6 years) who underwent isolated operative repair of coarctation between 1946 and 2005 at the Mayo Clinic. The survival rates were 93%, 86%, and 74% at 10, 20, and 30 years after primary repair, respectively, which were significantly lower than age- and sex-matched controls.[47] The most common cause of late death was coronary artery disease, followed by sudden death, heart failure, cerebrovascular accident, and ruptured aortic aneurysm. Coronary artery disease does not seem to be independently predicted by coarctation alone and likely mediated by other coexistent risk factors.[48,49] However, when patients with coarctation do experience myocardial infarction, it occurs at a significantly younger age than in those without coarctation.[50] Therefore, it is imperative that those who have undergone repair are monitored longitudinally for the development of complications and that risk factors for atherosclerosis are aggressively treated and managed.

Systemic Hypertension

Surgical and transcatheter repair of aortic coarctation decreases hypertension and use of antihypertensive medication.[44,51–53] However, systemic hypertension is one of the major long-term morbidities after repair of aortic coarctation. Persistent or recurrent hypertension and exercise-induced hypertension can develop after repair, especially in patients whose repairs are performed later in life, older age at follow-up, and those with residual narrowing.[47] A risk factor for exercise-induced hypertension is hypoplastic aortic arch or mild coarctation, even in the absence of a significant gradient.[54] When combining resting blood pressure, ambulatory blood pressure monitoring, and exercise testing, systemic hypertension has been reported in as many as 70% of patients after coarctation repair.[55]

Abnormalities of vascular function, including decreased compliance of the aortic wall, endothelial dysfunction, and dysregulation of the renin-angiotensin system are factors that contribute to hypertension.[56] Regardless of type of repair, vascular stiffness and decreased compliance remain.[19,57] In a small, randomized crossover study in 20 normotensive patients with repaired aortic coarctation, Ramipril improved maximum hyperemic forearm blood flow and decreased circulating levels of proinflammatory cytokines (interleukin-6) and molecules (sVCAM-1 and sCD40 L), suggesting that targeting the renin-angiotensin pathway could be used as a treatment for vascular dysfunction in repaired coarctation.[58] However, there are no guidelines regarding specific antihypertensive agent for the treatment of hypertension in coarctation (see **Table 2**).

When hypertension is detected at rest, recoarctation must be excluded by physical examination (brachial/femoral pulse delay, arm/leg blood pressure gradient), Doppler echocardiography, and/or CMR or cardiac CTA. Recoarctation should be evaluated and candidacy for transcatheter therapy (ie, stent angioplasty) should be determined. If there is no evidence of recoarctation, medical management for hypertension is indicated. Assessment of activity-related hypertension is performed with a 24-hour ambulatory blood pressure monitor or exercise study to determine peak systolic blood pressure at maximal exercise and should be a component of long-term care (**Table 3**).

Recoarctation

Recurrent coarctation refers to restenosis after an initially successful intervention. Symptoms suggestive of recoarctation are headaches or claudication, although many patients are asymptomatic and present with hypertension. The rate of recoarctation is up to 34% after surgery[37] and is seen primarily in children, usually due to inadequate aortic wall growth at the site of repair when surgery is performed before the aorta has reached adult size. In addition to end-to-end repair, restenosis can also be seen in patients who have undergone subclavian flap arterioplasty as residual ductal tissue is left behind and interposition graft for long-segment stenosis. Following balloon angioplasty, children are also at greater risk for recoarctation compared with adults, with rates up to 50% in infants and neonates compared with 9% in young adults likely due to higher elastic recoil in younger patients.[59,60]

Indications for intervention for recoarctation are similar to those for native coarctation and include hypertension, a peak instantaneous pressure gradient across the coarctation of ≥20 mm Hg, and/or imaging evidence of collateral circulation.[32,61] Discrete coarctation in older children and adults is treated with percutaneous balloon angioplasty, often with stent therapy, although surgical repair may be necessary for complex cases, including long-segment recoarctation, hypoplastic aortic arch, and associated aneurysm or pseudoaneurysm.

Table 3
Guidelines for routine follow-up and testing intervals in aortic coarctation

Frequency of Routine Follow-Up and Testing	Physiologic Stage A[a] (mo)	Physiologic Stage B[a] (mo)	Physiologic Stage C[a] (mo)	Physiologic Stage D[a] (mo)
Outpatient ACHD cardiologist	24	24	6–12	3–6
ECG	24	24	12	12
TTE[b]	24	24	12	12
CMR[c]/Cardiac CT[d]	36–60	36–60	12–24	12–24
Exercise test[e]	36	24	24	12

Abbreviations: ACHD, adult congenital heart disease; CMR, cardiovascular magnetic resonance imaging; CoA, coarctation of the aorta; CPET, cardiopulmonary exercise; CT, computed tomography; ECG, electrocardiogram; NYHA, New York Heart Association; TTE, transthoracic echocardiogram.

[a] Physiologic Stage A: NYHA FC I, no hemodynamic or anatomic sequelae, normal exercise capacity. Physiologic Stage B: NYHA FC II, mild hemodynamic sequelae (mild aortic enlargement, ventricular dysfunction, or valve disease), abnormal exercise function testing. Physiologic Stage C: NYHA FC III, at least moderate aortic enlargement, ventricular dysfunction, or valve disease, end-organ dysfunction responsive to therapy. Physiologic Stage D: NYHA FC IV, severe aortic enlargement, refractory end-organ dysfunction.

[b] Routine TTE may be unnecessary in a year when CMR imaging is performed unless clinical indications warrant otherwise.

[c] CMR may be indicated for assessment of aortic size and aortic arch/coarctation repair site anatomy. Baseline study is recommended with periodic follow-up CMR, with frequency of repeat imaging determined by anatomic and physiologic findings.

[d] CT may be used if CMR is not feasible and to evaluate cross-sectional imaging status–post-stent therapy for coarctation of the aorta; the frequency should be weighed against radiation exposure.

[e] Six-minute walk test or CPET, depending on the clinical indication.

Adapted from Stout KK, Daniels CJ, Aboulhosn JA, et al. 2018 AHA/ACC Guideline for the Management of Adults With Congenital Heart Disease: A Report of the American College of Cardiology/American Heart Association Task Force on Clinical Practice Guidelines. J Am Coll Cardiol. 2019;73:1494-1563.

Aortic Aneurysm/Pseudoaneurysm and Dissection

Diagnosis and surveillance for late aortic complications after coarctation repair, either surgical or percutaneous, requires intermittent 3D assessment of the coarctation site, including CMR or CTA to assess for aneurysm, pseudoaneurysm, recoarctation, stent fracture, and/or migration.

An aortic aneurysm may develop at the site of previous coarctation years after surgery (especially after patch angioplasty), balloon dilation, or stent implantation of native coarctation and can occur despite relief of systemic hypertension or residual/recurrent coarctation. The rate of aneurysm formation ranges between 3% and 20%.[47,62,63] Risk factors for postrepair aneurysms are older age at the time of coarctation repair, patch angioplasty technique, and bicuspid aortic valve.[64,65]

Pseudoaneurysms at the coarctation repair site demonstrate an area of weakening with outpouching of the adventitia thin layer of the aorta, usually along the suture line. At increased risk for rupture, pseudoaneurysms should be considered for repair at the time of diagnosis. Vascular dysfunction may be the underlying mechanism contributing to the development of aneurysm or pseudoaneurysm associated with repaired coarctation of the aorta.

For most patients, aneurysm or pseudoaneurysm repair requires surgical intervention with resection of the aneurysm and graft placement. Alternatively, endovascular stent grafts have been used with more frequency. The COAST II trial published results on the Cheatham-Platinum stent covered with an expandable sleeve of ePTFE in 158 children and adults with aortic coarctation and either evidence of aortic wall injury or risk factors for such. The theoretic benefits of a covered stent to prevent aortic wall injury have been documented.[66] The COAST II trial has shown efficacy in the use of covered endovascular stents for aortic wall injury, including aneurysm and pseudoaneurym.[45]

Reintervention

Of the 819 patients operated on at the Mayo Clinic described above, there were 175 reinterventions in 124 patients. Freedom from reintervention of the descending aorta were 97%, 92%, and 89% at 10, 20, and 30 years with older age and end-to-end anastomosis technique independently associated with lower rate of reintervention. In fact, the highest rate of reintervention was in patients less than 5 years at the time of repair. The most common reason for any cardiac reintervention (not just the descending aorta), however, was aortic valve surgery.[47]

Left Ventricular Dysfunction

With increased aortic stiffness, there is evidence to support impaired ventriculo-arterial coupling, which impacts left ventricular performance. Despite successful repair and normotension, patients with aortic coarctation have been shown to have increased left ventricular mass[67] and diastolic dysfunction.[68] Global longitudinal and radial strain are decreased late after coarctation repair in the face of normal left ventricular ejection fraction, suggestive of subtle impairment of left ventricular function.[69,70] Left ventricular contractile reserve in response to exercise is also abnormal and related to exaggerated blood pressure response to exercise.[71] Left ventricular fibrosis has been demonstrated in an animal model of repaired coarctation,[72] which may also play a role in the development of ventricular dysfunction and predisposition toward heart failure in this population.

Cerebral Aneurysm and Stroke

Intracranial aneurysm is found in approximately 10% of patients with aortic coarctation as diagnosed by CTA and magnetic resonance imaging with older age as a risk factor.[73,74] It occurs with a frequency of 5-fold compared with the general population.[75]

High rates of cerebrovascular accidents are a historical morbidity associated with unrepaired coarctation and hypertension. The prevalence of stroke in patients with aortic coarctation is not well described but these patients experience both hemorrhagic and ischemic stroke at significantly younger age compared with the general population.[76] Hemorrhagic stroke is related to intracranial aneurysm but the relationship between these aneurysms, coarctation, and stroke are not entirely clear.

The association of intracranial aneurysm and coarctation is thought to be related to either developmental abnormalities of the arterial wall or pathologic changes as a result of mechanical forces attributable to hypertension.[77] Just as aortic endothelial dysfunction has been demonstrated, there is evidence that the cerebral vasculature of those with aortic coarctation have increased stiffness and less vasoreactivity.[78] Furthermore, reduced aortic distensibility has been shown to result in greater transmission of aortic forward wave energy into the carotid artery on vascular studies of young adults with repaired coarctation, which may contribute to cerebrovascular disease.[18]

Vascular abnormalities, including vertebral artery hypoplasia and incomplete posterior circle of Willis, are associated with increased cerebral vascular resistance. There is a significantly higher prevalence of both of these cerebral vascular abnormalities in aortic coarctation patients compared with the general population and is an independent risk factor for hypertension, highlighting another potential mechanism linking stroke and hypertension in aortic coarctation.[79]

Many of these intracranial aneurysms are small and do not require treatment but there is no consensus on screening and surveillance of such aneurysms when found. The current American Heart Association/American College of Cardiology Guidelines on the management of adults with congenital heart disease state that it may be reasonable to screen for intracranial aneurysm giving it a class IIb recommendation with level of evidence B.[32] In the authors' institutions, consideration is given to patient age, risk factors, presence of new headache, and/or plans for systemic anticoagulation in the setting of cardiopulmonary bypass.

PREGNANCY

Because medical, surgical, and catheter-based therapies have advanced, the number of women living into adulthood and reaching childbearing years has grown. Preconception counseling is crucial to provide the most well-informed risk assessment for the individual patient. This includes up-to-date cardiac imaging, ECG, cardiopulmonary exercise test to evaluate functional capacity, review of medications that may pose a risk to a fetus, and discussion of potential for familial/genetic influence on a fetus. All women with congenital heart disease should undergo a fetal echocardiogram to screen for congenital heart disease in the fetus at ~20 weeks' gestation.

Women with aortic coarctation, repaired or unrepaired, are at risk for untoward cardiovascular outcomes and specifically are at increased risk for hypertensive disorders of pregnancy.[80] The frequency of a hypertensive complication was 24.1% ± 3.3% for women with coarctation compared with 8.0% ± 0.1% for women without coarctation in a study examining pregnancy outcomes in a nationally representative sample.[81] Aortic dimensions appear to correlate with adverse cardiovascular outcome in pregnancy. In a study of women who underwent CMR examinations before pregnancy, women with an aortic diameter of 12 mm (7 mm/m^2) or less were more likely to experience hypertensive complications.[82]

For these reasons, women with repaired coarctation are classified as World Health Organization (WHO) category II–III, which is defined as moderate increase for maternal morbidity and mortality.[83] In this case, pregnancy is not contraindicated but monitoring should take place throughout the pregnancy by both the adult congenital heart disease provider as well as with high-risk obstetrics/maternal fetal medicine. Patients with severe, native coarctation are considered WHO category IV or high risk for maternal morbidity and mortality and pregnancy is contraindicated.[83] If unplanned pregnancy occurs discussion regarding termination should take place.

There are numerous hemodynamic changes that occur throughout pregnancy in the woman with congenital heart disease. These hemodynamic changes can abruptly change during delivery and the postpartum period. During the second stage of labor, pushing is essentially a Valsalva maneuver that can impair venous return thereby decreasing cardiac output. In those with coarctation (native or recurrent), this drop in cardiac output can be severe and life-threatening. Therefore, a detailed delivery plan that includes an assisted second stage (use of forceps or vacuum) to minimize time spent pushing is recommended. An arterial line may also be placed to monitor blood pressure continuously. Ultimately, care should be individualized within the context of a multidisciplinary team. Women with repaired coarctation can undergo a successful pregnancy and delivery with appropriate preconception evaluation and careful monitoring.[83]

SUMMARY

Although often a simple discrete lesion, there can be a wide spectrum of aortic arch anatomy in aortic coarctation. The evolution in treatment of aortic coarctation over the past 3 decades has demonstrated improvements in survival for this condition but, despite successful repair, adults with aortic coarctation continue to experience excess morbidity and premature mortality associated with hypertension, heart failure, cerebrovascular accident, coronary artery disease, and aortic dissection/rupture. The understanding of aortic coarctation as a diffuse aortopathy may explain some of these long-term morbidities. This ongoing hazard warrants lifelong surveillance and follow-up with specialists in congenital heart disease to screen for and monitor late-onset complications.

DISCLOSURE

The authors have nothing to disclose.

REFERENCES

1. Beekman RH. Coarctation of the aorta. In: Allen HD, Driscoll D, Shaddy RE, et al, editors. Moss and Adams's heart disease in infants, children and adolescents: including the fetus and young adult, vol. 2, 8 edition. Lippincott Williams & Wilkins; 2013.
2. Hoffman JI, Kaplan S. The incidence of congenital heart disease. J Am Coll Cardiol 2002;39(12):1890–900.
3. Teo LL, Cannell T, Babu-Narayan SV, et al. Prevalence of associated cardiovascular abnormalities in 500 patients with aortic coarctation referred for cardiovascular magnetic resonance imaging to a tertiary center. Pediatr Cardiol 2011;32(8):1120–7.
4. Shone JD, Sellers RD, Anderson RC, et al. The developmental complex of "parachute mitral valve," supravalvular ring of left atrium, subaortic stenosis, and coarctation of aorta. Am J Cardiol 1963;11:714–25.
5. Freylikhman O, Tatarinova T, Smolina N, et al. Variants in the NOTCH1 gene in patients with aortic coarctation. Congenit Heart Dis 2014;9(5):391–6.
6. McBride KL, Zender GA, Fitzgerald-Butt SM, et al. Linkage analysis of left ventricular outflow tract malformations (aortic valve stenosis, coarctation of the aorta, and hypoplastic left heart syndrome). Eur J Hum Genet 2009;17(6):811–9.
7. Lalani SR, Ware SM, Wang X, et al. MCTP2 is a dosage-sensitive gene required for cardiac outflow tract development. Hum Mol Genet 2013;22(21):4339–48.
8. Sanchez-Castro M, Eldjouzi H, Charpentier E, et al. Search for rare copy-number variants in congenital heart defects identifies novel candidate genes and a potential role for FOXC1 in patients with coarctation of the aorta. Circ Cardiovasc Genet 2016;9(1):86–94.
9. Bayer ML, Frommelt PC, Blei F, et al. Congenital cardiac, aortic arch, and vascular bed anomalies in PHACE syndrome (from the International PHACE Syndrome Registry). Am J Cardiol 2013;112(12):1948–52.
10. Edwards JE, Christensen NA. Pathologic considerations of coarctation of the aorta. Proc Staff Meet Mayo Clin 1948;23(15):324–32.
11. Kennedy A, Taylor DG, Durrant TE. Pathology of the intima in coarctation of the aorta: a study using light and scanning electron microscopy. Thorax 1979;34(3):366–74.
12. Jimenez M, Daret D, Choussat A, et al. Immunohistological and ultrastructural analysis of the intimal thickening in coarctation of human aorta. Cardiovasc Res 1999;41(3):737–45.

13. Isner JM, Donaldson RF, Fulton D, et al. Cystic medial necrosis in coarctation of the aorta: a potential factor contributing to adverse consequences observed after percutaneous balloon angioplasty of coarctation sites. Circulation 1987; 75(4):689–95.

14. Yokoyama U, Ishiwata R, Jin MH, et al. Inhibition of EP4 signaling attenuates aortic aneurysm formation. PLoS One 2012;7(5):e36724.

15. Gardiner HM, Celermajer DS, Sorensen KE, et al. Arterial reactivity is significantly impaired in normotensive young adults after successful repair of aortic coarctation in childhood. Circulation 1994;89(4): 1745–50.

16. de Divitiis M, Pilla C, Kattenhorn M, et al. Vascular dysfunction after repair of coarctation of the aorta: impact of early surgery. Circulation 2001;104(12 Suppl 1):I165–70.

17. Brili S, Tousoulis D, Antoniades C, et al. Evidence of vascular dysfunction in young patients with successfully repaired coarctation of aorta. Atherosclerosis 2005;182(1):97–103.

18. Kowalski R, Lee MGY, Doyle LW, et al. Reduced aortic distensibility is associated with higher aorto-carotid wave transmission and central aortic systolic pressure in young adults after coarctation repair. J Am Heart Assoc 2019;8(7):e011411.

19. Schafer M, Morgan GJ, Mitchell MB, et al. Impact of different coarctation therapies on aortic stiffness: phase-contrast MRI study. Int J Cardiovasc Imaging 2018;34(9):1459–69.

20. Brili S, Oikonomou E, Antonopoulos AS, et al. ^{18}F-Fluorodeoxyglucose positron emission tomography/computed tomographic imaging detects aortic wall inflammation in patients with repaired coarctation of aorta. Circ Cardiovasc Imaging 2018;11(1): e007002.

21. Brili S, Tousoulis D, Antonopoulos AS, et al. Effects of atorvastatin on endothelial function and the expression of proinflammatory cytokines and adhesion molecules in young subjects with successfully repaired coarctation of aorta. Heart 2012;98(4): 325–9.

22. Campbell M. Natural history of coarctation of the aorta. Br Heart J 1970;32(5):633–40.

23. Whelton PK, Carey RM, Aronow WS, et al. 2017 ACC/AHA/AAPA/ABC/ACPM/AGS/APhA/ASH/ASPC/NMA/PCNA guideline for the prevention, detection, evaluation, and management of high blood pressure in adults: executive summary: a report of the American College of Cardiology/American Heart Association Task Force on Clinical Practice Guidelines. Circulation 2018;138(17):e426–83.

24. Tacy TA, Baba K, Cape EG. Effect of aortic compliance on Doppler diastolic flow pattern in coarctation of the aorta. J Am Soc Echocardiogr 1999;12(8): 636–42.

25. Seifert BL, DesRochers K, Ta M, et al. Accuracy of Doppler methods for estimating peak-to-peak and peak instantaneous gradients across coarctation of the aorta: an in vitro study. J Am Soc Echocardiogr 1999;12(9):744–53.

26. Krieger EV, Stout KK, Grosse-Wortmann L. How to image congenital left heart obstruction in adults. Circ Cardiovasc Imaging 2017;10(5).

27. Hedgire SS, Baliyan V, Ghoshhajra BB, et al. Recent advances in cardiac computed tomography dose reduction strategies: a review of scientific evidence and technical developments. J Med Imaging (Bellingham) 2017;4(3):031211.

28. Julsrud PR, Breen JF, Felmlee JP, et al. Coarctation of the aorta: collateral flow assessment with phase-contrast MR angiography. AJR Am J Roentgenol 1997;169(6):1735–42.

29. Hom JJ, Ordovas K, Reddy GP. Velocity-encoded cine MR imaging in aortic coarctation: functional assessment of hemodynamic events. Radiographics 2008;28(2):407–16.

30. Padang R, Dennis M, Semsarian C, et al. Detection of serious complications by MR imaging in asymptomatic young adults with repaired coarctation of the aorta. Heart Lung Circ 2014;23(4):332–8.

31. Nielsen JC, Powell AJ, Gauvreau K, et al. Magnetic resonance imaging predictors of coarctation severity. Circulation 2005;111(5):622–8.

32. Stout KK, Daniels CJ, Aboulhosn JA, et al. 2018 AHA/ACC guideline for the management of adults with congenital heart disease: executive summary: a report of the American College of Cardiology/American Heart Association Task Force on Clinical Practice Guidelines. J Am Coll Cardiol 2019; 73(12):1494–563.

33. Wendell DC, Friehs I, Samyn MM, et al. Treating a 20 mm Hg. gradient alleviates myocardial hypertrophy in experimental aortic coarctation. J Surg Res 2017;218:194–201.

34. Kvitting JP, Olin CL. Clarence Crafoord: a giant in cardiothoracic surgery, the first to repair aortic coarctation. Ann Thorac Surg 2009;87(1):342–6.

35. Dodge-Khatami A, Backer CL, Mavroudis C. Risk factors for recoarctation and results of reoperation: a 40-year review. J Cardiovasc Surg 2000;15(6): 369–77.

36. Cramer JW, Ginde S, Bartz PJ, et al. Aortic aneurysms remain a significant source of morbidity and mortality after use of Dacron((R)) patch aortoplasty to repair coarctation of the aorta: results from a single center. Pediatr Cardiol 2013;34(2):296–301.

37. Choudhary P, Canniffe C, Jackson DJ, et al. Late outcomes in adults with coarctation of the aorta. Heart 2015;101(15):1190–5.

38. Waldhausen JA, Nahrwold DL. Repair of coarctation of the aorta with a subclavian flap. J Thorac Cardiovasc Surg 1966;51(4):532–3.

39. Amato JJ, Rheinlander HF, Cleveland RJ. A method of enlarging the distal transverse arch in infants with hypoplasia and coarctation of the aorta. Ann Thorac Surg 1977;23(3):261–3.

40. Lock JE, Bass JL, Amplatz K, et al. Balloon dilation angioplasty of aortic coarctations in infants and children. Circulation 1983;68(1):109–16.

41. Harris KC, Du W, Cowley CG, et al, Congenital Cardiac Intervention Study Consortium. A prospective observational multicenter study of balloon angioplasty for the treatment of native and recurrent coarctation of the aorta. Catheter Cardiovasc Interv 2014;83(7):1116–23.

42. Cowley CG, Orsmond GS, Feola P, et al. Long-term, randomized comparison of balloon angioplasty and surgery for native coarctation of the aorta in childhood. Circulation 2005;111(25):3453–6.

43. O'Laughlin MP, Perry SB, Lock JE, et al. Use of endovascular stents in congenital heart disease. Circulation 1991;83(6):1923–39.

44. Forbes TJ, Kim DW, Du W, et al. Comparison of surgical, stent, and balloon angioplasty treatment of native coarctation of the aorta: an observational study by the CCISC (Congenital Cardiovascular Interventional Study Consortium). J Am Coll Cardiol 2011;58(25):2664–74.

45. Taggart NW, Minahan M, Cabalka AK, et al. Immediate outcomes of covered stent placement for treatment or prevention of aortic wall injury associated with coarctation of the aorta (COAST II). JACC Cardiovasc Interv 2016;9(5):484–93.

46. Lee MGY, Babu-Narayan SV, Kempny A, et al. Long-term mortality and cardiovascular burden for adult survivors of coarctation of the aorta. Heart 2019; 105(15):1190–6.

47. Brown ML, Burkhart HM, Connolly HM, et al. Coarctation of the aorta: lifelong surveillance is mandatory following surgical repair. J Am Coll Cardiol 2013; 62(11):1020–5.

48. Roifman I, Therrien J, Ionescu-Ittu R, et al. Coarctation of the aorta and coronary artery disease: fact or fiction? Circulation 2012;126(1):16–21.

49. Egbe AC, Rihal CS, Thomas A, et al. Coronary artery disease in adults with coarctation of aorta: incidence, risk factors, and outcomes. J Am Heart Assoc 2019;8(12):e012056.

50. Pickard SS, Gauvreau K, Gurvitz M, et al. A national population-based study of adults with coronary artery disease and coarctation of the aorta. Am J Cardiol 2018;122(12):2120–4.

51. Hager A, Kanz S, Kaemmerer H, et al. Coarctation Long-term Assessment (COALA): significance of arterial hypertension in a cohort of 404 patients up to 27 years after surgical repair of isolated coarctation of the aorta, even in the absence of restenosis and prosthetic material. J Thorac Cardiovasc Surg 2007;134(3):738–45.

52. Holzer R, Qureshi S, Ghasemi A, et al. Stenting of aortic coarctation: acute, intermediate, and long-term results of a prospective multi-institutional registry—Congenital Cardiovascular Interventional Study Consortium (CCISC). Catheter Cardiovasc Interv 2010;76(4):553–63.

53. Morgan GJ, Lee KJ, Chaturvedi R, et al. Systemic blood pressure after stent management for arch coarctation implications for clinical care. JACC Cardiovasc Interv 2013;6(2):192–201.

54. Egbe AC, Allison TG, Ammash NM. Mild coarctation of aorta is an independent risk factor for exercise-induced hypertension. Hypertension 2019;74(6): 1484–9.

55. Canniffe C, Ou P, Walsh K, et al. Hypertension after repair of aortic coarctation—a systematic review. Int J Cardiol 2013;167(6):2456–61.

56. Parker FB Jr, Streeten DH, Farrell B, et al. Preoperative and postoperative renin levels in coarctation of the aorta. Circulation 1982;66(3):513–4.

57. Martins JD, Zachariah J, Selamet Tierney ES, et al. Impact of treatment modality on vascular function in coarctation of the aorta: the LOVE - COARCT Study. J Am Heart Assoc 2019;8(7):e011536.

58. Brili S, Tousoulis D, Antoniades C, et al. Effects of ramipril on endothelial function and the expression of proinflammatory cytokines and adhesion molecules in young normotensive subjects with successfully repaired coarctation of aorta: a randomized cross-over study. J Am Coll Cardiol 2008;51(7):742–9.

59. Adjagba PM, Hanna B, Miro J, et al. Percutaneous angioplasty used to manage native and recurrent coarctation of the aorta in infants younger than 1 year: immediate and midterm results. Pediatr Cardiol 2014;35(7):1155–61.

60. Chen SS, Dimopoulos K, Alonso-Gonzalez R, et al. Prevalence and prognostic implication of restenosis or dilatation at the aortic coarctation repair site assessed by cardiovascular MRI in adult patients late after coarctation repair. Int J Cardiol 2014;173(2): 209–15.

61. Baumgartner H, Bonhoeffer P, De Groot NM, et al. ESC Guidelines for the management of grown-up congenital heart disease (new version 2010). Eur Heart J 2010;31(23):2915–57.

62. Cohen M, Fuster V, Steele PM, et al. Coarctation of the aorta. Long-term follow-up and prediction of outcome after surgical correction. Circulation 1989; 80(4):840–5.

63. Jenkins NP, Ward C. Coarctation of the aorta: natural history and outcome after surgical treatment. QJM 1999;92(7):365–71.

64. Oliver JM, Gallego P, Gonzalez A, et al. Risk factors for aortic complications in adults with coarctation of the aorta. J Am Coll Cardiol 2004;44(8):1641–7.

65. Oliver JM, Alonso-Gonzalez R, Gonzalez AE, et al. Risk of aortic root or ascending aorta complications

in patients with bicuspid aortic valve with and without coarctation of the aorta. Am J Cardiol 2009;104(7):1001–6.

66. Tzifa A, Ewert P, Brzezinska-Rajszys G, et al. Covered Cheatham-Platinum stents for aortic coarctation: early and intermediate-term results. J Am Coll Cardiol 2006;47(7):1457–63.

67. Ong CM, Canter CE, Gutierrez FR, et al. Increased stiffness and persistent narrowing of the aorta after successful repair of coarctation of the aorta: relationship to left ventricular mass and blood pressure at rest and with exercise. Am Heart J 1992;123(6):1594–600.

68. Voges I, Kees J, Jerosch-Herold M, et al. Aortic stiffening and its impact on left atrial volumes and function in patients after successful coarctation repair: a multiparametric cardiovascular magnetic resonance study. J Cardiovasc Magn Reson 2016;18(1):56.

69. Menting ME, van Grootel RW, van den Bosch AE, et al. Quantitative assessment of systolic left ventricular function with speckle-tracking echocardiography in adult patients with repaired aortic coarctation. Int J Cardiovasc Imaging 2016;32(5):777–87.

70. Kutty S, Rangamani S, Venkataraman J, et al. Reduced global longitudinal and radial strain with normal left ventricular ejection fraction late after effective repair of aortic coarctation: a CMR feature tracking study. Int J Cardiovasc Imaging 2013;29(1):141–50.

71. Li VW, Chen RH, Wong WH, et al. Left ventricular contractile reserve in young adults long-term after repair of coarctation of the aorta. Am J Cardiol 2015;115(3):348–53.

72. Liu J, Drak D, Krishnan A, et al. Left ventricular fibrosis and systolic hypertension persist in a repaired aortic coarctation model. Ann Thorac Surg 2017;104(3):942–9.

73. Curtis SL, Bradley M, Wilde P, et al. Results of screening for intracranial aneurysms in patients with coarctation of the aorta. AJNR Am J Neuroradiol 2012;33(6):1182–6.

74. Donti A, Spinardi L, Brighenti M, et al. Frequency of intracranial aneurysms determined by magnetic resonance angiography in children (mean age 16) having operative or endovascular treatment of coarctation of the aorta (mean age 3). Am J Cardiol 2015;116(4):630–3.

75. Cook SC, Hickey J, Maul TM, et al. Assessment of the cerebral circulation in adults with coarctation of the aorta. Congenit Heart Dis 2013;8(4):289–95.

76. Pickard SS, Gauvreau K, Gurvitz M, et al. Stroke in adults with coarctation of the aorta: a national population-based study. J Am Heart Assoc 2018;7(11):e009072.

77. Singh PK, Marzo A, Staicu C, et al. The effects of aortic coarctation on cerebral hemodynamics and its importance in the etiopathogenesis of intracranial aneurysms. J Vasc Interv Neurol 2010;3(1):17–30.

78. Wong R, Ahmad W, Davies A, et al. Assessment of cerebral blood flow in adult patients with aortic coarctation. Cardiol Young 2017;27(8):1606–13.

79. Rodrigues JCL, Jaring MFR, Werndle MC, et al. Repaired coarctation of the aorta, persistent arterial hypertension and the selfish brain. J Cardiovasc Magn Reson 2019;21(1):68.

80. Vriend JW, Drenthen W, Pieper PG, et al. Outcome of pregnancy in patients after repair of aortic coarctation. Eur Heart J 2005;26(20):2173–8.

81. Krieger EV, Landzberg MJ, Economy KE, et al. Comparison of risk of hypertensive complications of pregnancy among women with versus without coarctation of the aorta. Am J Cardiol 2011;107(10):1529–34.

82. Jimenez-Juan L, Krieger EV, Valente AM, et al. Cardiovascular magnetic resonance imaging predictors of pregnancy outcomes in women with coarctation of the aorta. Eur Heart J Cardiovasc Imaging 2014;15(3):299–306.

83. Canobbio MM, Warnes CA, Aboulhosn J, et al. Management of pregnancy in patients with complex congenital heart disease: a scientific statement for healthcare professionals from the American Heart Association. Circulation 2017;135(8):e50–87.

Ebstein Anomaly in the Adult Patient

Margaret M. Fuchs, MD*, Heidi M. Connolly, MD

KEYWORDS

- Ebstein anomaly • Tricuspid valve • Cone repair • Pregnancy • Accessory pathway

KEY POINTS

- Ebstein anomaly is a congenital malformation involving primarily apical displacement of the tricuspid valve and right ventricular myopathy.
- Typical presenting symptoms in the adult patient are palpitations, exertional limitation, and cyanosis.
- Echocardiography is the key imaging modality for diagnosis and demonstrates tricuspid valve findings, including apical displacement of the septal leaflet and tethering of the valve to the right ventricular myocardium.
- Tricuspid valve repair is the ideal operative approach and should be considered when there is exertional limitation, cyanosis, and/or progressive right ventricular dilation or dysfunction.
- Pregnancy generally is well tolerated, with risk of right heart failure, arrhythmia, prematurity, and congenital heart disease in the offspring.

INTRODUCTION

Ebstein anomaly was first described by Wilhelm Ebstein in 1866 in a 19 year old with cardiac cachexia and cyanosis.[1] It is a rare form of congenital heart disease involving primarily the tricuspid valve and right ventricle. It has a wide spectrum of anatomic involvement and clinical presentation. This article focuses on the presentation and management of the adult with Ebstein anomaly.

EPIDEMIOLOGY

Ebstein anomaly is estimated to occur at a rate of 0.17 to 0.72 per 10,000 live births and has no correlation with gender or race.[2,3] An association with maternal age and multiple gestation pregnancy has been observed in some epidemiologic series but not in others.[2–4] Antenatal exposure to lithium historically has been believed to be a cause of Ebstein anomaly[5]; however, the impact of lithium exposure more recently has been challenged.[6,7]

Ebstein anomaly has been observed to occur at higher rates in some families, including identical twins, suggesting there may be a genetic etiology in a minority of cases.[4,8,9] Mutations in genes encoding sarcomere proteins, including MYH7 and α-tropomyosin, have been identified in other affected patients, providing a possible genetic link between Ebstein anomaly and occasionally co-occurring left ventricular noncompaction.[10,11] Most cases of Ebstein anomaly, however, are without identifiable genetic explanation.

ANATOMY

Ebstein anomaly primarily is characterized by abnormalities of both the tricuspid valve and the right ventricle. There is a wide spectrum of tricuspid valve anatomic derangements possible, and attention to valve morphology is critical to optimally planning surgical intervention and patient management.

Department of Cardiovascular Medicine, Mayo Clinic, 200 First Street Southwest, Rochester, MN 55905, USA
* Corresponding author.
E-mail address: fuchs.margaret@mayo.edu

Cardiol Clin 38 (2020) 353–363
https://doi.org/10.1016/j.ccl.2020.04.004
0733-8651/20/© 2020 Elsevier Inc. All rights reserved.

Tricuspid Valve

Formation of the tricuspid valve in utero requires delamination of the valve leaflets, or separation of the leaflet tissue from the underlying myocardium. The tricuspid valve leaflets in Ebstein anomaly demonstrate varying degrees of failure of delamination, leaving them adherent to the right ventricle.[12] The septal and posterior leaflets typically are affected most severely, sometimes with little functional tissue present.[12] The anterior leaflet can be large and sail-like or tethered by fibrous tissue with reduced mobility.[12] Very mobile anterior leaflets often lack appropriate chordal attachment, whereas tethered leaflets may have insertion directly to a papillary muscle or the myocardium.[13] Fenestrations often are present in the anterior leaflet, contributing to tricuspid regurgitation.[14]

In addition to abnormality in the shape and size of the leaflets, the annular attachment of the septal and posterior leaflets is displaced apically, with the point of maximal displacement at the commissure of these 2 leaflets.[13] The functional tricuspid valve orifice thereby is shifted anteroapically toward the right ventricular outflow tract.[12] In most cases, there is severe tricuspid regurgitation related to inability of the abnormal tricuspid leaflets to effectively coapt.[12] Rarely, excessive attachment of the anterior leaflet directly to the myocardium results in tricuspid stenosis or even an imperforate tricuspid valve.[13]

Right Ventricle

Displacement of the tricuspid valve results in 2 portions of the right ventricle. The inlet right ventricle, between the anatomic (nondisplaced) tricuspid annulus and the functional right ventricle, often is referred to as the atrialized right ventricle.[13] This portion tends to become very dilated and often dyskinetic.[12] The atrialized right ventricle receives the tricuspid regurgitation volume load and has to-and-fro flow with the anatomic right atrium, given the lack of a valve between these 2 structures. The resulting volume overload leads to progressive dilation of both chambers.[12] Pathologic specimens frequently demonstrate very thin walls in the atrialized right ventricle that are fibrotic and sometimes entirely lacking in muscular tissue.[13]

The functional right ventricle typically is smaller than normal and sometimes contains only the right ventricular outflow tract.[12] Although its function is better than the atrialized right ventricle, there is an inherent myopathy in patients with Ebstein anomaly, such that even the functional right ventricle may be enlarged and have declining function over time.[15] In the setting of severe right ventricular enlargement, the ventricular septum can be pushed left-ward, causing left ventricular compression, which may contribute to impairment of left ventricular function.[12]

Associated Defects

The most common associated congenital anomaly is atrial septal defect and patent foramen ovale, occurring in more than 80% of patients.[16] Ventricular septal defects and pulmonary stenosis also are observed.[16] Left heart disease of some form occurs in a significant number of patients, in 1 series close to 40%.[17] This includes findings consistent with left ventricular noncompaction (most common, with a potential genetic link, described previously), abnormalities of left ventricular systolic or diastolic function, and left-sided valve disease, including mitral valve prolapse and bicuspid aortic valve.[17] Left-sided valve disease has been observed to occur at rates above the general population, suggesting a nonrandom association. Accessory conduction pathways occur frequently in Ebstein anomaly, in 5% to 25% of patients,[18] and Wolff-Parkinson-White syndrome is associated more commonly with Ebstein anomaly than any other form of congenital heart disease.[19]

CLINICAL MANIFESTATIONS
Symptoms

Although often diagnosed by prenatal ultrasound or in early childhood, many patients present with a new diagnosis of Ebstein anomaly in adulthood. Palpitations are a common presenting symptom. One series of adults with unoperated Ebstein anomaly demonstrated arrhythmia in 51% at the time of presentation.[20] Some adult patients report symptoms of heart failure, including dyspnea, fatigue, and lower extremity edema.[12] Exercise intolerance can occur due to reduced right ventricular function and severe tricuspid regurgitation or related to exercise-induced cyanosis from right-to-left shunting across the atrial septum. Paradoxic embolism through an atrial septal defect or patent foramen ovale also can occur, especially in the setting of severe tricuspid regurgitation, and present as stroke or transient ischemic attack, brain abscess, or myocardial infarction.[21]

Physical Examination

The physical examination, like the clinical presentation, is dictated in large part by the severity of pathology. Young children with severe disease present with signs of heart failure and severe cyanosis.[12] Adults generally have a milder phenotype than children and less profound symptoms. Careful attention to the physical examination can provide clues to the diagnosis.

Despite the presence of severe tricuspid regurgitation in most cases, the jugular venous pulse typically is normal, without prominent V wave. This is related to the very large right atrium and atrialized right ventricle accommodating tricuspid regurgitation without transmitting pressure to the jugular vein.[22] Failure of the right ventricle may lead to rise in the mean jugular venous pressure, but a prominent V wave and systolic pulsation of the liver are not expected.[23] Additionally, despite significant right ventricular enlargement, the parasternal impulse of the right ventricle typically is subtle.[22]

On auscultation, the first heart sound usually is split with delayed tricuspid valve closure (T1), due to both a right bundle branch block and the large anterior leaflet, which takes longer to fully close.[23] T1 typically is loud, related to increased tension in the anterior leaflet as it reaches its fully closed position; this often is referred to as the sail sound.[23,24] If the anterior leaflet is very mobile, there can be multiple closure sounds that mimic ejection clicks.[12] The second heart sound is split, again due to right bundle branch block. There often is a third and/or fourth heart sound present.[23]

Tricuspid regurgitation results in a holosystolic murmur at the lower left sternal border that increases with inspiration. Paradoxically, many adults have a very soft or absent systolic murmur due to severe regurgitation with rapid equalization of pressure across the tricuspid valve. A diastolic murmur of increased flow across the tricuspid valve occasionally can be appreciated,[24] although clinically this is heard infrequently in adult patients.

DIAGNOSTIC FEATURES
Electrocardiogram

The electrocardiogram (ECG) of a patient with Ebstein anomaly can reveal multiple abnormal findings (Fig. 1), including the following:

- Right atrial enlargement, with the so-called Himalayan P waves[22]
- Right bundle branch block, often with fragmented QRS complexes (a second QRS complex attached to the related to infra-Hisian conduction disturbance and abnormal activation of the atrialized right ventricle[25]
- PR prolongation, resulting from atrial dilation and delayed intra-atrial conduction[26]
- Low-voltage QRS in right-sided chest leads, secondary to generalized right ventricular myopathy[27]
- Supraventricular tachycardia and atrial arrhythmias

Apical displacement of the septal tricuspid valve leaflet results in discontinuity of the central fibrous body and septal atrioventricular (AV) ring.[23] This disruption of the AV connection creates the potential for accessory pathways.[25] In these cases, pathologic specimens demonstrate muscular tissue that passes through the fibrous tissue at the hinge of the tricuspid leaflet, thereby forming a bridge from the atrial wall to the ventricular

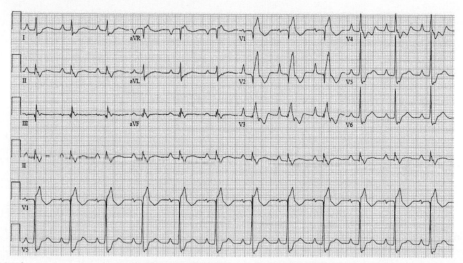

Fig. 1. ECG of a 43-year-old man with Ebstein anomaly, demonstrating right atrial enlargement (as seen by the tall, peaked P waves), first-degree AV block (PR interval 224 ms), and right bundle branch block with fragmented QRS complex (fragmentation defined as >2 notches in the R or S wave in 2 contiguous leads). (*From* Das MK, Zipes DP. Fragmented QRS: a predictor of mortality and sudden cardiac death. *Heart Rhythm.* 2009;6(3 Suppl):S8-14.)

myocardium.[28] In Ebstein patients with reentrant tachycardia, 30% are found to have more than 1 accessory pathway.[18] Electrographically, patients with accessory pathways may demonstrate evidence of preexcitation, with left bundle branch block and predominant S wave in the right precordial leads (**Fig. 2**).[25] In other cases, preexcitation can be subtle, with short PR interval and loss of the typical right bundle branch block.[18]

In addition to accessory pathway–mediated tachycardia, patients with Ebstein anomaly have a high incidence of atrial arrhythmias. ECG in these cases may reveal atrial fibrillation, typical atrial flutter, atrial tachycardia (incisional, after repair), or, less commonly, AV nodal reentrant tachycardia.[18,19] Although relatively uncommon, sudden death related to ventricular arrhythmias recently has been recognized to occur in this patient population more frequently than realized previously.[29] It is important to differentiate wide complex tachycardia related to aberrantly conducted atrial fibrillation from ventricular tachycardia.[18]

Chest Radiograph

Chest radiograph findings vary depending on the severity of disease. In cases of significant right heart enlargement, chest radiograph demonstrates right atrial enlargement and marked cardiomegaly with a globular contour[22] (**Fig. 3**). The great arteries generally are small with a subtle aortic shadow, creating a narrow vascular pedicle.[22,23]

Echocardiogram

Transthoracic echocardiography is the test of choice for the evaluation of a patient with suspected Ebstein anomaly. Echocardiogram can confirm the diagnosis, assess the severity of disease, and identify other associated anomalies. The echocardiographic diagnosis of Ebstein anomaly involves demonstrating apical displacement of the septal leaflet, which is best assessed in an apical 4-chamber view (**Fig. 4**D). Calculation of the displacement index involves measuring the distance between the mitral and septal tricuspid hinge points, which then is indexed to body surface area. A displacement index greater than 8 mm/m^2 has been demonstrated to be a sensitive predictor of Ebstein anomaly.[30]

In addition to apical displacement, echocardiography in Ebstein anomaly demonstrates evidence of failure of delamination of the tricuspid valve leaflets. Leaflet tethering, defined as 3 or more attachments to the ventricular wall that impede leaflet motion, is expected and usually affects the septal and inferior leaflets more than the anterior leaflet.[15,31] In severely affected valves, there may be little mobility of the septal and inferior leaflet. It is important to use multiple echo imaging windows to completely assess the tricuspid valve anatomy (**Fig. 4**). The anterior and septal leaflets often are viewed best in the apical 4-chamber view, whereas the inferior leaflet may be better assessed using an right ventricular inflow view.[15] Due to distortion of valve anatomy, nonstandard imaging planes may be needed to adequately

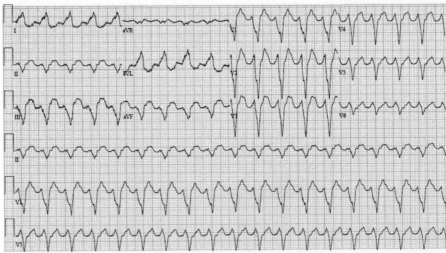

Fig. 2. ECG of a 16-year-old girl with Ebstein anomaly, Wolff-Parkinson-White syndrome, and prior pathway ablation, presenting with palpitations. ECG demonstrates wide complex tachycardia with left bundle branch block morphology and prominent S wave in the right precordial leads. The patient was found to be in supraventricular tachycardia.

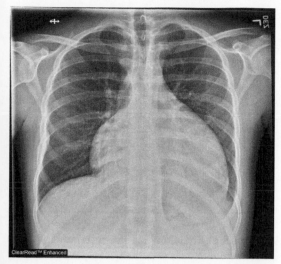

Fig. 3. Chest radiograph of a 19-year-old man with Ebstein anomaly demonstrating marked cardiomegaly with clear lung fields and subtle aortic shadow.

assess all 3 valve leaflets. When anticipating surgical repair of the tricuspid valve, thorough visualization and description of all 3 leaflets are important to allow for appropriate surgical planning.[14]

The demonstration and quantification of tricuspid regurgitation can be challenging. Distorted valve anatomy means that the origin of the regurgitant jet may be very near the apex in an apical 4-chamber view, and therefore can be missed by placing the color Doppler box closer to the anatomic annulus. There often are multiple jets of tricuspid regurgitation and they may be oriented inferiorly, because the valve orifice frequently is angled toward the right ventricular outflow tract.[15] In this case, regurgitation may be best demonstrated in the parasternal short axis or subcostal view.[15] Quantification methods used for other forms of tricuspid regurgitation are less helpful in cases of Ebstein anomaly. The large, compliant right atrium and atrialized right ventricle, as well as right ventricular dysfunction, result in a low-velocity tricuspid regurgitation signal with rapid equalization of pressures.[23] Systolic reversal of flow in the hepatic veins is not common due to the compliant right atrium accommodating regurgitant flow.[15] In the setting of multiple jets of regurgitation, quantification with vena contracta and proximal isovelocity surface area is challenging. Optimal assessment, therefore, involves careful 2-dimensional (2-D) assessment of valve structure, color Doppler interrogation of visualized coaptation defects, and semiquantitative grading of all regurgitant jets.[15]

Attention also should be paid to the size and function of the right heart. An enlarged right atrium is expected, and in some cases can be severely enlarged.[22] The atrialized right ventricle is myopathic, appearing dilated, thin, and dysfunctional.[15] Traditional echocardiographic assessments of right ventricular function, including

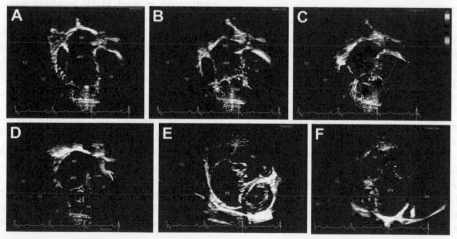

Fig. 4. Transthoracic echocardiographic images from a patient with Ebstein anomaly. Apical 4-chamber view (apex down format) in diastole (*A*), systole (*B*), and color Doppler (*C*), showing severe right heart enlargement, apical displacement of the septal leaflet, tethering of the anterior leaflet, coaptation defect (*B* [*arrowhead*]) and the origin of tricuspid regurgitation (*C*). (*D*) Measurement of apical displacement of the septal leaflet in a modified apical 4-chamber view. (*E*) Parasternal short axis view at the midventricle showing large, tethered anterior leaflet and rudimentary septal leaflet with coaptation defect (*arrowhead*). (*F*) Parasternal RV inflow view demonstrates anterior and inferior leaflets. AL, anterior tricuspid valve leaflet; aRV, atrialized right ventricle; IL, inferior tricuspid valve leaflet; LV, left ventricle; RA, right atrium; RV, right ventricle; SL, septal tricuspid valve leaflet.

lateral tissue Doppler and tricuspid annular plane systolic excursion, are of limited use in the assessment of the Ebstein ventricle, because the small functional right ventricle is primarily responsible for systolic function.[15] Qualitative visual assessment of the ventricular size (relative to the left ventricle) and function generally is used.

Echocardiography may demonstrate other associated anomalies. Careful inspection of the atrial septum should be performed, given the high incidence of atrial septal defect and patent foramen ovale. If imaging is suboptimal, agitated saline can be used to detect the presence of a right-to-left atrial-level shunt.[32] Close assessment of left ventricular function is important. Left ventricular dysfunction can occur in patients with Ebstein anomaly, either due to inherent myopathy or related to marked right ventricular dilation.[17]

Transesophageal echocardiogram generally is not required for diagnosis and evaluation of Ebstein anomaly. It can be helpful to better delineate tricuspid valve and atrial septal anatomy when transthoracic imaging is suboptimal due to limited acoustic windows.[15] It is used routinely during surgical intervention to assess anatomy prior to and after operation.

Cardiac Magnetic Resonance Imaging

Data obtained from cardiac magnetic resonance imaging (MRI) in patients with Ebstein anomaly are complementary to echocardiographic assessment, and both modalities often are appropriate to evaluate these patients. Cardiac MRI can quantify right heart size and function more easily,[33] which may be of use when deciding on a management strategy for a particular patient. When comparing the assessment of right ventricular function by echocardiography and MRI, only 2-D global longitudinal right ventricular strain correlates with cardiac MRI–derived right ventricular ejection fraction.[34] Cardiac MRI also can better demonstrate the inferior tricuspid leaflet anatomy in some patients.[33] Echocardiography remains the test of choice to evaluate the degree of tricuspid regurgitation and to identify other associated cardiac anomalies.[15] For patients who cannot undergo MRI, cardiac computed tomography also can be utilized to assess ventricular volumes and ejection fraction.[15] It also is useful for the preoperative assessment of the coronary arteries.

TESTING AFTER DIAGNOSIS
Exercise Test

Exercise testing in patients with Ebstein anomaly can provide an objective measure of functional capacity[35] and is helpful especially in adult patients with no reported symptoms. Exercise performance has been demonstrated to decline in patients with Ebstein anomaly and at least grade 2 tricuspid regurgitation who are managed medically.[36] Monitoring oxygen saturation at rest and during exercise also provides important information. Resting oxygen saturation is a major predictor of maximal oxygen uptake with exercise as well as peak exercise oxygen saturation.[37] Exercise-induced cyanosis may be demonstrated in the presence of right-to-left shunt and can be a major cause of exertional symptoms.

Cardiac Catheterization

Cardiac catheterization is not required for the diagnosis of Ebstein anomaly, and hemodynamic assessment usually is not necessary when making management decisions.[22] In select cases of bidirectional cavopulmonary shunt considered, hemodynamic catheterization may be indicated to assess left ventricular end-diastolic pulmonary artery pressures.[12] Coronary angiography should be performed prior to surgical repair for patients with an intermediate or high pretest probability of coronary disease.[35]

Electrophysiology Evaluation

The need for specialized electrophysiology evaluation is dependent on historical features and noninvasive testing. Due to the high rate of atrial arrhythmias in Ebstein anomaly, both a resting ECG and an ambulatory ECG monitor should be performed as part of the baseline assessment.[35] Patients with a history of unexplained syncope, documented supraventricular tachycardia (excluding atrial fibrillation), sustained ventricular tachycardia, or ventricular preexcitation should be seen by a congenital electrophysiologist and may benefit from an electrophysiologic study.[38] In addition, an electrophysiology study often is performed as part of preoperative planning prior to tricuspid valve repair or replacement.[35] Sudden death increasingly has been recognized as a threat to this patient population, with risk factors including prior ventricular tachycardia, heart failure, syncope, and pulmonic stenosis.[29] Some patients should be considered for primary prevention implantable cardioverter-defibrillator (ICD).

MANAGEMENT

All adults with Ebstein anomaly should be followed at a center with expertise in caring for adults with congenital heart disease. Patient management involves monitoring over time as well as consideration of surgical intervention and arrhythmia treatment, depending on an individual patient's course.

Monitoring

Most patients with Ebstein anomaly should be seen annually in an adult congenital heart disease clinic, with assessment of heart failure, cyanosis, and arrhythmia. Testing at the annual visit should include pulse oximetry, ECG, and echocardiogram. Patients with moderate or greater functional limitation should have annual Holter monitoring and an exercise test; it may be appropriate for patients with no or mild cardiac symptoms to be tested every 2 years to 3 years. Cardiac MRI, assessing right heart size and function as well as tricuspid valve anatomy and regurgitation, should be performed every 1 year to 2 years in patients with significant functional impairment and every 3 years to 5 years in patients with no or mild symptoms.[35]

Medical therapy does not have a prominent role in the management of patients with Ebstein anomaly; those patients with symptoms should be referred for surgical intervention. Despite the high prevalence of right ventricular dysfunction and not infrequent associated left ventricular dysfunction, there are no studies to date supporting the use of traditional heart failure medications in Ebstein anomaly.[39] Diuretics can be used to manage heart failure prior to surgery or if a patient is not a surgical candidate. Pharmacologic management of rhythm disturbances can be considered where otherwise indicated. Endocarditis prophylaxis is indicated if the patient has cyanosis, a prosthetic heart valve, or a history of endocarditis.[35]

Indication for Surgery

Surgery is recommended for adults with Ebstein anomaly who have significant tricuspid regurgitation as well as one of the following: heart failure symptoms, worsening exercise capacity, and progressive right ventricular dysfunction. Surgery also can be considered in the setting of progressive right ventricular enlargement, cyanosis from right-to-left shunt, paradoxic embolism, and atrial arrhythmia.[35]

Surgical Management

Tricuspid valve repair is the goal of operative intervention where possible.[14] Repair techniques have undergone significant evolution since first performed in the 1970s. Early repairs by Danielson and colleagues[40] and Carpentier and colleagues[41] involved using the anterior leaflet to create a monocuspid valve. The current repair technique is the cone reconstruction, introduced by da Silva and colleagues in 2007[42] and subsequently modified by Dearani.[43] This technique involves mobilizing the septal and posterior leaflet tissue as well as the anterior leaflet, creating a 360° cone that is reattached at the true annulus.[14,42] Relative contraindications to tricuspid valve repair include technical factors (absent septal leaflet, poor delamination of the anterior leaflet, and severe dilation of the tricuspid annulus) as well as clinical factors (age >55–60 years, moderate pulmonary hypertension, and left ventricular ejection fraction <30%).[12] When tricuspid valve repair is not feasible, tricuspid valve replacement should be performed. Bioprosthetic valve is favored over mechanical prosthesis. Tricuspid valve bioprosthesis in Ebstein anomaly have demonstrated good durability.[44] Compared with Ebstein patients with mechanical prostheses, those with a bioprosthesis have similar operation-free survival and better overall 20-year survival.[45] Because tricuspid valve replacement can be performed quickly without cross-clamp, it is an attractive option for patients with poor biventricular function.[12] The tricuspid prosthesis often is placed above the anatomic annulus in the right atrium in an effort to avoid injury to the conduction tissue and the right coronary artery, leaving the coronary sinus to drain into the right ventricle.[12] This is an important consideration should biventricular pacing be pursued in the future.

In the setting of severe right ventricular dilation and dysfunction, a 1.5-ventricle repair with creation of a bidirectional cavopulmonary shunt can be pursued to off-load the right ventricle. Although uncommon in Ebstein anomaly, pulmonary hypertension should be excluded prior to shunt creation, especially in patients where left ventricular diastolic dysfunction is suspected.[14] Shunt creation also can be considered for patients with tricuspid valve stenosis after repair. Data from a high-volume center demonstrate that patients undergoing bidirectional cavopulmonary shunt creation have very good long-term survival and a low rate of reoperation.[46] Caution should be exercised when combining bioprosthetic tricuspid valve replacement and bidirectional cavopulmonary shunt due to concern for bioprosthetic valve thrombosis, which occurs with increased frequency in patients with a large prosthesis and low-flow state.[46]

If present, atrial septal defect or patent foramen ovale should be closed at the time of operative intervention. This primarily is to address the risk of paradoxic embolism. In patients with severe right ventricular dysfunction, leaving an atrial septal fenestration is sometimes employed to provide a pop-off for the dysfunctional right ventricle. Although useful in infants and young children, this generally should be avoided in the adult patient.[12]

Outcomes of tricuspid valve repair vary based on patient characteristics, the operative repair strategy, and where the surgery is performed. A European multicenter study of 150 patients undergoing a variety of surgical approaches at different centers cited an overall operative mortality of 13.3%, although all mortalities were in children under the age of 10, many of whom underwent palliative surgical procedures.[47] Patients in that series had a 76% complication rate, most commonly postoperative arrhythmia, delayed sternal closure, and low cardiac output. In contrast, a review of 539 patients undergoing operative management at Mayo Clinic, with mean age 24 years, revealed an overall 30-day mortality of 5.9%, improving to 2.7% for those undergoing surgery after 2001.[16] A later series reviewing 235 Mayo Clinic patients who underwent cone repair demonstrates very low early mortality (0.4%) and 98% freedom from reoperation at 6 years.[43] The findings of both series demonstrate that at an experienced center valve repair or replacement is safe, and most patients do well long term. Risk factors for poor surgical outcome include right or left ventricular systolic dysfunction, right ventricular outflow tract obstruction, and elevated hemoglobin and hematocrit.[16] For patients undergoing operative intervention, survival free of reoperation is 74% at 10 years and 46% at 20 years, with most patients reporting good functional status.[48]

Atrial Septal Defect Device Closure

In most cases, an atrial septal defect or patent foramen ovale should be addressed surgically at the time of tricuspid valve intervention. Uncommonly, a patient with Ebstein anomaly has tricuspid regurgitation but prominent right-to-left shunting across the atrial septum at rest or with exercise. In this case, percutaneous device closure of the atrial septal defect or patent foramen ovale can be considered. Studies have demonstrated that this is feasible and safe and that most patients have improvement in exertional capacity.[49,50] In the setting of significant right ventricular dysfunction, careful hemodynamic assessment with balloon test occlusion is required to ensure that shunt closure is tolerated.[49]

Indication for Reoperation

In a patient with prior tricuspid valve repair, reoperation should be considered for severe tricuspid regurgitation with declining exercise capacity, progressive right ventricular dilation or dysfunction, or the onset or progression of atrial or ventricular arrhythmia.[22] Patients with a tricuspid bioprosthesis should be considered for re-replacement in the setting of significant regurgitation with associated symptoms, severe stenosis (mean gradient >12–15 mm Hg), or progressive, nonsevere stenosis in the presence of symptoms.[22]

As an alternative to operative intervention, patients with a tricuspid valve prosthesis can consider percutaneous valve-in-valve implantation. An international multicenter registry of 81 Ebstein patients undergoing valve-in-valve replacement demonstrated successful deployment in all patients with no procedural mortality.[51] There was a 5% rate of acute valve thrombosis and of endocarditis, with 8 patients requiring reintervention (percutaneous or surgical) to address valve dysfunction. The long-term outcomes in this cohort of patients are not yet known.

Arrhythmia Management

As reviewed previously, all patients with Ebstein anomaly should have baseline ECG and ambulatory ECG monitor due to the high incidence of cardiac arrhythmias in this population. Those patients with symptomatic rhythm disturbances, unexplained syncope, or documented ventricular preexcitation should be referred for electrophysiologic study.[35,38] A series of patients undergoing cone repair revealed that, in those having preoperative electrophysiologic studies, 69% had a significant electrophysiologic finding, even in the absence of symptoms or ventricular preexcitation.[52] Because of the high prevalence of (sometimes multiple) accessory pathways in this patient population, it is recommended that electrophysiology study be considered prior to surgical intervention for symptomatic patients. Pathway ablation, if required, is performed more easily prior to tricuspid valve surgery. Additionally, the identification of atrial fibrillation or flutter allows for operative planning of surgical atrial ablation.

Although most atrial arrhythmias in Ebstein patients are amenable to catheter ablation, these ablations can be challenging due to presence of multiple pathways and related to technical issues around the dysplastic tricuspid valve and annulus. In a multicenter series of 32 Ebstein patients undergoing catheter ablation, procedural success rates were 80% to 100%, but 56% of the cohort ultimately required repeat ablation of the same or a different rhythm disturbance.[53] If catheter ablation is unsuccessful or not technically feasible, surgical ablation can be pursued at the time of tricuspid valve operation, in some series with high success rates and few operative complications.[19,54]

A single-center series of 968 patients with Ebstein anomaly demonstrated the 70-year cumulative incidence of sudden death to be 14.6%.[29] Predictors of sudden death in this population were history of ventricular tachycardia, heart failure, tricuspid valve surgery, syncope, pulmonic stenosis, and hemoglobin greater than 15 g/dL. To date, there are no guidelines regarding primary prevention ICD in this patient population[38]; however, risk stratification and individualized decision making are appropriate.

Pregnancy

The normal hemodynamic changes of pregnancy involve an increase in cardiac output and blood volume up to 50% above baseline by 32 weeks of pregnancy. The inability to augment cardiac output in the setting of right ventricular systolic dysfunction and tricuspid regurgitation predisposes patients with Ebstein anomaly to heart failure, especially in the third trimester of pregnancy.[55] Arrhythmias can occur, driven by both an underlying predisposition and hemodynamic and hormonal changes.[56] In patients with atrial-level shunt, cyanosis can occur or worsen and contribute to symptomatic limitation as well as fetal growth restriction.[55] Paradoxic embolism is a concern given enhanced hypercoagulability during pregnancy and potential immobility during pregnancy or after delivery.

Despite the potential morbidity, most patients with Ebstein anomaly tolerate pregnancy without significant complications. A single-center series of 111 pregnancies in 44 women (including 20 with atrial-level shunt and 16 with cyanosis) found no maternal mortality or significant adverse cardiac events.[57] A multicenter series reviewing only the hospitalization for delivery demonstrated that, compared with patients without Ebstein anomaly, Ebstein patients had more frequent major adverse cardiac events, most commonly heart failure and atrial arrhythmias, with an incidence of approximately 10%.[58]

Obstetric and fetal outcomes also are a consideration. Most series suggest that preterm delivery is more common in patients with Ebstein anomaly compared to the general population, with preterm delivery rates reported as 20% to 27%.[57,58] Maternal cyanosis is known to contribute to low fetal birth weight and mortality.[57,59] There is increased risk of congenital heart disease in the fetus when the mother has Ebstein anomaly, observed to be 4% to 6%, depending on the series.[48,59] The impact of paternal Ebstein anomaly is less certain but may contribute to slightly increased risk of fetal congenital heart disease.[57] Pregnancies complicated by parental Ebstein anomaly should be managed with fetal echocardiogram at approximately 20 weeks of pregnancy.[35]

SUMMARY

Ebstein anomaly is a rare congenital malformation that involves primarily abnormalities of the tricuspid valve and a right ventricular myopathy. Echocardiography is the diagnostic procedure of choice, demonstrating the myocardium, tricuspid valve anatomy, and regurgitation. Common associated lesions include atrial septal defect and patent foramen ovale. Other right and left heart congenital anomalies are associated with Ebstein anomaly, including ventricular septal defect, pulmonary stenosis, left ventricular noncompaction, and left heart valve abnormalities. Tricuspid valve cone repair is the optimal surgical approach when valve anatomy is suitable, and intermediate follow-up data suggest that this approach can provide a durable repair in most patients. Bidirectional cavopulmonary shunt can off-load the right ventricle and allow for repair in patients with severe right ventricular dysfunction. Arrhythmias are common in Ebstein anomaly, including accessory-pathway and atrial arrhythmias, and patients have a lifelong risk of sudden cardiac death. Electrophysiology study should be performed in the setting of symptoms, preferably prior to operative intervention. Pregnancy generally is well tolerated, and the risk of congenital heart disease in the fetus is approximately 4%. Patients with Ebstein anomaly require lifelong follow-up at a specialized adult congenital heart disease center.

DISCLOSURE

The authors have nothing to disclose.

REFERENCES

1. van Son JAM, Konstantinov IE, Zimmermann V. Wilhelm ebstein and ebstein's malformation. Eur J Cardiothoracic Surg 2001;20:1082–5.
2. Pradat P, Francannet C, Harris JA, et al. The epidemiology of cardiovascular defects, part I: a study based on data from three large registries of congenital malformations. Pediatr Cardiol 2003;24(3):195–221.
3. Lupo PJ, Langlois PH, Mitchell LE. Epidemiology of Ebstein anomaly: prevalence and patterns in Texas, 1999-2005. Am J Med Genet A 2011;155A(5):1007–14.

4. Correa-Villasenor A, Ferencz C, Neill CA, et al. Ebstein's malformation of the tricuspid valve: genetic and environmental factors. Teratology 1994;50: 137–47.

5. Nora JJ, Nora AH, Toews WH. Letter: lithium, Ebstein's anomaly, and other congenital heart defects. Lancet 1974;304(7880):594–5.

6. Diav-Citrin O, Shechtman S, Tahover E, et al. Pregnancy outcome following in utero exposure to lithium: a prospective, comparative, observational study. Am J Psychiatry 2014;171(7):785–94.

7. Boyle B, Garne E, Loane M, et al. The changing epidemiology of Ebstein's anomaly and its relationship with maternal mental health conditions: a European registry-based study. Cardiol Young 2017; 27(4):677–85.

8. Benson DW, Silberbach GM, Kavanaugh-McHugh A, et al. Mutations in the cardiac transcription factor NKX2.5 affect diverse cardiac developemntal pathways. J Clin Invest 1999; 104(11):1567–73.

9. Giannakou A, Sicko RJ, Zhang W, et al. Copy number variants in Ebstein anomaly. PLoS One 2017; 12(12):e0188168.

10. van Engelen K, Postma AV, van de Meerakker JB, et al. Ebstein's anomaly may be caused by mutations in the sarcomere protein gene MYH7. Neth Heart J 2013;21(3):113–7.

11. Kelle AM, Bentley SJ, Rohena LO, et al. Ebstein anomaly, left ventricular non-compaction, and early onset heart failure associated with a de novo alpha-tropomyosin gene mutation. Am J Med Genet A 2016;170(8):2186–90.

12. Dearani JA, Mora BN, Nelson TJ, et al. Ebstein anomaly review: what's now, what's next? Expert Rev Cardiovasc Ther 2015;13(10):1101–9.

13. Anderson KR, Zuberbuhler JR, Anderson RH, et al. Morphologic spectrum of Ebstein's anomaly of the heart: a review. Mayo Clin Proc 1979;54:174–80.

14. Holst KA, Connolly HM, Dearani JA. Ebstein's anomaly. Methodist Debakey Cardiovascluar J 2019; 15(2):138–44.

15. Qureshi MY, O'Leary PW, Connolly HM. Cardiac imaging in Ebstein anomaly. Trends Cardiovasc Med 2018;28(6):403–9.

16. Brown ML, Dearani JA, Danielson GK, et al. The outcomes of operations for 539 patients with Ebstein anomaly. J Thorac Cardiovasc Surg 2008;135(5): 1120–36, 1136.e1-7.

17. Attenhofer Jost CH, Connolly HM, O'Leary PW, et al. Left heart lesions in patients with Ebstein anomaly. Mayo Clin Proc 2005;80(3):361–8.

18. Hebe J. Ebstein's anomaly in adults. Arrhythmias: diagnosis and therapeutic approach. Thorac Cardiovasc Surg 2000;48(4):214–9.

19. Khositseth A, Danielson GK, Dearani JA, et al. Supraventricular tachyarrhythmias in Ebstein anomaly:

management and outcome. J Thorac Cardiovasc Surg 2004;128(6):826–33.

20. Attie F, Rosas M, Rijlaarsdam M, et al. The adult patient with Ebstein anomaly: outcome in 72 unoperated patients. Medicine 2000;79(1):27–36.

21. Attenhofer Jost CH, Connolly HM, Scott CG, et al. Increased risk of possible paradoxical embolic events in adults with ebstein anomaly and severe tricuspid regurgitation. Congenit Heart Dis 2014;9:30–7.

22. Warnes CA, Williams RG, Bashore TM, et al. ACC/AHA 2008 guidelines for the management of adults with congenital heart disease: a report of the American College of Cardiology/American Heart Association Task Force on Practice Guidelines (writing committee to develop guidelines on the management of adults with congenital heart disease). Circulation 2008;118(23):e714–833.

23. Perloff JK, Marelli AJ. Ebstein's anomaly of the tricuspid valve. In: Perloff JK, Marelli AJ, editors. Clinical recognition of congenital heart disease. 6th edeition edition. Philadelphia: Saunders; 2012. p. 176–95.

24. Crews TL, Pridie RB, Benham R, et al. Auscultatory and phonocardiographic findings in Ebstein's anomaly: correlation of first heart sound with ultrasonic records of tricuspid valve movement. Br Heart J 1972; 34:681–7.

25. Attenhofer Jost CH, Connolly HM, Dearani JA, et al. Ebstein's anomaly. Circulation 2007;115(2):277–85.

26. Sherwin ED, Abrams DJ. Ebstein anomaly. Card Electrophysiol Clin 2017;9(2):245–54.

27. Van Lingen B, Bauersfeld SR. The electrocardiogram in ebstein's anomaly of the tricuspid valve. Am Heart J 1955;50(1):13–23.

28. Ho SY, Goltz D, McCarthy K, et al. The atrioventricular junctions in Ebstein malformation. Heart 2000; 83:444–9.

29. Attenhofer Jost CH, Tan NY, Hassan A, et al. Sudden death in patients with Ebstein anomaly. Eur Heart J 2018;39(21):1970–1977a.

30. Shiina A, Seward JB, Edwards WD, et al. Two-dimensional echocardiographic spectrum of ebstein's anomaly: detailed anatomic assessment. J Am Coll Cardiol 1984;3(2):356–70.

31. Roberson DA, Silverman NH. Ebstein's anomaly: echocardiographic and clinical features in the fetus and neonate. J Am Coll Cardiol 1989;14(5):1300–7.

32. Saric M, Armour AC, Arnaout MS, et al. Guidelines for the use of echocardiography in the evaluation of a cardiac source of embolism. J Am Soc Echocardiogr 2016;29(1):1–42.

33. Attenhofer Jost CH, Edmister WD, Julsrud PR, et al. Prospective comparison of echocardiography versus cardiac magnetic resonance imaging in patients with Ebstein's anomaly. Int J Cardiovasc Imaging 2012;28(5):1147–59.

34. Kuhn A, Meierhofer C, Rutz T, et al. Non-volumetric echocardiographic indices and qualitative

assessment of right ventricular systolic function in Ebstein's anomaly: comparison with CMR-derived ejection fraction in 49 patients. Eur Heart J Cardiovasc Imaging 2016;17(8):930–5.

35. Stout KK, Daniels CJ, Aboulhosn JA, et al. 2018 AHA/ACC guideline for the management of adults with congenital heart disease: a report of the American College of Cardiology/American heart association Task Force on clinical Practice guidelines. J Am Coll Cardiol 2019;73(12):e81–192.

36. Muller J, Kuhn A, Tropschuh A, et al. Exercise performance in Ebstein's anomaly in the course of time - Deterioration in native patients and preserved function after tricuspid valve surgery. Int J Cardiol 2016;218:79–82.

37. MacLellan-Tobert SG, Driscoll DJ, Mottram CD, et al. Exercise tolerance in patients with Ebstein's anomaly. J Am Coll Cardiol 1997;29(7):1615–22.

38. Khairy P, Van Hare GF, Balaji S, et al. PACES/HRS expert consensus statement on the recognition and management of arrhythmias in adult congenital heart disease: developed in partnership between the Pediatric and congenital electrophysiology Society (PACES) and the heart rhythm Society (HRS). Endorsed by the governing bodies of PACES, HRS, the American College of Cardiology (ACC), the American heart association (AHA), the European heart rhythm association (EHRA), the Canadian heart rhythm Society (CHRS), and the international Society for adult congenital heart disease (ISACHD). Heart Rhythm 2014;11(10):e102–65.

39. Stout KK, Broberg CS, Book WM, et al. Chronic heart failure in congenital heart disease: a scientific statement from the American Heart Association. Circulation 2016;133(8):770–801.

40. Danielson GK, Maloney JD, Devloo RA. Surgical repair of Ebstein's anomaly. Mayo Clin Proc 1979; 54(3):185–92.

41. Carpentier A, Chauvaud S, Mace L, et al. A new reconstructive operation for Ebstein's anomaly of the tricuspid valve. J Thorac Cardiovasc Surg 1988;96(1):92–101.

42. da Silva JP, Baumgratz JF, da Fonseca L, et al. The cone reconstruction of the tricuspid valve in Ebstein's anomaly. The operation: early and midterm results. J Thorac Cardiovasc Surg 2007;133(1):215–23.

43. Holst KA, Dearani JA, Said S, et al. Improving results of surgery for Ebstein anomaly: where are we after 235 cone repairs? Ann Thorac Surg 2018;105(1):160–8.

44. Kiziltan HT, Theodoro DA, Warnes CA, et al. Late results of bioprosthetic tricuspid valve replacement in Ebstein's anomaly. Ann Thorac Surg 1998;66:1539–45.

45. Brown ML, Dearani JA, Danielson GK, et al. Comparison of the outcome of porcine bioprosthetic versus mechanical prosthetic replacement of the tricuspid valve in the Ebstein anomaly. Am J Cardiol 2009;103(4):555–61.

46. Raju V, Dearani JA, Burkhart HM, et al. Right ventricular unloading for heart failure related to Ebstein malformation. Ann Thorac Surg 2014;98(1):167–73 [discussion: 173–4].

47. Sarris GE, Giannopoulos NM, Tsoutsinos AJ, et al. Results of surgery for ebstein anomaly: a multicenter study from the European congenital heart Surgeons association. J Thorac Cardiovasc Surg 2006;132(1): 50–7.

48. Brown ML, Dearani JA, Danielson GK, et al. Functional status after operation for Ebstein anomaly: the Mayo Clinic experience. J Am Coll Cardiol 2008;52(6):460–6.

49. Jategaonkar SR, Scholtz W, Horstkotte D, et al. Interventional closure of atrial septal defects in adult patients with Ebstein's anomaly. Congenit Heart Dis 2011;6:374–81.

50. Silva M, Teixeira A, Menezes I, et al. Percutaneous closure of atrial right-to-left shunt in patients with Ebstein's anomaly of the tricuspid valve. Eurointervention 2012;8(1):94–7.

51. Taggart NW, Cabalka AK, Eicken A, et al. Outcomes of transcatheter tricuspid valve-in-valve implantation in patients with ebstein anomaly. Am J Cardiol 2018; 121(2):262–8.

52. Shivapour JK, Sherwin ED, Alexander ME, et al. Utility of preoperative electrophysiologic studies in patients with Ebstein's anomaly undergoing the Cone procedure. Heart Rhythm 2014;11(2):182–6.

53. Roten L, Lukac P, Deg N, et al. Catheter ablation of arrhythmias in ebstein's anomaly: a multicenter study. J Cardiovasc Electrophysiol 2011;22(12): 1391–6.

54. Stulak JM, Sharma V, Cannon BC, et al. Optimal surgical ablation of atrial tachyarrhythmias during correction of Ebstein anomaly. Ann Thorac Surg 2015;99(5):1700–5 [discussion 1705].

55. Regitz-Zagrosek V, Roos-Hesselink JW, Bauersachs J, et al. 2018 ESC guidelines for the management of cardiovascular diseases during pregnancy. Eur Heart J 2018;39(34):3165–241.

56. Kounis NG, Zavras GM, Papadaki PJ, et al. Pregnancy-induced increase of supraventricular arrhythmias in wolff-Parkinson-white syndrome. Clin Cardiol 1995;18(3):137–40.

57. Connolly HM, Warnes CA. Ebstein's anomaly: outcome of pregnancy. J Am Coll Cardiol 1994; 23(5):1194–8.

58. Lima FV, Koutrolou-Sotiropoulou P, Yen TY, et al. Clinical characteristics and outcomes in pregnant women with Ebstein anomaly at the time of delivery in the USA: 2003-2012. Arch Cardiovasc Dis 2016; 109(6–7):390–8.

59. Drenthen W, Pieper PG, Roos-Hesselink JW, et al. Outcome of pregnancy in women with congenital heart disease: a literature review. J Am Coll Cardiol 2007;49(24):2303–11.

Tetralogy of Fallot

Eric V. Krieger, MD[a], Anne Marie Valente, MD[b],*

KEYWORDS

- Repaired tetralogy of Fallot • Congenital heart disease • Pulmonary valve replacement
- Surgical pulmonary valve replacement

KEY POINTS

- Repaired tetralogy of Fallot (rTOF) is one of the most common conditions managed by adult congenital heart disease providers.
- Early studies identified several risk factors for death relating to timing and types of surgical repair, and the major causes of death were sudden and heart failure related.
- Echocardiography is a reliable tool to evaluate for many important late complications of rTOF, including the presence of residual ventricular septal defect, left ventricular systolic dysfunction, aortic root dilation, tricuspid regurgitation severity, and quantification of right ventricular (RV) outflow gradients and RV systolic pressure.
- Cardiac magnetic resonance imaging allows for quantification of right ventricular size and function, pulmonary regurgitation severity, and evaluation of fibrosis.
- Patients with rTOF are at risk for ventricular arrhythmias. Sudden cardiac death remains a leading cause of cardiac death for adults with rTOF, second only to heart failure.

 Video content accompanies this article at http://www.cardiology.theclinics.com.

Repaired tetralogy of Fallot (rTOF) is one of the most common conditions managed by adult congenital heart disease providers. Recent comprehensive review articles and book chapters are devoted to this topic. The purpose of this article is to address several common clinical questions encountered in the management of patients with rTOF. These answers are not intended to supplant Practice Guidelines.

WHAT IS THE CONTEMPORARY NATURAL HISTORY OF REPAIRED TETRALOGY OF FALLOT?

The anatomy of tetralogy of Fallot (TOF) was first described by Stetson in 1671, and it was more than a century before Fallot published in 1888.[1] The first management strategies involved establishing a reliable source of pulmonary blood flow with palliative procedures, such as the Blalock-Taussig shunt in the mid 1940s, followed by the first intracardiac repair in 1954. Surgical strategies evolved, and primary neonatal repair began in the 1970s. Innovations over the past several decades have progressed at a much more rapid pace, with the advent of valve-sparing surgical approaches and more recently the widespread application of transcatheter techniques for pulmonary valve replacement (PVR). These advances in management have resulted in improved outcomes. However, the impact of current management strategies will not be fully recognized for several decades.

The mortality for rTOF in the early surgical experience was high, with a hospital mortality of 40% in the initial surgical experience, reported by Lillehei and colleagues.[2] However, survival improved as surgical experience increased. The natural history

---

[a] Division of Cardiology, Department of Medicine, University of Washington School of Medicine, University of Washington Medical Center, Seattle Children's Hospital, 1959 Northeast Pacific Street, Box 356422, Seattle, WA 98195, USA; [b] Department of Cardiology, Boston Children's Hospital, Division of Cardiology, Department of Medicine, Brigham and Women's Hospital, Harvard Medical School, Bader 208, Boston, MA 02115, USA
* Corresponding author.
E-mail address: Anne.Valente@CARDIO.CHBOSTON.ORG

Cardiol Clin 38 (2020) 365–377
https://doi.org/10.1016/j.ccl.2020.04.009

of rTOF has improved over time as well. Initially patients were older at the time of initial repair (median age 10–12 years), and many had undergone prior palliative shunts (23%–40%).[3,4] Early studies identified several risk factors for death relating to timing and types of surgical repair, and the major causes of death were sudden and heart failure related. As the population of rTOF patients has increased and grown older, the mode of death has changed; now patients are more likely to die of noncardiac comorbidities.[5] In 2014, Cuypers and colleagues[6] published results of prospective follow-up of 72 adults repaired between 1968 and 1980; the mean age of repair was 4.6 years. The 40-year survival was 72%. Interestingly, 40% of this cohort had undergone a subsequent PVR, and 50% had been hospitalized in the past decade.

The predominant hemodynamic sequela following repair of TOF is pulmonary regurgitation (PR), although rTOF patients may also have some degree of residual right ventricular outflow tract (RVOT) obstruction. The amount of regurgitation or obstruction is often directly related to the initial anatomy and surgical approach. The surgical approaches have evolved over time to current strategies, which attempt to preserve pulmonary valve function, so-called valve-sparing repairs.[7] Nonetheless, most patients with rTOF have residual PR. The optimal timing of PVR following rTOF remains one of the core challenges in the management of rTOF and is discussed more later. Furthermore, as patients with rTOF age, the incidence of ventricular dysfunction increases.[8] It is unclear at this time how guideline-directed management and therapy might affect the prevalence of heart failure in rTOF patients. In addition, patients with rTOF have an electromechanical cardiomyopathy and are predisposed to both atrial and ventricular arrhythmias. Risk factors for arrhythmia are discussed in greater detail later.[9,10]

Answer: The current late outcomes of TOF patients reflect management strategies performed in a prior era. However, the lessons learned from these patients are extremely important to guide current therapies.

IS ECHOCARDIOGRAPHY A RELIABLE WAY OF EVALUATING RIGHT VENTRICULAR FUNCTION OR PULMONARY REGURGITATION IN PATIENTS WITH REPAIRED TETRALOGY OF FALLOT?

Despite the high reproducibility and accuracy of CMR, transthoracic echocardiography (TTE) remains the primary imaging modality used to follow patients with rTOF because of advantages of accessibility, comparatively low cost, patient comfort, and practicality in patients with implanted metallic hardware. Echocardiography is a reliable tool to evaluate for many important late complications of rTOF, including the presence of residual ventricular septal defect, left ventricular systolic dysfunction, aortic root dilation, tricuspid regurgitation severity, and quantification of right ventricular (RV) outflow gradients and RV systolic pressure.[11]

Practice guidelines recommend elective PVR for patients with at least moderate PR who have severe RV dilation or RV dysfunction. For this reason, if TTE is to be useful in determining which patients require PVR, it is important to determine whether TTE can reliably measure PR severity, RV size, or RV systolic function.

Transthoracic Echocardiography Evaluation of Pulmonary Regurgitation Severity

Various methods have been proposed to evaluate PR severity by echocardiography, but none has reliably been shown to correlate with cardiac magnetic resonance (CMR) quantification of regurgitation volume or regurgitation fraction. Qualitatively, PR severity can be evaluated by color Doppler. However, in patients with rTOF and free PR, the jet can be low velocity, laminar, and relatively brief, which can make severe PR appear unimpressive by color Doppler. Vena contracta width and proximal isovelocity surface area radius have not been validated in grading of PR and are not typically used. Numerous investigators have attempted to correlate the pressure half-time (PHT) of the PR jet with PR severity. In general, a shorter PHT correlates with more severe PR. However, because PHT is also impacted by ventricular compliance, PHT has modest linear correlation with PR percentage as measured by CMR. Most investigators have found that patients with a long PHT (>100–130 milliseconds) are unlikely to have hemodynamically significant PR.[12–14] Other investigators have studied the correlation between the diastolic-systolic time-velocity integral (DSTVI) and CMR-derived PR severity, with higher DSTVI values correlating with worse PR. Again, the results of these studies have been highly variable in whether this TTE feature can identify severe PR.[12,13,15] An experienced congenital echocardiographer can accurately integrate qualitative data to identify mild, moderate, or severe PR as measured by CMR.[15,16]

Transthoracic Echocardiography Evaluation of Right Ventricular Size and Function

RV volume and ejection fraction (EF) cannot be routinely calculated from 2-dimensional TTE. RV size is usually determined qualitatively, or from basal dimension. RV function is typically assessed qualitatively or using surrogates for EF, such as fractional area change (FAC), tricuspid annular plane systolic excursion (TAPSE), tissue-Doppler derived tricuspid annulus systolic velocity (S'), and myocardial performance index. These parameters were not developed to evaluate patients with rTOF and do not take into account the aneurysmal and dyskinetic outflow portions of the RV, which are common in patients with rTOF.

Multiple investigators have studied whether echocardiographic measurements of RV size and function correlate with CMR-derived RV volume or RV EF. Overall, the results have been inconsistent. RV end-diastolic area from an apical 4-chamber view seems to have better correlation with CMR-derived RV end-diastolic volume than does the basal RV diameter.[16]

Egbe and colleagues[17] reported that a TAPSE less than 17 mm had the strongest sensitivity and specificity for detecting an RV EF less than 40% and outperformed visual assessment of RV function. However, others have found poor or modest correlation between TAPSE and RV EF, perhaps because patients with rTOF have relatively less functional contribution from the basal portions of the RV and more from the apex.[15,18–21] Correlation between RV FAC% and RV EF has been similarly inconsistent.[16,17] Myocardial performance index is less frequently performed in routine TTE, but has some correlation with RV EF, although misclassification is common.[15,17]

In situations whereby image quality is adequate, software and processing expertise is available, and postprocessing is feasible, 3-dimensional (3D) echocardiography has promise for the determination of RV size and function. However, high-quality analyzable images are uncommon in adult patients and those with multiple sternotomies, limiting the applicability in the adult population with rTOF.[22] Measurement of RV free wall strain may provide additional information, but clinical data remain limited.[23,24]

Answer: Echocardiography remains important for the longitudinal follow-up for patients with rTOF, but no parameters are consistently and strongly associated with PR severity or RV size and function. Qualitative evaluation by experienced congenital imagers is necessary.

BEYOND PULMONARY REGURGITATION VOLUME AND VENTRICULAR FUNCTION, WHAT ELSE CAN WE LEARN FROM CARDIAC MRI?

CMR is ideally suited for assessment of rTOF because it allows comprehensive assessment of cardiovascular morphology and physiology, is independent of acoustic windows, and avoids ionizing radiation, which makes it ideally suited for longitudinal follow-up of rTOF patients.[25] Bokma and colleagues[26] published the use of CMR in the noninvasive risk stratification in 575 adults with rTOF, highlighting thresholds of ventricular dysfunction below which result in worse clinical outcomes. Patient-specific 3D models may be created to facilitate increased understanding of the spatial relationships of the anatomy (**Fig. 1**; Video 1). CMR is useful to determine the geometry of the RVOT and identify potential candidates for percutaneous PVR.[27] Delineation of the coronary artery course is essential before any RVOT intervention, because 5% to 7% of patients with rTOF have an anomalous left coronary artery that may course across the RVOT, which can complicate both surgical and transcatheter pulmonic valve implantation (**Fig. 2**). Cardiac and respiratory-gated magnetic resonance angiogram images have sufficient spatial resolution to assess the origins and proximal coronary artery courses. CMR is also superior to echocardiography to evaluate the branch pulmonary artery anatomy, and with phase-contrast imaging, it is possible to determine the percentage of blood flow to each lung. The ability to quantify blood flow to each lung is particularly important because patients with rTOF may have residual branch pulmonary artery stenosis that may result in unequal pulmonary blood flow distribution. CMR is often able to delineate the mechanism and severity of tricuspid valve regurgitation. Ascending aortic dilation is common in patients with rTOF, and CMR allows for reproducible measurements for longitudinal follow. Late gadolinium enhancement is able to identify areas of nonviable myocardium in these patients,

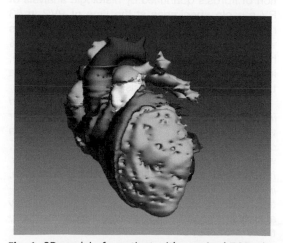

Fig. 1. 3D model of a patient with repaired TOF who has undergone a PVR created from CMR images.

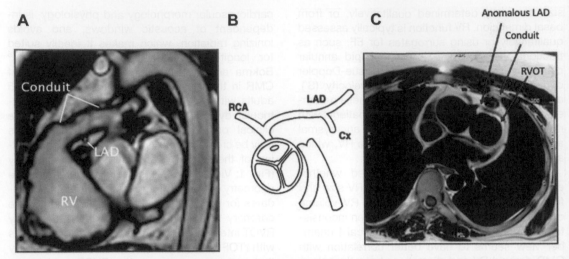

Fig. 2. (*A*) Bright-blood CMR of an rTOF patient with an anomalous left anterior descending artery (LAD) located just posterior to the RV-to-pulmonary artery conduit. (*B*) Short-axis diagram of this coronary anomaly, which is the most common coronary artery anomaly in rTOF. (*C*) Dark-blood axial CMR of an rTOF with the same anatomy, demonstrating the LAD coursing between the conduit and the native RV outflow tract. Cx, circumflex; RCA, right coronary artery.

which occurs at prior surgical sites as well as in areas remote from interventions.

The CMR technique of T1 mapping allows for measurement of the extracellular volume (ECV) fraction, a marker of extracellular matrix remodeling. Several investigators have demonstrated an association between diffuse myocardial fibrosis as measured by this technique in patients with rTOF and ventricular arrhythmias.[28,29] In addition, a linear relationship between left ventricular and RV ECV exists, implying an adverse ventricular-ventricular interaction at the tissue level.[30,31] Yamamura and colleagues[32] reported the association of fibrosis quantified by histologic analysis of RV muscle specimens at the time of PVR in 53 rTOF patients and CMR parameters. PVR patients with a collagen fibrosis volume greater than 11% had increased indexed RV end-systolic volume, increased RV mass, and larger right atrial area than those with less fibrosis.

Answer: In addition to being the gold-standard imaging test for quantification of PR and ventricular volumes in patients with rTOF, CMR provides a complete anatomic assessment of the RVOT, which is necessary for subsequent interventions. It produces accurate and reproducible flow data, including branch pulmonary artery flow distribution. CMR techniques, such as T1 mapping, may also prove to act as prognostic indicators in patients with rTOF.

WHAT CLINICAL AND IMAGING FEATURES DETERMINE TIMING OF PULMONARY VALVE REPLACEMENT?

The indications for PVR in rTOF patients continue to be refined. Historically, the decision to replace a pulmonary valve was driven by symptoms.[33] However, over the past several decades, this practice has been called into question because of the evidence that PVR may be offered to rTOF patients too late.[34] This reasoning was based on the observation that patients with an RV EF less than 40% at the time of PVR had little chance of recovery of RV function following the procedure. Therefore, current guidelines now include considerations for asymptomatic patients who have certain objective imaging or exercise criteria. **Table 1** lists the 2018 American College of Cardiology/American Heart Association Guidelines for PVR in patients with rTOF.[35] It is important to recognize that much of the imaging data used in this decision focuses on identifying a pre-PVR threshold value of RV size that predicts normalization of RV volumes following PVR. Massive RV dilation is unlikely to resolve following PVR and is more likely to be seen in patients with late primary repair and nonwhite race.[36] However, it has been shown that post-PVR RV size is not predictive of adverse clinical outcomes in rTOF patients, and new criteria need to be defined.[37] Although the guidelines suggest RV volumes above which

Table 1
American College of Cardiology/American Heart Association guideline criteria for pulmonary valve replacement in patients with repaired tetralogy of Fallot and at least moderate pulmonary regurgitation[35]

Class I	Class IIa (Any 2 of the Following)	Class IIb
Symptoms	RV or LV dysfunction RVEDVi $\geq$160 mL/m^2, RVESVi $\geq$80 mL/m^2, or RVEDVi $\geq$LVEDVi RVSP (due to RVOT obstruction) $\geq$2/3 systemic pressure Objective reduction in exercise tolerance	Sustained tachyarrhythmias Residual lesions requiring surgery

Abbreviations: EDV, end-diastolic volume; ESV, end-systolic volume; LV, left ventricular; LVEDVi, left ventricular end-diastolic volume index; RVEDVi, right ventricular end-diastolic volume index; RVESVi, right ventricular end-systolic volume index; RVSP, right ventricular systolic pressure.

patients could be considered for PVR, there is not a clear consensus that has been reached regarding the absolute values.[38–40] Ventricular dysfunction remains a strong criterion for consideration of PVR. In rTOF patients with severe right or left ventricular dysfunction, consultation with an advanced heart disease team for considerations of mechanical support following PVR should be addressed before the procedure.[41]

The goal of timing of PVR should be to do the intervention at a time before deleterious effects of residual disease, yet not so premature that it would lead to recurrent procedures in the future. This "sweet spot" for timing of PVR is a moving target and may be different for individualized patients whether they have a more volume-loading (PR) or pressure-loading (residual RVOT obstruction) lesion.[42] Separate criteria may also need to be defined for transcatheter versus surgical PVR in TOF patients.

Answer: Indications for timing of PVR now include considerations for the asymptomatic rTOF patient with significant ventricular dilation, any degree of ventricular dysfunction, and exercise limitations. There are increasing data that suggest an individualized approach to PVR is advisable.

HOW DOES PULMONARY VALVE REPLACEMENT AFFECT VENTRICULAR FUNCTION AND CLINICAL STATUS?

Although there are many studies relating to various clinical outcomes in rTOF patients, no randomized studies have been performed comparing PVR with conservative medical therapy. In a metaanalysis of 657 adults with rTOF who underwent PVR in 10 studies, the pooled incidence rate of death was 1% per year (95% confidence interval [CI]: 0% to 1% per year), and the pooled incidence rate of sustained ventricular arrhythmias was 1% per year (95% CI: 1% to 2% per year).

PVR results in beneficial reverse remodeling of the RV.[43,44] Although there is a significant reduction in RV volumes following PVR, there is evidence that RV volumes gradually return to near preoperative values 7 to 10 years following PVR.[45] Despite gains in RV size early after PVR, there is no beneficial effect on ventricular function.[43,44,46]

Most adults with rTOF experience symptomatic improvement following PVR. A systematic review showed that New York Heart Association (NYHA) functional class improves by nearly 1 functional class following PVR, but this benefit was attenuated in patients with very large preoperative RV volumes.[43] However, most studies included in the analysis were retrospective studies and all were unblended, so bias may contribute to the perceived improvement in functional status following PVR. A metaanalysis that accompanied the Canadian Cardiovascular Society guidelines confirmed that PVR did improve symptoms as reported by NYHA class (odds ratio: 0.08; 95% CI: 0.03–0.24).[44] A separate metaanalysis found no significant improvement in peak oxygen consumption (Vo$_2$) following PVR.[47]

There is no evidence that PVR lessens mortality or reduces the risk of ventricular arrhythmias in rTOF patients.[48] Geva and colleagues[49] identified pre-PVR risk factors that are associated with a shorter time to postoperative death and sustained ventricular tachycardia (VT) in 452 rTOF patients from 4 centers. These predictors included age at PVR $\geq$28 years, preoperative RV mass-to-volume ratio $\geq$0.45 g/mL, and an RV EF less than 40%. The threshold of age at PVR at which there may be a mortality benefit has been confirmed by a retrospective study of 707 patients in the National Institute for Outcomes Research in the United Kingdom, which reported a 5.6-fold increase in 10-year mortality following PVR in rTOF patients who were older than 35 years at the time of PVR.[50]

Answer: PVR results in improved symptomatic status and reduced RV size. However, there is no evidence that PVR reduces mortality or lessens ventricular arrhythmias in rTOF patients. Age at PVR is an important determinant of long-term outcomes.

WHAT ARE THE ADVANTAGES AND DISADVANTAGES OF A TRANSCATHETER PULMONARY VALVE REPLACEMENT COMPARED WITH A SURGICAL PULMONARY VALVE REPLACEMENT?

Transcatheter pulmonary valve replacement (TPVR) was introduced in 2000 as an alternative to surgical pulmonary valve replacement (SPVR), and its use has expanded dramatically over the last 2 decades. In the modern era, commercially available TPVR is an option for implantation into surgically placed RV to pulmonary artery conduits or dysfunctional bioprosthetic pulmonary valves. In some patients with favorable anatomy, approved devices can be placed in a native RVOT. There are ongoing clinical trials of devices designed to fit in aneurysmal outflow tracts typical for patients with rTOF. TPVR can be used to treat both RVOT obstruction and regurgitation. A comprehensive review of the use of transcatheter valves in congenital heart disease is published elsewhere in this issue (see article by Aboulhosn in this issue).

At experienced centers, both SPVR and TPVR can be performed with very low mortality and few complications.[51,52] Because there has been no randomized trial comparing TPVR and SPVR, it is not possible to draw definitive conclusions on the relative safety of either approach. Observed differences may be related to patient selection because there are differences in the patients referred for TPVR compared with those referred for SPVR.

One advantage to TPVR is reduced length of stay and reduced patient discomfort. One study by Steinberg and colleagues[53] performed a risk-adjusted propensity score to compare TPVR with SPVR. After adjusting for baseline differences, mortality and major morbidity were the same between the 2 groups. However, as would be expected, patients treated with TPVR had shorter hospitalization. There is a paucity of data comparing patient-related quality of life in the immediate or long term after TPVR or SPVR. Comparative data on the durability of TPVR versus SPVR are lacking, but publications suggest good valve durability of TPVR placed inside a conduit or bioprosthetic valve.[54]

Clinical experience and recent publications suggest that the Melody valve is susceptible to endocarditis.[55] It is not known whether this risk extends to other models of TPVR. A prospective registry of more than 300 Melody valve implantations performed in clinical trials showed an annualized endocarditis incidence rate of 3.1% per patient-year; 5-year freedom from endocarditis was 89% in patients treated with a Melody valve. Patients with a postimplant peak gradient $\geq$15 mm Hg were at higher risk for endocarditis.[56]

There should be a high suspicion for TPVR-related endocarditis for patients presenting with infectious or constitutional symptoms. As always, if endocarditis is suspected, multiple sets of blood cultures should be obtained before initiation of antibiotics. It is very difficult, and often impossible, to visualize a vegetation on a TPVR using TTE or transesophageal echocardiogram. However, these modalities are important to exclude vegetations the other valves, and to evaluate for new TPVR dysfunction. Intracardiac echocardiography is the most reliable way to assess for TPVR endocarditis. Approximately half of patients can be treated medically without needing valve explantation.[56]

Answer: TPVR is a reasonable alternative to SPVR in those with previously surgically implanted valves or conduits, or favorable native RVOT anatomy. Transcatheter valves result in shorter hospital stays but a higher late risk of endocarditis. There are insufficient data to suggest either type of valve has advantages in terms of operative safety or valve durability.

WHICH PATIENTS WITH TETRALOGY OF FALLOT REQUIRE A PRIMARY PREVENTION DEFIBRILLATOR?

Patients with rTOF are at risk for ventricular arrhythmias. Sudden cardiac death remains a leading cause of cardiac death for adults with rTOF, second only to heart failure.[5] Up to 10% of patients with rTOF have clinical sustained VT, and the likelihood of lethal ventricular arrhythmias ranges between 1.6% and 6% per year and increases with age.[10,57]

Despite the high rate of VT in patients with rTOF, it is challenging to decide which patients with repaired TOF benefit from a primary prevention implantable cardioverter-defibrillator (ICD). It would be inappropriate to implant a primary prevention ICD in all adults with rTOF because the costs-benefit ratio would not support that approach: compared with patients with dilated cardiomyopathy, patients with rTOF have more device-related complications and are less likely to receive appropriate therapy from ICDs. Patients with rTOF have high rates of oversensing, inappropriate antitachycardia pacing, and inappropriate shocks. In addition, rTOF patients have a higher incidence of lead failure and device-related infection.[58–60] The rate of inappropriate shocks in patients with rTOF ranges between 6% and 10% per year, a rate that is much higher than that seen in dilated cardiomyopathy. Inappropriate shocks are associated with reduced quality of life. The increased device-related complication rates may be related to the fact that rTOF patients are younger and have a high incidence of atrial arrhythmias, both of which are risk factors for device-related complications. In addition to higher complication rates, patients with rTOF are less likely to receive appropriate shocks than those with other forms of heart disease.[58,59,61] Because adults with rTOF have a high rate of VT but indiscriminate implantation of ICDs would be associated with high rates of complications, it is important to identify high-risk patients who would benefit from ICDs.

Risk Factors for Ventricular Tachycardia in Tetralogy of Fallot

Numerous investigators have described clinical features that are associated with an increased risk of ventricular arrhythmias. Some of the more strongly validated are listed as follows:

1. QRS duration greater than 180 milliseconds[10,62,63]
2. Fragmentation of the QRS complex[64–66] (**Fig. 3**)
3. Left ventricular or RV systolic or diastolic dysfunction[8,61,63,67–69]

4. RV hypertrophy or extensive scar seen on CMR[5,28,48,49,70]
5. History of VT[48,61,69]
6. Inducible sustained VT or high-risk substrate seen at electrophysiology (EP) study[59,69,71,72]

Overall, ventricular function (both systolic and diastolic) and electrocardiogram abnormalities are more predictive of VT than is the degree of PR or RV dilation.

Predicting Risk in Patients Undergoing Pulmonary Valve Replacement

There remains no consensus as to which combination of risk factors warrants implantation of an ICD. Patients with none of the risk factors listed above are unlikely to benefit from a primary prevention ICD, and ICD is not recommended in this context.[73] For patients with at least one or 2 risk factors, ICD can be considered. Invasive EP study with programmed ventricular stimulation has the ability to reclassify intermediate-risk patients for whom ICD is being considered.[74]

Answer: Patients with multiple risk factors for VT, or risk factors plus a positive ventricular stimulation study, should be offered a defibrillator.

WHAT IS THE IMPACT OF ABLATION IN PREVENTING VENTRICULAR TACHYCARDIA IN PATIENTS WITH REPAIRED TETRALOGY OF FALLOT?

Most VT in rTOF is related to macro-reentry circuits and depends on slow conduction through a limited number of discrete anatomic isthmuses

A

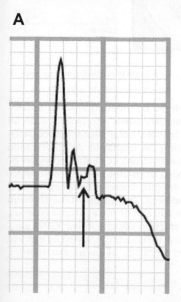

B

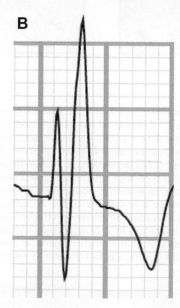

Fig. 3. Right bundle branch block (RBBB) with and without QRS fragmentation. Lead V2 of an ECG in a patient with TOF (*A*) with RBBB and evident fragmentation (*arrows*) of the prolonged QRS complexes compared with a patient with TOF (*B*) with a wide RBBB without fragmentation of prolonged QRS complexes. (*From* Bokma JP, Winter MM, Vehmeijer JT, et al. QRS fragmentation is superior to QRS duration in predicting mortality in adults with tetralogy of Fallot. Heart. 2017;103(9):666-671; with permission.)

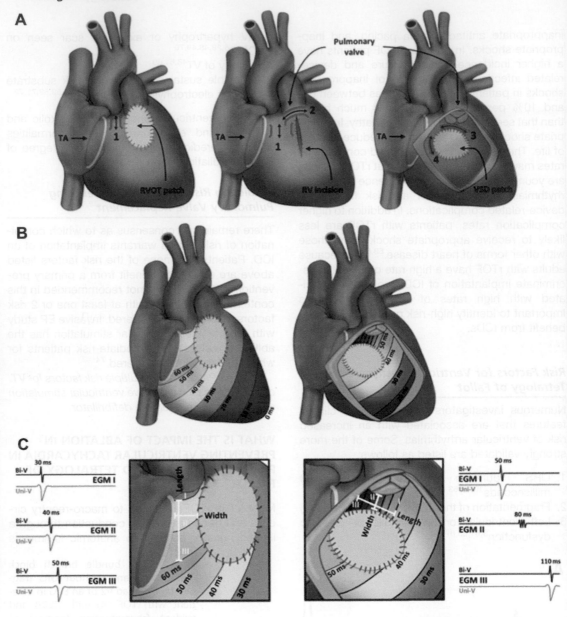

Fig. 4. (A) The 4 potential anatomic isthmuses (*blue brackets*): isthmus 1 bordered by tricuspid annulus and RV outflow tract patch/RV incision; isthmus 2 bordered by RV incision and pulmonary valve; isthmus 3 bordered by pulmonary valve and ventricular septal defect patch; isthmus 4 bordered by ventricular septal defect patch and tricuspid annulus. (B) Schematic activation of the right ventricle during SR displayed as color-coded isochronal (10 milliseconds) map from red (early activation) to purple (latest activation). (C) Enlarged views of anatomic isthmus 1 (*left*) and 3 (*right*) with corresponding electrograms recorded from sites I–II–III, as indicated. Isthmus width, distance between unexcitable anatomic boundaries; isthmus length, distance between normal electrograms (I and III) recorded at entrance and exit site of the anatomic isthmus. Conduction time through the anatomic isthmus, difference in local activation time between the entrance and exit of the anatomic isthmus. Conduction velocity index calculated as indicated. Bi-V, biventricular; CVi, conduction velocity index; EGM, electrogram. (*From* Kapel GF, Sacher F, Dekkers OM, et al. Arrhythmogenic anatomical isthmuses identified by electroanatomical mapping are the substrate for ventricular tachycardia in repaired Tetralogy of Fallot. Eur Heart J. 2017;38(4):268-276; with permission.)

Table 2
Selected studies of ventricular tachycardia ablation in patients with repaired tetralogy of Fallot[8,60,77–79]

Author, Year	Number of TOF Patients Ablated	Acute Success Rate, %	Follow-Up, mo	Results
Zeppenfeld et al,[78] 2007	9	100	30.4 ± 29.3	No recurrence of VT
Kriebel et al,[79] 2007	10	80	35.4 (range 3–52)	Recurrence in 25% of acutely successful ablations
Kapel et al,[60] 2015	28	75	46 ± 28	No recurrence of VT in patients with procedural success
van Zyl et al,[77] 2016	21	57	33 ± 7	No recurrence of VT if successful block. No events in 95%
Laredo et al,[80] 2017	34	82	112 ± 62	18% VT recurrence, including sudden death in 2

(**Fig. 4**). These features make VT in rTOF appealing for catheter ablation because creation of a conduction block across the isthmus can eliminate the substrate for VT. Because the isthmuses usually appear in predictable locations, ablation can be possible using substrate mapping, even for hemodynamically unstable VTs, which cannot be mapped with entrainment techniques.[72,75,76]

Several investigators have reported on the outcomes of catheter-based VT ablation. Results of selected studies are shown in **Table 2**.[60,77–80] Overall, the data suggest that most patients who undergo an ablation have an acutely successful procedure with achievement of block. In addition, most patients who had an acutely successful ablation are free of arrhythmia over the next 3 to 5 years. Importantly, however, ablation is not 100% reliable in preventing late VT, even in those who were thought to have a successful procedure, as shown in **Table 2**.

It is common for patients being considered for PVR to be evaluated for VT at the time of surgical referral. Many centers perform an EP study before surgical PVR on patients who are thought to be at increased risk for VT. The rationale for this approach is to facilitate surgical cryoablation at the time of PVR. One advantage of performing ablation at the time of surgery is that it allows for complete exposure and targeted ablation of the defined anatomic isthmuses. However, performing ablation at the time of surgery does not allow for the confirmation of block or demonstration of noninducibility of VT. For this reason, postoperative

EP studies are required to confirm success of the surgical ablation. Two series that studied the outcomes of patients who underwent surgical ablation at the time of PVR documented that a substantial number of patients (16%–45%) remained inducible for VT during a postoperative EP study.[81,82]

In summary, it appears that patients who are inducible for VT and have a successful catheter ablation are at low risk for future clinical VT, but the risk is eliminated. Patients who have a surgical ablation need to have successful block confirmed on a follow-up EP study.

Answer: Catheter ablation is not a replacement for a secondary prevention ICD in patients with a history of clinical VT. Ablation can be complementary to an ICD to reduce shocks in patients with clinical VT. It remains uncertain whether patients with a positive EP study and a successful ablation require a primary prevention ICD following an acutely successful catheter-based VT ablation.

SUMMARY

The authors have addressed some of the common clinical questions encountered in the management of adults with rTOF. Echocardiography remains important for the longitudinal follow-up for patients with rTOF, and CMR is a gold-standard imaging tool for quantification of RV size, function, and PR. Whereas traditionally the indication for PVR involved symptomatic patients, the recommendations now include intervention for asymptomatic rTOF patients with significant ventricular dilation, any degree of ventricular dysfunction, and exercise limitations. PVR results in improved symptomatic status and reduced RV size, but does not reduce mortality. Age at PVR appears to be an important determinant of long-term outcomes. Choice of PVR now includes not only surgical options but also transcatheter delivery. There are insufficient data to suggest either type of valve has advantages in terms of operative safety or valve durability. Risk stratification for rTOF patients is important, and patients with multiple risk factors for VT, or risk factors plus a positive ventricular stimulation study, should be offered a defibrillator. Catheter ablation can be complementary to an ICD to reduce shocks in patients with clinical VT.

SUPPLEMENTARY DATA

Supplementary data related to this article can be found online at https://doi.org/10.1016/j.ccl.2020.04.009.

REFERENCES

1. Van Praagh R. Etienne-Louis Arthur Fallot and his tetralogy: a new translation of Fallot's summary and a modern reassessment of this anomaly. Eur J Cardiothorac Surg 1989;3(5):381–6.

2. Lillehei CW, Varco RL, Cohen M, et al. The first open heart corrections of tetralogy of Fallot. A 26-31 year follow-up of 106 patients. Ann Surg 1986;204(4):490–502.

3. Murphy JG, Gersh BJ, Mair DD, et al. Long-term outcome in patients undergoing surgical repair of tetralogy of Fallot. N Engl J Med 1993;329(9):593–9.

4. Nollert G, Fischlein T, Bouterwek S, et al. Long-term survival in patients with repair of tetralogy of Fallot: 36-year follow-up of 490 survivors of the first year after surgical repair. J Am Coll Cardiol 1997;30(5):1374–83.

5. Valente AM, Gauvreau K, Assenza GE, et al. Contemporary predictors of death and sustained ventricular tachycardia in patients with repaired tetralogy of Fallot enrolled in the INDICATOR cohort. Heart 2014;100(3):247–53.

6. Cuypers JA, Menting ME, Konings EE, et al. Unnatural history of tetralogy of Fallot: prospective follow-up of 40 years after surgical correction. Circulation 2014;130(22):1944–53.

7. Bove T, Francois K, Van De Kerckhove K, et al. Assessment of a right-ventricular infundibulum-sparing approach in transatrial-transpulmonary repair of tetralogy of Fallot. Eur J Cardiothorac Surg 2012;41(1):126–33.

8. Broberg CS, Aboulhosn J, Mongeon FP, et al. Prevalence of left ventricular systolic dysfunction in adults with repaired tetralogy of fallot. Am J Cardiol 2011;107(8):1215–20.

9. Gatzoulis MA, Till JA, Somerville J, et al. Mechanoelectrical interaction in tetralogy of Fallot. QRS prolongation relates to right ventricular size and predicts malignant ventricular arrhythmias and sudden death. Circulation 1995;92(2):231–7.

10. Khairy P, Aboulhosn J, Gurvitz MZ, et al. Arrhythmia burden in adults with surgically repaired tetralogy of Fallot: a multi-institutional study. Circulation 2010;122(9):868–75.

11. Valente AM, Cook S, Festa P, et al. Multimodality imaging guidelines for patients with repaired tetralogy of Fallot: a report from the American Society of Echocardiography: developed in collaboration with the Society for Cardiovascular Magnetic Resonance and the Society for Pediatric Radiology. J Am Soc Echocardiogr 2014;27(2):111–41.

12. Bansal N, Gupta P, Joshi A, et al. Utility of Doppler echocardiography to estimate the severity of pulmonary valve regurgitation fraction in patients with repaired tetralogy of Fallot. Pediatr Cardiol 2019;40(2):404–11.

13. Beurskens NEG, Gorter TM, Pieper PG, et al. Diagnostic value of Doppler echocardiography for identifying hemodynamic significant pulmonary valve regurgitation in tetralogy of Fallot: comparison with cardiac MRI. Int J Cardiovasc Imaging 2017;33(11):1723–30.

14. Silversides CK, Veldtman GR, Crossin J, et al. Pressure half-time predicts hemodynamically significant pulmonary regurgitation in adult patients with repaired tetralogy of Fallot. J Am Soc Echocardiogr 2003;16(10):1057–62.

15. Mercer-Rosa L, Yang W, Kutty S, et al. Quantifying pulmonary regurgitation and right ventricular function in surgically repaired tetralogy of Fallot: a comparative analysis of echocardiography and magnetic resonance imaging. Circ Cardiovasc Imaging 2012;5(5):637–43.

16. Brown DW, McElhinney DB, Araoz PA, et al. Reliability and accuracy of echocardiographic right heart evaluation in the U.S. Melody Valve Investigational Trial. J Am Soc Echocardiogr 2012;25(4):383–92.e4.

17. Egbe AC, Pislaru SV, Kothapalli S, et al. The role of echocardiography for quantitative assessment of right ventricular size and function in adults with repaired tetralogy of Fallot. Congenit Heart Dis 2019;14(5):700–5.

18. Morcos P, Vick GW 3rd, Sahn DJ, et al. Correlation of right ventricular ejection fraction and tricuspid annular plane systolic excursion in tetralogy of Fallot by magnetic resonance imaging. Int J Cardiovasc Imaging 2009;25(3):263–70.

19. Koestenberger M, Nagel B, Ravekes W, et al. Systolic right ventricular function in pediatric and adolescent patients with tetralogy of Fallot: echocardiography versus magnetic resonance imaging. J Am Soc Echocardiogr 2011;24(1):45–52.

20. Mercer-Rosa L, Parnell A, Forfia PR, et al. Tricuspid annular plane systolic excursion in the assessment of right ventricular function in children and adolescents after repair of tetralogy of Fallot. J Am Soc Echocardiogr 2013;26(11):1322–9.

21. D'Anna C, Caputi A, Natali B, et al. Improving the role of echocardiography in studying the right ventricle of repaired tetralogy of Fallot patients: comparison with cardiac magnetic resonance. Int J Cardiovasc Imaging 2018;34(3):399–406.

22. Renella P, Marx GR, Zhou J, et al. Feasibility and reproducibility of three-dimensional echocardiographic assessment of right ventricular size and function in pediatric patients. J Am Soc Echocardiogr 2014;27(8):903–10.

23. Arroyo-Rodriguez C, Fritche-Salazar JF, Posada-Martinez EL, et al. Right ventricular free wall strain predicts functional capacity in patients with repaired tetralogy of Fallot. Int J Cardiovasc Imaging 2020;36(4):595–604.

24. Yim D, Hui W, Larios G, et al. Quantification of right ventricular electromechanical dyssynchrony in relation to right ventricular function and clinical outcomes in children with repaired tetralogy of Fallot. J Am Soc Echocardiogr 2018;31(7):822–30.

25. Valente AM, Geva T. How to image repaired tetralogy of Fallot. Circ Cardiovasc Imaging 2017;10(5) [pii:e004270].

26. Bokma JP, de Wilde KC, Vliegen HW, et al. Value of cardiovascular magnetic resonance imaging in noninvasive risk stratification in tetralogy of Fallot. JAMA Cardiol 2017;2(6):678–83.

27. Ferrari I, Shehu N, Mkrtchyan N, et al. Different CMR imaging modalities for native and patch-repaired right ventricular outflow tract sizing: impact on percutaneous pulmonary valve replacement planning. Pediatr Cardiol 2020;41(2):382–8.

28. Hanneman K, Crean AM, Wintersperger BJ, et al. The relationship between cardiovascular magnetic resonance imaging measurement of extracellular volume fraction and clinical outcomes in adults with repaired tetralogy of Fallot. Eur Heart J Cardiovasc Imaging 2018;19(7):777–84.

29. Broberg CS, Huang J, Hogberg I, et al. Diffuse LV myocardial fibrosis and its clinical associations in adults with repaired tetralogy of Fallot. JACC Cardiovasc Imaging 2016;9(1):86–7.

30. Chen CA, Dusenbery SM, Valente AM, et al. Myocardial ECV fraction assessed by CMR is associated with type of hemodynamic load and arrhythmia in repaired tetralogy of Fallot. JACC Cardiovasc Imaging 2016;9(1):1–10.

31. Geva T. Diffuse myocardial fibrosis in repaired tetralogy of Fallot: linking pathophysiology and clinical outcomes. Circ Cardiovasc Imaging 2017;10(3) [pii:e006184].

32. Yamamura K, Yuen D, Hickey EJ, et al. Right ventricular fibrosis is associated with cardiac remodelling after pulmonary valve replacement. Heart 2019;105(11):855–63.

33. Ebert PA. Second operations for pulmonary stenosis or insufficiency after repair of tetralogy of Fallot. Am J Cardiol 1982;50(3):637–40.

34. Therrien J, Siu SC, McLaughlin PR, et al. Pulmonary valve replacement in adults late after repair of tetralogy of Fallot: are we operating too late? J Am Coll Cardiol 2000;36(5):1670–5.

35. Stout KK, Daniels CJ, Aboulhosn JA, et al. 2018 AHA/ACC guideline for the management of adults with congenital heart disease: executive summary: a report of the American College of Cardiology/American Heart Association Task Force on clinical practice guidelines. J Am Coll Cardiol 2019;73(12):1494–563.

36. Cochran CD, Yu S, Gakenheimer-Smith L, et al. Identifying risk factors for massive right ventricular dilation in patients with repaired tetralogy of Fallot. Am J Cardiol 2020;125(6):970–6.

37. Pastor TA, Geva T, Lu M, et al. Relation of right ventricular dilation after pulmonary valve replacement to outcomes in patients with repaired tetralogy of Fallot. Am J Cardiol 2020;125(6):977–81.

38. Bokma JP, Winter MM, Oosterhof T, et al. Preoperative thresholds for mid-to-late haemodynamic and clinical outcomes after pulmonary valve replacement in tetralogy of Fallot. Eur Heart J 2016;37(10):829–35.

39. Geva T. Indications for pulmonary valve replacement in repaired tetralogy of Fallot: the quest continues. Circulation 2013;128(17):1855–7.

40. Alvarez-Fuente M, Garrido-Lestache E, Fernandez-Pineda L, et al. Timing of pulmonary valve replacement: how much can the right ventricle dilate before it looses its remodeling potential? Pediatr Cardiol 2016;37(3):601–5.

41. Givertz MM, DeFilippis EM, Landzberg MJ, et al. Advanced heart failure therapies for adults with congenital heart disease: JACC state-of-the-art review. J Am Coll Cardiol 2019;74(18):2295–312.

42. Gorter TM, van Melle JP, Hillege HL, et al. Ventricular remodelling after pulmonary valve replacement: comparison between pressure-loaded and volume-loaded right ventricles. Interact Cardiovasc Thorac Surg 2014;19(1):95–101.

43. Ferraz Cavalcanti PE, Sa MP, Santos CA, et al. Pulmonary valve replacement after operative repair of tetralogy of Fallot: meta-analysis and meta-regression of 3,118 patients from 48 studies. J Am Coll Cardiol 2013;62(23):2227–43.

44. Mongeon FP, Ben Ali W, Khairy P, et al. Pulmonary valve replacement for pulmonary regurgitation in adults with tetralogy of Fallot: a meta-analysis–a report for the writing committee of the 2019 update of the Canadian Cardiovascular Society Guidelines for the management of adults with congenital heart disease. Can J Cardiol 2019; 35(12):1772–83.

45. Hallbergson A, Gauvreau K, Powell AJ, et al. Right ventricular remodeling after pulmonary valve replacement: early gains, late losses. Ann Thorac Surg 2015;99(2):660–6.

46. Ho JG, Schamberger MS, Hurwitz RA, et al. The effects of pulmonary valve replacement for severe pulmonary regurgitation on exercise capacity and cardiac function. Pediatr Cardiol 2015;36(6): 1194–203.

47. Sabate Rotes A, Johnson JN, Burkhart HM, et al. Cardiorespiratory response to exercise before and after pulmonary valve replacement in patients with repaired tetralogy of Fallot: a retrospective study and systematic review of the literature. Congenit Heart Dis 2015;10(3):263–70.

48. Bokma JP, Geva T, Sleeper LA, et al. A propensity score-adjusted analysis of clinical outcomes after pulmonary valve replacement in tetralogy of Fallot. Heart 2018;104(9):738–44.

49. Geva T, Mulder B, Gauvreau K, et al. Preoperative predictors of death and sustained ventricular tachycardia after pulmonary valve replacement in patients with repaired tetralogy of Fallot enrolled in the INDICATOR cohort. Circulation 2018; 138(19):2106–15.

50. Dorobantu DM, Sharabiani MTA, Taliotis D, et al. Age over 35 years is associated with increased mortality after pulmonary valve replacement in repaired tetralogy of Fallot: results from the UK National Congenital Heart Disease Audit database. Eur J Cardiothorac Surg 2020. [Epub ahead of print].

51. Babu-Narayan SV, Diller GP, Gheta RR, et al. Clinical outcomes of surgical pulmonary valve replacement after repair of tetralogy of Fallot and potential prognostic value of preoperative cardiopulmonary exercise testing. Circulation 2014;129(1):18–27.

52. Plessis J, Hascoet S, Baruteau A, et al. Edwards SAPIEN transcatheter pulmonary valve implantation: results from a French registry. JACC Cardiovasc Interv 2018;11(19):1909–16.

53. Steinberg ZL, Jones TK, Verrier E, et al. Early outcomes in patients undergoing transcatheter versus surgical pulmonary valve replacement. Heart 2017; 103(18):1455–60.

54. Cheatham JP, Hellenbrand WE, Zahn EM, et al. Clinical and hemodynamic outcomes up to 7 years after transcatheter pulmonary valve replacement in the US Melody valve investigational device exemption trial. Circulation 2015;131(22):1960–70.

55. Van Dijck I, Budts W, Cools B, et al. Infective endocarditis of a transcatheter pulmonary valve in comparison with surgical implants. Heart 2015;101(10): 788–93.

56. McElhinney DB, Sondergaard L, Armstrong AK, et al. Endocarditis after transcatheter pulmonary valve replacement. J Am Coll Cardiol 2018;72(22): 2717–28.

57. Silka MJ, Hardy BG, Menashe VD, et al. A population-based prospective evaluation of risk of sudden cardiac death after operation for common congenital heart defects. J Am Coll Cardiol 1998; 32(1):245–51.

58. Witte KK, Pepper CB, Cowan JC, et al. Implantable cardioverter-defibrillator therapy in adult patients with tetralogy of Fallot. Europace 2008;10(8): 926–30.

59. Egbe AC, Miranda WR, Madhavan M, et al. Cardiac implantable electronic devices in adults with tetralogy of Fallot. Heart 2019;105(7):538–44.

60. Kapel GF, Reichlin T, Wijnmaalen AP, et al. Re-entry using anatomically determined isthmuses: a curable ventricular tachycardia in repaired congenital heart disease. Circ Arrhythm Electrophysiol 2015;8(1): 102–9.

61. Khairy P, Harris L, Landzberg MJ, et al. Implantable cardioverter-defibrillators in tetralogy of Fallot. Circulation 2008;117(3):363–70.

62. Gatzoulis MA, Balaji S, Webber SA, et al. Risk factors for arrhythmia and sudden cardiac death late after repair of tetralogy of Fallot: a multicentre study. Lancet 2000;356(9234):975–81.

63. Ghai A, Silversides C, Harris L, et al. Left ventricular dysfunction is a risk factor for sudden cardiac death in adults late after repair of tetralogy of Fallot. J Am Coll Cardiol 2002;40(9):1675–80.

64. Bokma JP, Winter MM, Vehmeijer JT, et al. QRS fragmentation is superior to QRS duration in predicting mortality in adults with tetralogy of Fallot. Heart 2017;103(9):666–71.

65. Heng EL, Gatzoulis MA. QRS fragmentation in tetralogy of Fallot: clinical utility and risk prediction. Heart 2017;103(9):645–6.

66. Egbe AC, Miranda WR, Mehra N, et al. Role of QRS fragmentation for risk stratification in adults with tetralogy of Fallot. J Am Heart Assoc 2018;7(24): e010274.

67. Broberg CS, Aboulhosn J, Mongeon FP, et al. Prevalence of left ventricular systolic dysfunction in adults with repaired tetralogy of Fallot. Am J Cardiol 2011;107(8):1215–20.

68. Diller GP, Kempny A, Liodakis E, et al. Left ventricular longitudinal function predicts life-threatening ventricular arrhythmia and death in adults with repaired tetralogy of Fallot. Circulation 2012;125(20): 2440–6.

69. Sabate Rotes A, Connolly HM, Warnes CA, et al. Ventricular arrhythmia risk stratification in patients with tetralogy of Fallot at the time of pulmonary valve replacement. Circ Arrhythm Electrophysiol 2015; 8(1):110–6.

70. Babu-Narayan SV, Kilner PJ, Li W, et al. Ventricular fibrosis suggested by cardiovascular magnetic resonance in adults with repaired tetralogy of Fallot and its relationship to adverse markers of clinical outcome. Circulation 2006;113(3): 405–13.

71. Khairy P, Landzberg MJ, Gatzoulis MA, et al. Value of programmed ventricular stimulation after tetralogy of Fallot repair: a multicenter study. Circulation 2004; 109(16):1994–2000.

72. Kapel GF, Sacher F, Dekkers OM, et al. Arrhythmogenic anatomical isthmuses identified by electroanatomical mapping are the substrate for ventricular tachycardia in repaired tetralogy of Fallot. Eur Heart J 2017;38(4):268–76.

73. Stout KK, Daniels CJ, Aboulhosn JA, et al. 2018 AHA/ACC guideline for the management of adults with congenital heart disease: a report of the American College of Cardiology/American Heart Association Task Force on clinical practice guidelines. J Am Coll Cardiol 2019;73(12):e81–192.

74. Khairy P. Programmed ventricular stimulation for risk stratification in patients with tetralogy of Fallot: a Bayesian perspective. Nat Clin Pract Cardiovasc Med 2007;4(6):292–3.

75. Walsh EP. The role of ablation therapy for ventricular tachycardia in patients with tetralogy of Fallot. Heart Rhythm 2018;15(5):686–7.

76. Brouwer C, Hazekamp MG, Zeppenfeld K. Anatomical substrates and ablation of reentrant atrial and ventricular tachycardias in repaired congenital heart disease. Arrhythm Electrophysiol Rev 2016;5(2): 150–60.

77. van Zyl M, Kapa S, Padmanabhan D, et al. Mechanism and outcomes of catheter ablation for ventricular tachycardia in adults with repaired congenital heart disease. Heart Rhythm 2016;13(7):1449–54.

78. Zeppenfeld K, Schalij MJ, Bartelings MM, et al. Catheter ablation of ventricular tachycardia after repair of congenital heart disease: electroanatomic identification of the critical right ventricular isthmus. Circulation 2007;116(20):2241–52.

79. Kriebel T, Saul JP, Schneider H, et al. Noncontact mapping and radiofrequency catheter ablation of fast and hemodynamically unstable ventricular tachycardia after surgical repair of tetralogy of Fallot. J Am Coll Cardiol 2007;50(22):2162–8.

80. Laredo M, Frank R, Waintraub X, et al. Ten-year outcomes of monomorphic ventricular tachycardia catheter ablation in repaired tetralogy of Fallot. Arch Cardiovasc Dis 2017;110(5):292–302.

81. Sandhu A, Ruckdeschel E, Sauer WH, et al. Perioperative electrophysiology study in patients with tetralogy of Fallot undergoing pulmonary valve replacement will identify those at high risk of subsequent ventricular tachycardia. Heart Rhythm 2018; 15(5):679–85.

82. Caldaroni F, Lo Rito M, Chessa M, et al. Surgical ablation of ventricular tachycardia in patients with repaired tetralogy of Fallot†. Eur J Cardiothorac Surg 2019;55(5):845–50.

The Adult Patient with a Fontan

Ahmed AlZahrani, MBBS[a], Rahul Rathod, MD[b], Ahmed Krimly, MBChB, FRCPC, ABIM[c,d,e], Yezan Salam, MBBS[f], AlJuhara Thaar AlMarzoog, RN, MSN[g], Gruschen R. Veldtman, MBChB, FRCP[h],*

KEYWORDS

- Fontan operation • Single ventricle physiology • Late outcomes • Arrhythmia
- Congenital heart disease • Exercise capacity • Fontan physiology

KEY POINTS

- Single ventricle physiology is a rare condition but is highly represented in clinical practice due to a high prevalence of late complications and comorbidities.
- The Fontan operation has undergone considerable modification over the past 5 decades and is now in a superior hydrodynamic form.
- Survival in the current era is very good, with operative mortality less than 1%, and expected 20-year survival around 89%.
- Fontan failure, and end-organ disease are, however, common and require ongoing surveillance and early intervention when feasible.
- Other late complications include cyanosis, arrhythmia, atrioventricular valve regurgitation, protein-losing enteropathy and plastic bronchitis.

OVERVIEW

The birth prevalence of patients with functional single ventricles (FSVs) is around 35 per 100,000 live births.[1] Before Fontan surgery being available, many infants with FSVs developed progressively severe and life-threatening hypoxemia or low-output cardiac shock. Staged palliation ultimately resulting in the Fontan operation (Fig. 1) specifically addressed these hemodynamic perils by allowing passive redirection of caval return to the pulmonary arteries without a subpulmonary ventricle. While enabling these patients to survive well into adulthood, this "unnatural physiology" results in significant comorbidities and increased mortality as these patients enter the second and third decades of life.[2] In this article the authors:

1. Define the key anatomic and physiologic characteristics of single ventricle (SV) physiology.
2. Define the physiologic and anatomic considerations before and after Fontan palliation.
3. Describe the late outcomes and potential therapeutic approaches.

a Adult Congenital Heart Disease Program, Paediatric Cardiology, Prince Sultan Cardiac Centre, PO Box 7897 - G352, Riyadh 11159, Saudi Arabia; b Department of Pediatrics, Harvard Medical School, Boston Children's Hospital, 300 Longwood Avenue, Boston, MA 02115, USA; c Department of Cardiology, King Faisal Cardiac Center, King Abdulaziz Medical City, Ministry of National Guard Health Affairs, 6412 Ibn Mashhur Street, Alsalama District, Jeddah 23436 2946, Saudi Arabia; d Department of Medical Research, King Abdullah International Medical Research Center, Jeddah, Saudi Arabia; e Department of Medical Research, King Saud Bin Abdulaziz University for Health Science, Jeddah, Saudi Arabia; f College of Medicine, Alfaisal University, Takhassusi Street, Riyadh-11533, Saudi Arabia; g Adult Congenital Heart Disease Service, King Faisal Specialist Hospital and Research Centre, Zahrawi Street, Al Maather, Al Maazer, Riyadh 12713, Saudi Arabia; h Adult Congenital Heart Disease, Heart Centre, King Faisal Specialist Hospital and Research Centre, Zahrawi Street, Al Maather, Al Maazer, Riyadh 12713, Saudi Arabia
* Corresponding author.
E-mail address: f1511919@kfshrc.edu.sa

Cardiol Clin 38 (2020) 379–401
https://doi.org/10.1016/j.ccl.2020.05.002
0733-8651/20/© 2020 Elsevier Inc. All rights reserved.

A

Fontan: Ventriculzation of the right atrium

B

Kreutzer: Anterior APA with fenestration

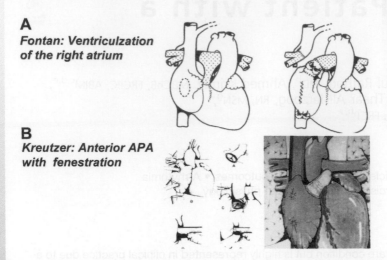

Fig. 1. The original Fontan operations described by Fontan (*A*) and Kreutzer (*B*) independently. (*Adapted from* Kreutzer, C., Kreutzer, J., & Kreutzer, G. O. (2013). Reflections on five decades of the Fontan Kreutzer procedure. Frontiers in pediatrics, 1, 45. https://doi.org/10.3389/fped.2013.00045.)

ANATOMIC SPECTRUM

Functional SV anatomy comprises a broad spectrum of anatomic defects resulting in the inability of the pulmonary and systemic circulations to function competently in parallel. This may be due to absence, hypoplasia, or gross functional impairment of one of the ventricles. It also includes ventricles not able to produce enough stroke volume due to systolic and/or diastolic dysfunction. Functional SV palliation is used in some patients in whom it is difficult to septate the circulation due to massive ventricular septal defects or complex atrioventricular (AV) or ventriculo-arterial (VA) relationships. Given these enormous anatomic variations of such affected hearts, a unifying sequential segmental approach to anatomic classification has generally been adopted[3] (**Fig. 2**).

Accordingly, FSV hearts have been classified as univentricular or biventricular AV connections. When univentricular AV connection is present, it

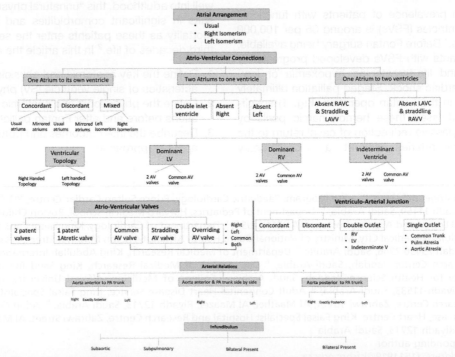

Fig. 2. Flow chart demonstrating sequential segmental cascade of complex congenital heart disease analysis and classification.

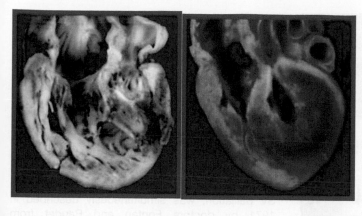

Fig. 3. Heart with hypoplastic left heart syndrome, that is biventricular with absent left AV connection (mitral atresia, hypoplastic left heart syndrome).

may be double inlet left ventricle (DILV), or double inlet right ventricle (RV). There may also be biventricular AV connection with absent left AV connection, such as in mitral atresia with hypoplastic left heart syndrome (HLHS), or absent right AV connection, such as in tricuspid atresia. Such complex cardiac malformation can be associated with heterotaxy syndromes where there is loss of chirality in the cardiac, thoracic, and abdominal organs. The univentricular spectrum of FSVs also includes extreme forms of Ebstein's anomaly in which the functional portion of the RV may be severely dysfunctional such that it cannot independently support the pulmonary circulation. The most commonly encountered FSV diagnoses include HLHS (**Fig. 3**), tricuspid atresia (**Fig. 4**), DILV (**Fig. 5**), and unbalanced AV canal defects (**Fig. 6**).

INITIAL PALLIATION
Palliative Procedures for Single Ventricle Physiology

Functionally, SV individuals undergo multistage palliations. The choice of initial palliation depends on the specific anatomic lesion and its hemodynamic consequences, as well as the pulmonary vascular physiology, which changes quite

profoundly in the first few weeks of life. The initial surgical options available include (**Fig. 7**):

1. Pulmonary artery banding for those with high or unrestricted pulmonary blood flow
2. Systemic to pulmonary artery (PA) shunt (Blalock-Taussig shunt) for those with reduced pulmonary blood flow see **Fig. 7**A and B
3. Stage I (Norwood procedure) with a systemic to PA shunt or ventricle to PA conduit, for those with HLHS or one of its variants
4. Glenn procedure—see **Fig. 7**E
5. Fontan operation

For the purposes of this article, the authors will focus on the Fontan procedure, and briefly discuss what the Glenn shunt is.

GLENN PROCEDURE

The classic Glenn shunt, in which the superior vena cava (SVC) is surgically connected to the right pulmonary artery (RPA) in an end-to-end fashion, was first reported in 1958 by William Glenn at Yale[4] (**Fig. 8**). In its subsequent modification, the bidirectional cavopulmonary anastomosis, the SVC is connected to the RPA in an end-to-side fashion while maintaining continuity between the right and left pulmonary arteries

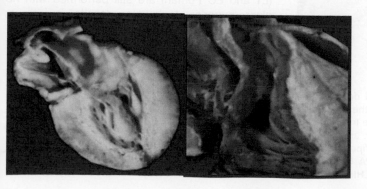

Fig. 4. Heart with absent right AV connection (tricuspid atresia) with concordant VA connection, which occurs in approximately 15% of cases with tricuspid atresia.

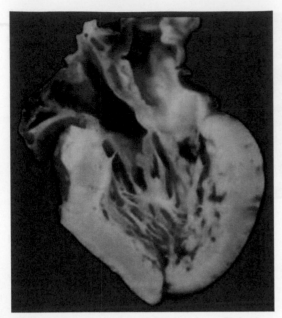

Fig. 5. Double inlet left ventricle.

(see **Fig. 7**E). After the Glenn procedure, pulmonary blood flow from the head and neck is driven by nonpulsatile low-pressure venous forces toward the pulmonary venous atrium, obliterating the previous arterial shunt physiology which in contrast provides continuous arterial blood flow into the pulmonary circulation. With this

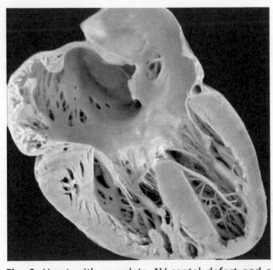

Fig. 6. Heart with complete AV septal defect and a common AV valve. (This image is from the Web Portal of the Archiving Working Group of The International Society for Nomenclature of Paediatric and Congenital Heart Disease (ISNPCHD) (http://ipccc-awg.net) and *courtesy of* Diane E. Spicer BS, PA (ASCP) (The Congenital Heart Institute of Florida [CHIF]).)

transformation, there is usually reduction in ventricular preload. Ventricular wall acutely thickens as the volume-to-wall thickness increases. This gradually remodels to a more normal wall mass in the weeks after the Glenn shunt.[5] Significant practice variation continues to exist with respect to the optimal age at which the Glenn shunt is performed.[23] However, generally this procedure is generally performed at around age 4 to 6 months.

FONTAN PROCEDURE

The "Fontan operation," the final planned stage in SV palliation, was simultaneously described in 1971 by doctors Fontan and Baudet from Bordeaux, France, and Dr Kreutzer from Buenos Aires, Argentina.[2,6] The operation was applied first in patients with tricuspid atresia. Fontan surgery increased survival for children born with FSVs. The Fontan connection is created by fashioning a new pathway for inferior caval return to the pulmonary arteries (see **Fig. 7**F–H).

Fontan Types and Modifications

The Fontan procedure has undergone numerous modifications over the past 6 decades. The older AV and atriopulmonary connections worked on the premise that ventricular or atrial contraction might provide adequate ventricularized preload to the pulmonary circulation and pulmonary venous atrium. Consistent with these conceptions, valved connections were used initially between the right atrium (RA) and RV, and the RV and PA, connections. However, these conduits invariably became stenosed[7] and the RA became massively dilated with huge energy losses.[8]

In 1988, Marc De Leval and colleagues[9] elegantly demonstrated the hydrodynamic and energy conservation superiority of the lateral tunnel (LT) Fontan (see **Fig. 7**G). Marcelletti and colleagues,[10] in 1988, introduced a valve-less extracardiac (EC) conduit between the inferior vena cava and the PA. It became known as the EC Fontan (see **Fig. 7**H). Today, although both procedures (LT and EC Fontan) are still performed with no clear superior technique despite numerous, mostly retrospective, analyses trying to answer this question. A further landmark in the evolution of the Fontan procedure was the introduction of a fenestration between the systemic venous return and the pulmonary venous atrium.[11] This effectively creates a controlled right-to-left shunt and augments ventricular preload and partially offloads systemic venous hypertension. Fenestration at the time of Fontan has been associated with a reduction in pleural drainage duration, and in post-Fontan hospital stay.[12] Other benefits of

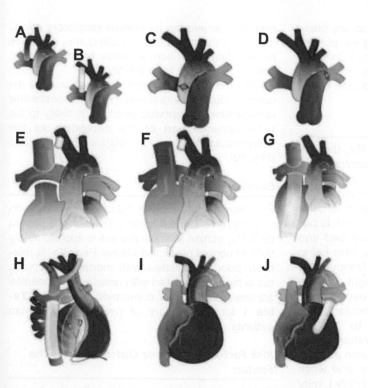

Fig. 7. Aortopulmonary shunts and variations of Fontan surgery: (*A*) the classic Blalock-Taussig shunt; (*B*) modified Blalock-Taussig shunt; (*C*) Waterston shunt; (*D*) Potts shunt; (*E*) bidirectional Glenn operation; (*F*) modified classic Fontan; (*G*) intracardiac lateral tunnel Fontan; (*H*) extracardiac Fontan; (*I*) Norwood stage I procedure; (*J*) Sano modification. (*From* Khairy P., Poirier N., Mercier L. Circulation: Univentricular Heart Wolters. Kluwer Health, Inc. 2007;115(6) 800-812.; with permission.)

fenestration are also becoming evident, such as improved infradiaphragmatic hemodynamics.[13]

Optimal Age for Fontan Completion

The most optimal age for performing the Fontan has long been controversial. Earlier age at Fontan brings forward the potential late complications as

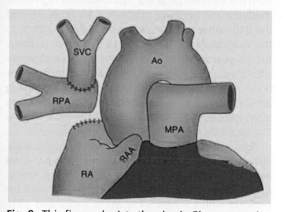

Fig. 8. This figure depicts the classic Glenn operation where the SVC is connected to the RPA in an end-to-end fashion, and the RPA is disconnected from the central pulmonary arteries. (Mazur W, Siegel MJ, Miszalski-Jamka T, Pelberg R. (2013) Norwood Procedures and Sano Modification. In: CT Atlas of Adult Congenital Heart Disease. Springer, London. Reprinted with permission.)

the Fontan clock starts ticking.[14] In contrast, later Fontan completion means longer duration of cyanosis and its neurodevelopmental risks, a greater likelihood of pulmonary arteriovenous malformations, greater degrees of ventricular hypertrophy, ventricular dysfunction, and AV valve regurgitation as volume load persists. Recent data have consistently suggested that the most optimal age for the Fontan operation is aged around 3 to 5 years.[15] There is a mortality benefit, greater exercise capacity, [16] lower rates of in-hospital mortality and procedure-related complications, as well as lower rates of nonroutine discharge when the operation is performed aged between 3 and 5 years.[15]

Good Versus Bad Fontan Candidacy

In 1978, Choussat and Fontan laid down fundamental ground rules for a successful Fontan operation[17] Although many of these principles have been neglected, modified, or revised, some important principles remain for a successful early and late outcome. These include unobstructed ventricular inflow, reasonable ventricular function, unobstructed ventricular outflow, unobstructed connection from the systemic venous system into the pulmonary arteries, good sized pulmonary arteries without distortion, a well-developed pulmonary vascular bed, normal pulmonary vascular resistance, and unobstructed pulmonary venous return. As a general rule, a transpulmonary pressure gradient (TPG) less than 6 mm Hg and pulmonary vascular resistance (PVR) <2 Wood Units are associated with reasonable outcomes. In patients living at high altitude higher TPG less than 8 mm Hg may be accepted.[18]

Normal Fontan Physiology

In the absence of a subpulmonary RV, there is obligatory increase in resting central and secondarily peripheral venous pressures. Commonly these pressures are around 10 to 15 mm Hg when the Fontan circulation is functioning optimally. The venous gradient exists between the peripheral venous capillary bed and the left atrium, with the dominant resistor being the pulmonary capillary bed.[19] Nonpulsatile flow through the PAs and the upright position exacerbate the pulmonary vascular dependence of the circulation. The pulmonary vascular bed is therefore commonly understood to be the "bottleneck" in the circulation, and relatively minor alterations in PVR, particularly when above 2 Wood units, and perhaps even less, and when combined with low cardiac index (<2.5 L/min/m^2) are associated with poor outcomes[20] (Fig. 9). Preload to the SV is therefore often low, and there is inherent limitation in ventricular filling, particularly during exercise and at higher heart rates.[21] The circulation is also fundamentally dependent on negative intrathoracic

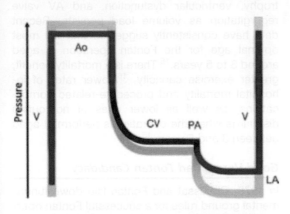

Fig. 9. Flow/pressure/saturation diagram of the Fontan circulation: changes over time. Fontan hemodynamics late (full color) superimposed on Fontan early (transparent): with time the ventricular end-diastolic pressure and pulmonary vascular resistance increase, resulting in overall decreased flow and increased caval vein pressure/congestion. A downward progressive spiral ensues. Ao, aorta; CV, caval veins; LA, left atrium; PA, pulmonary artery; V, single ventricle.

pressure generation by normal ventilatory effort, as well as the peripheral muscle pump, the latter contributing as much as 30% toward cardiac output generation from the SV.[22]

After the Fontan operation venous volume increases due to angiotensin II and aldosterone upregulation. Lymphatic overflow is likely to be a fundamental part of the circulation as the microcirculation has a relative "exit block" (Fig. 10).

Exercise Capacity

Exercise capacity is often reduced in patients with a Fontan (see Table 1 below). The average pooled peak Vo$_2$ across multiple studies is approximately 50% of normal predicted values. Peak Vo$_2$ is relatively poorly correlated with mortality outcomes but is highly correlated with unscheduled hospital admissions and other comorbidities.[23,24] See Table 1 for a summary of peak Vo$_2$ in Fontan patients.

Risk Factors for a Poor Outcome After the Fontan

Risk factors for late outcomes after the Fontan operation are summarized in Table 2 below.

Era effect: Fontan surgical epochs can be categorized into early era (1971–1990), the middle era (1991–2000), and the current era. Operative mortality in the early era was around 17%,[25–27] in the middle era 4% to 9%, and in the current era operative mortality is now generally less than 1%.

Atriopulmonary Fontans: patients who have undergone atriopulmonary Fontan (APF) hail mostly from the early surgical era, with relatively high initial mortality and ongoing mortality over time. Among the 215 patients who underwent APF operation in the Australian and New Zealand Fontan registry, the 28-year freedom from death, death and transplantation, and Fontan failure (death, transplantation, takedown, conversion, protein-losing enteropathy (PLE), or plastic bronchitis, NYHA class III/IV) were 69% (95% CI, 61–78), 64% (95% CI, 56–74), and 45% (95% CI, 36–55), respectively.[28]

Total cavopulmonary connection Fontans: Individuals who undergo lateral tunnel Fontans have excellent survival prospects. In a recent meta-analysis of 3330 patients, the pooled survival for patients with LT was 94% at 10 years and 89% at 20 years.[29] Factors known to influence late mortality include presence of AV valve regurgitation, ventricular dilation, thromboembolism, arrhythmia, heart failure, PLE, late operative reintervention, and end-organ dysfunction. See Table 2 for a summary of risk factors for the Fontan procedure. Fontan See Fig. 11.

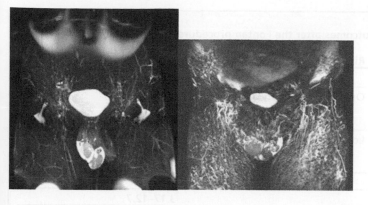

Fig. 10. Lymphatic overload and dysfunction in a patient with a Fontan circulation. Lower limb and pelvic lymphatics in a normal individual on the left and an asymptomatic Fontan patient on the right. (*Courtesy of* Vibeke Hjortdal, MD, Norway, Copenhagen.)

Fontan Circulatory Failure

Fontan circulatory failure is said to occur when cardiac output is insufficient for daily cardiovascular needs and when there is evolving venous congestion. Presentation may be with deteriorating exercise intolerance, as well as peripheral and/or central edema. A myriad of potential hemodynamic causes may contribute, including systolic or diastolic ventricular dysfunction, increased pulmonary vascular resistance, pathway obstruction, AV valve regurgitation or stenosis, restrictive interatrial septum, and a wide array of arrhythmias. Lymphatic dysfunction, such as PLE and plastic bronchitis, may also herald the presence of circulatory failure.[30] Pathway narrowing with pullback gradients at cardiac catheterization of as little as 1 mm Hg may represent significant obstruction.

Fontan circulatory failure has been clinically categorized to aid management:[31]

- Type I: Fontan failure with low ejection fraction
- Type II: Fontan failure with preserved ejection fraction
- Type III: Fontan failure with normal intracardiac pressures
- Type IV: Fontan failure with abnormal lymphatics

See **Table 3** for hemodynamic characteristics of the different types of Fontan failure.

Type I: Fontan failure with low ejection fraction (systolic dysfunction)

In FSVs, an ejection fraction less than 30% is generally considered significant. Frank pulmonary edema due to low ejection fraction is uncommon; however, with the exception of end-stage PLE where patients may be volume sensitive, and during the pediatric years where it may occur during

Table 1
A summary of peak exercise performance of Fontan patients

| Author/ Study | Peak Vo₂; (mL/kg/min) | | | | Peak Vo₂ Percent of Predicted Sample Size | | | | Sample Size | Age (SD) |
	Mean	SD	25th Percentile	75th Percentile	Mean	SD	25th Percentile	75th Percentile		
Diller et al[75]	22.8	7.4	17.842	27.758	51.7	15.4	41.382	62.018	321	21 ± 9
Fernandes et al[76]	21.2	6.2	17.046	25.354	57.1	14.1	47.6S3	66.547	146	21.5 (range 16.0)
Ohuchi et al[77]	27.1	7.4	22.142	32.058	61.0	15.0	50.95	71.05	335	18 ± 9
Nathan et al[78]	23.5	6.9	18.877	28.123	59.7	14.3	50.119	69.281	253	19 ± 9
Egbe et al[79]	22.7	5.4	19.082	26.318	63.0	11.0	55.63	70.37	145	24 + 3
Atz et al[80]	–	–			61.0	16.0	50.28	71.72	334	21 ± 4
Cunningham et al[81]	22.0	5.7	18.181	25.819	60.9	13.7	51.721	70.079	130	26.6 ± 9.5
	–	–	–	–	–	–	–	–	1664	0

Courtesy of Tarek Alsaied, MD, Cincinnati, OH.

Table 2
Summary of risk factors for poor outcomes after the Fontan procedure

Risk Factor	Risk	Pooled Hazard
Preoperative risk factors		
Operative era after 2001	Operative mortality and late mortality and late Fontan failure	0.12–0.85
Preoperative evidence of lymphatic dysfunction	Longer postoperative stay and late Fontan failure	50% vs 4% for type 4 lymphatic abnormality vs types 1 and 2
Age above 7 at Fontan		
Heterotaxy syndromes		3.17–12.7
Hypoplastic left heart syndrome	Operative and late mortality and Fontan Failure	2.8–10.1
Multiple cardiac catheter interventions or surgical reinterventions before Fontan	Early Fontan failure and postoperative complications	
Perioperative risk factors		
Prolonged cardiopulmonary bypass and/or cross-clamp times	Early Fontan failure	
AV valve replacement at the time of Fontan	Mortality	4.02
Postoperative RA press > 20 mm HG	Greater mortality Greater likelihood of transplantation	2.29
Pleural drainage >3 wk	Late mortality in hospital survivors	1.2
Postoperative and late risk factors		
Hemodynamic factors: PA pressure > 15, post-Fontan pressure > 20 and presence of diastolic dysfunction	Mortality	1.14–3.5
Presence of heart failure	Heart transplantation, mortality	1.58–9.2
Postoperative arrhythmia	Mortality, thrombo-embolism	1.8–6
Lack of thromboprophylaxis	Sudden death; congestive heart failure	4.76
Moderate or severe AV valve regurgitation	Fontan failure, mortality	
Protein-losing enteropathy	Mortality or transplantation	1.97–8.5
End-organ disease include chronic kidney disease and Fontan-associated liver disease	Mortality	2.5–19
Ventricular dilation >125 mL/BSA[74]	Mortality or transplantation	7.7

Data from Alsaied T, Bokma JP, Engel ME, et al. Factors associated with long-term mortality after Fontan procedures: A systematic review. Heart. 2017;103(2). https://doi.org/10.1136/heartjnl-2016-310108 and Alsaied T, Bokma JP, Engel ME, et al. Predicting long-term mortality after Fontan procedures: A risk score based on 6707 patients from 28 studies. Congenit Heart Dis. 2017;12(4). https://doi.org/10.1111/chd.12468.

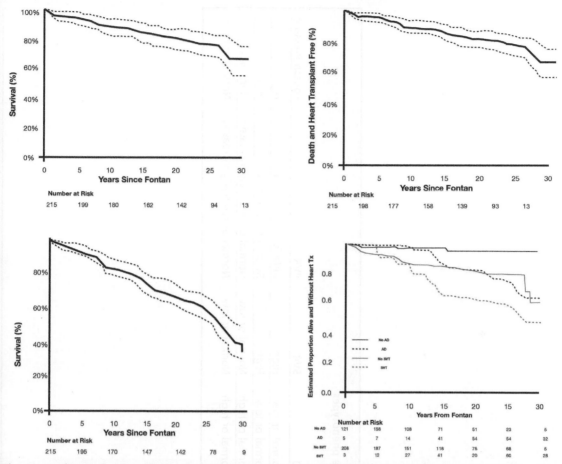

Fig. 11. Kaplan Meier curve for survival (1), freedom from death and heart transplantation (2), freedom from Fontan failure (3) and freedom from death and transplantation with/without atrial dilation (AD) and arrhythmia (SVT) (4). (*From* Poh CL, Zannino D, Weintraub RG, et al. Three decades later: The fate of the population of patients who underwent the Atriopulmonary Fontan procedure. Int J Cardiol 2017;231;99-104 https://doi.org/10.1016/j.ijcard.2017.01.057.)

interstage palliation. Prognosis is poor once symptomatic and when fluid retention is present.

Type II: Fontan failure with preserved ejection fraction (diastolic dysfunction)

Type II Fontan failure resembles heart failure with preserved ejection fraction. Diagnosis is currently cardiac catheterization based with resting or acute rise in wedge or LVED pressure greater than 12 mm Hg following a 15 mL/kg fluid volume challenge.[32] Patients with right ventricular morphology and APF are at greater risk. (23) Up to 28% of Fontan patients have myocardial fibrosis, and these individuals are more likely to have ventricular tachycardia, and increased end-diastolic pressures (24).

Type III: Fontan failure with normal intracardiac pressures (high-output cardiac failure)

The clinical picture resembles right-sided heart failure and there is usually evidence of multisystem involvements (liver cirrhosis and renal impairment), but characteristically Fontan pressures are in the normal range. The underlying physiology is believed to be due to an inadequate augmentation in stroke volume in the presence of cirrhosis-driven systemic vasodilation.

Type IV: Fontan failure with abnormal lymphatics (lymphatic abnormalities)

Lymphatic abnormalities may present as PLE, plastic bronchitis, ascites, chylous pleural, and pericardial effusions. Fluid retention itself is a manifestation of insufficiency of the lymphatic system.[31,33]

Protein-Losing Enteropathy

In PLE there is pathologic enteric protein loss usually due to liver lymphatic overload decompressing into the small bowel. It can be diagnosed from

Table 3
Hemodynamic characteristics of the different types of Fontan failure phenotypes

	Systolic Function	Ventricular End-Diastolic Pressure	CO	SVR	PVR	Fontan Pressure
Type I	Low	High	Normal or low	High	Relatively increased	High
Type II	Normal	High	Normal or low	High	Relatively increased	High
Type III	Normal	Normal	Normal or high	Normal or low	Normal or relatively increased	Normal
Type IV	Normal	Normal or low	Normal or high	Normal or low	Normal or relatively increased	Normal or high

fecal α1 antitrypsin (spot >54 mg/dL, α1 antitrypsin clearance >27 mL/24 hours without diarrhea and >56 mL/24 hours with diarrhea) or by nuclear scintigraphy using technetium-99m–labeled albumin and documenting bowel loss. PLE, when decompensated, manifests with hypoalbuminemia and an edematous state. Up to 12% of Fontan patients can be affected.[34,35] Treatment strategies focus on fluid management, hemodynamic optimization, nutritional support, and anti-inflammatory management of the gut. More recently, lymphatic intervention in the catheterization lab and surgically has been practiced with promising effect.[36,37] See **Fig. 12** for treatment strategies of PLE.

Plastic Bronchitis

Plastic bronchitis is another manifestation of lymphatic dysfunction. It is characterized by the leakage of lymphatic fluid rich in proteinaceous material into the airways, causing intermittent expectoration of bronchial casts (**Fig. 13**). Treatment is focused on pulmonary measures and cardiovascular measures. Cardiovascular interventions, including optimization of the Fontan circulatory hemodynamics, and primary lymphatic intervention.[38,39]

Arrhythmia

Atrial tachyarrhythmia is the most common late cardiovascular complication after Fontan surgery. Prevalence ranges between 30% and 60% at 20 years after Fontan surgery, APF connections being the most commonly affected. Among 996 Fontan patients with no history of arrhythmia before Fontan operation, 29% developed arrhythmia at 10 years, 58% at 20 years, and 76% at 30 years after the operation. Risk factors include longer duration of the Fontan circuit, poor Fontan hemodynamics, heterotaxy syndromes, and the presence of dextrocardia. Of note, early postoperative arrhythmia does not predict the onset of late arrhythmia.

Arrhythmia mechanisms

Multiple potential arrhythmia mechanisms are documented in Fontan patients, frequently overlapping in presence (**Fig. 14**).[40]

1. Macro reentrant atrial tachycardia—the most common resulting nonconductive scar tissue, suture lines, or anatomic structures, such as crista terminalis and AV valve and caval orifices

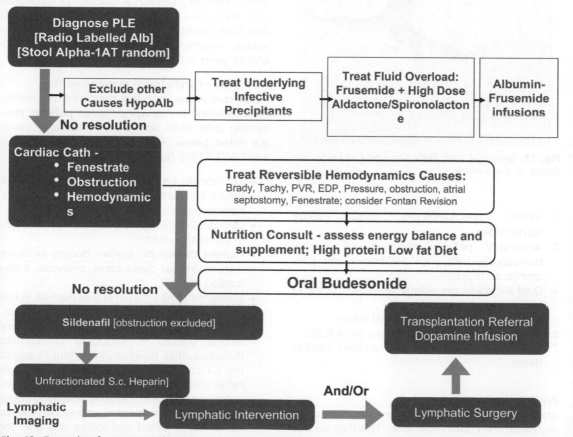

Fig. 12. Example of treatment algorithm for PLE in the current era.

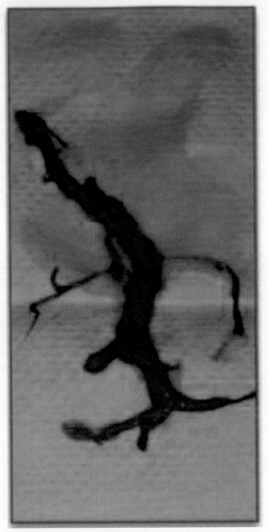

Fig. 13. Bronchial cast. Note the cast has taken the shape of the airways.

2. AVNRT (atrioventricular nodal reentry tachycardia)
3. Accessory pathway-mediated AV reentry tachycardia with both antidromic and prodromic conduction
4. Dual AV nodal physiology (especially in those with heterotaxy syndromes)
5. Typical as well as atypical atrial flutter
6. Atrial fibrillation with and without atrial flutter
7. Ventricular tachycardia and sudden cardiac death

Bradyarrhythmias

Bradycardia syndromes also are relatively common after the Fontan operation. This may be due to sinus node dysfunction, AV nodal disease, and heart block. Tachy-Brady syndromes may coexist.[41]

Outcomes after arrhythmia

The development of atrial tachyarrhythmia often marks a general decline in Fontan circulatory physiology, and not surprisingly morbid event rates following first arrhythmia event prevail[42] (**Figs. 15** and **16**). Fontan pressures are often high, usually around 16 mm Hg, but often are above 20 mm Hg.[43] In a series of 153 tachyarrhythmia patients, 33 subsequently died, 12 went on to have heart transplantation, 3 Fontan takedown, 12 PLE, 25 had NYHA functional class III or IV, and overall 84 met criteria for Fontan failure. Thromboembolic events after atrial tachyarrhythmia are highly prevalent.[44,45] Overall the risk ranges from 5% to 33%. Those with an APF, and/or not receiving anticoagulation, and those with an ejection fraction less than 35%, are at greatest risk for developing thromboembolic.

Atrial tachyarrhythmia in its own right may also precipitate decline in Fontan hemodynamics. For example, persistent tachycardia rates of as low as 105 to 110 bpm may precipitate tachymyopathy and heart failure in Fontan patients. This in turn may unleash a cascade of functional and end-organ (gastrointestinal tract, kidneys, and liver) decline. Once the first arrhythmia develops, freedom of death and transplant at 10 and 15 years is 68% and 63%, respectively.[42]

Principles of arrhythmia management

Acute care A few important principles are worthy of considering in managing Fontan patients presenting with atrial tachyarrhythmias and these are listed below. For more detailed guidelines see PACES/HRS guideline.[46]

- TEE should be performed as a general rule before any cardioversion, unless in the acute hemodynamically compromised situation.
- CHA2DS2-VASc score is not sensitive enough to be reliably used.
- Highest thrombotic burden occurs in those with ventricular dysfunction, cyanosis, intracardiac devices.
- Sustained atrial arrhythmia less than 48, is not a secure marker of the absence of thrombus.
- Cardiac computed tomography (CT) is a very helpful adjunct in excluding intracardiac thrombus. It is, however, important to adjust the CT protocol (approximately 2 to 3 mL/s rather than the usual 5 to 6 mL/s given for coronary imaging), and acquiring images at about 80 seconds from the start of injection allows for mixing of blood and iodine and also for inferior vena cava blood returning to the heart

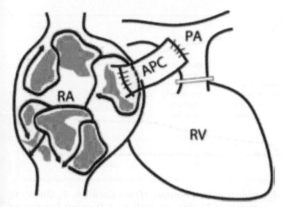

Fig. 14. The cardiac anatomy of a patient with a Fontan circulation. In the enlarged atria there are multiple corridors bordered by areas of scar tissue. Hence, there are numerous circuits possible, as indicated by the red arrows. APC, atriopulmonary conduit; PA, pulmonary artery; RA, right atrium; RV, right ventricle. (*From* de Groot NMS, Bogers AJJC. Development of Tachyarrhythmias Late After the Fontan Procedure: The Role of Ablative Therapy. Card Electrophysiol Clin. 2017. https://doi.org/10.1016/j.ccep.2017.02.009.)

to be properly opacified. For patients with lateral tunnel or extracardiac Fontan this almost invariably works (**Fig. 17**).

- There is emerging evidence for the safety of DOACs,[47–49] but current guideline recommendations favor vitamin K antagonism.[46]
- Following acute and intermediate management of the arrhythmia, detailed hemodynamic assessment of the Fontan circulation should be undertaken.
- Restoration of sinus rhythm is preferred, but the onset of persistent atrial tachycardias and particularly atrial fibrillation often herald advanced atriopathy and atrial scarring, resistant to medical therapy aimed at restoring sinus rhythm.

- Ablation therapy has a 33% to 100% success rate (i.e., 33%–100%), but recurrence is similar to success rate at 3 years.[50]
- Before ablation, detailed appraisal of native cardiac anatomy, surgically modified anatomy, and previous devices and interventional procedures is essential to safe procedural practice.

Fontan Conversion Surgery

Fontan conversion is performed in patients with atriopulmonary connections, and sometimes in those with very dilated lateral tunnel connections with the intent of alleviating energy losses in the massively dilated atrium, and reduce atrial arrhythmia burden. Surgery consists of a modified Cox-Maze III adjusted to each anatomic lesion, pacemaker placement (usual atrial lead), and establishing an EC tube connection (**Fig. 18**).

Indications for Fontan conversion include recalcitrant arrhythmias, atrial thrombus, adverse hemodynamics, such as AV valve regurgitation, atrial septal restriction, or outlet obstruction from within the ventricle or in the aortic arch. Fontan conversion surgery carries a high mortality risk in inexperienced teams. A prerequisite for successful outcomes is the presence of an integrated multidisciplinary team of ACHD cardiologists, electrophysiologists, anesthetists, surgeons experienced in arrhythmia surgery, and excellent Fontan-specific postoperative intensive care unit management. Pooled data suggest an overall procedural mortality of around 9% (41) and generally good acute and intermediate arrhythmia relief and 10-year arrhythmia-free survival of 77%.[51] Functional class often improves after the procedure. In a Mayo Clinic review of 70 patients, early mortality was 10%, and 84% improved compared with NYHA I or II or less during a mean follow-up of 5 years; only 8 patients (15%) had recurrence of atrial tachyarrhythmia.[52]

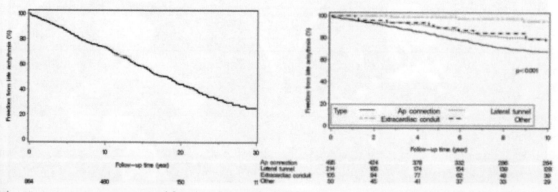

Fig. 15. Long-term outcomes and freedom from arrhythmia.

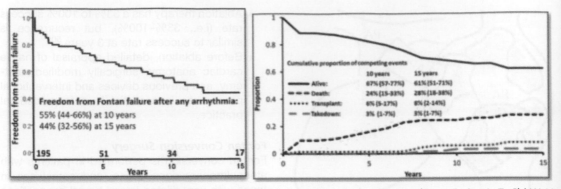

Fig. 16. Long-Term outcomes after first onset arrhythmia in patients with a Fontan. (*From* Carins A. T., Shi W. Y., Iyengar J. A., et al. Long-term outcomes after first-onset arrhythmia in Fontan physiology. J Thoracic Cardiovasc Surg 2016;152(5)1355-1363.)

Cyanosis

Arterial saturation in Fontan patients is usually around 92% and rarely more than 95% at rest. Saturations may drop during exercise, when below 88% it may contribute to exercise-related dyspnea. For many patients these shunts are small without a significant impact on oxygen saturations. They can serve as a physiologic pop-off in the setting of pulmonary stressors, such as lower respiratory tract infections, to maintain ventricular preload and cardiac output. The benefits and risks of closing these right-to-left shunts remains controversial. The most common causes are intracardiac return of coronary venous return, intrapulmonary ventilation-perfusion mismatch, since the nonpulsatile pulmonary flow favors the gravitation-dependent lower lung segment.[53] Additional causes include fenestrated baffles or

decompressing veno-venous collaterals that drain to the pulmonary venous atrium. The latter presents a "natural" fenestration and preload supplementation to the systemic SV. They are often seen in the early phases postpartum. When arterial saturations are very low (low 80s), and when the patient presents with related exertional symptoms or stroke, further evaluation and treatment may be necessary. The development of veno-venous collateralization may coincide with rising pulmonary vascular resistance or local Fontan pathway obstruction, or the development of diastolic heart disease. Understanding the pathophysiology helps formulate positive indications for structural intervention. Routine occlusion of veno-venous collaterals has been associated with a poorer outcome.[54] Other causes for cyanosis include pulmonary arteriovenous malformation, which may

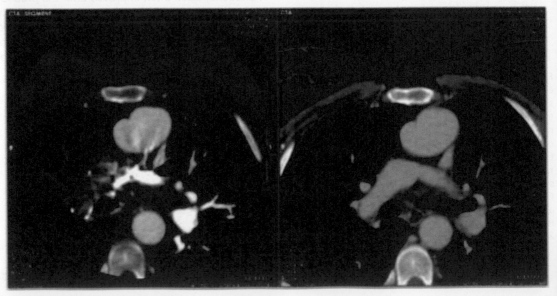

Fig. 17. CT scan demonstrating intrapulmonary thrombus.

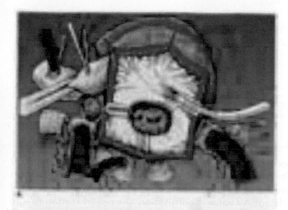

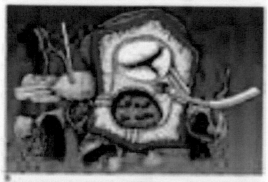

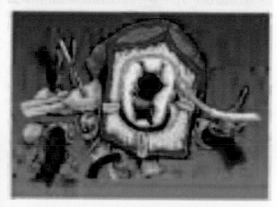

Fig. 18. These are a series of illustrations of the use of cryoablation in patients undergoing Fontan conversion. (*A*) The modified right-sided maze procedure in a patient with tricuspid atresia. (*B*) The modified right-sided maze procedure in a patient with double outlet right ventricle and mitral atresia. (*C*) The modified right atrial maze procedure in a patient with a functionally univentricular heart (unbalanced AV septal defect). (*Adapted from* Mavroudis C, Backer CL, Deal BJ, et al. Total cavopulmonary conversion and maze procedure for patients with failure of the Fontan operation. J Thorac Cardiovasc Surg 2001;122:863-871.; with permission.)

be due to macro-arteriovenous or to micro circulatory connections. The former is often amenable to percutaneous occlusion, whereas the latter is not, and requires redirection of hepatic effluent toward the affected lung segments. This has been alluded to as the protective effect of the "hepatic factor or factors."[55,56]

Atrioventricular Valvular Regurgitation

Atrioventricular valve regurgitation is relatively common in patients with a single ventricle. Almost 1 in 10 Fontan patients had required AV intervention the New Zealand and Australian Fontan registry at some point in their surgical history[57,58] (**Fig. 19**). The origins of regurgitation can often be traced back to initial palliation resulting in prolonged volume loading (arterial shunts), and dynamic interaction between the systemic AV valve anatomy, ventricular geometry, and underlying hemodynamic pressures. Systemic tricuspid valves (TCVs) in hypoplastic left heart syndrome may become regurgitant because of leaflet prolapse, annular dilation, leaflet dysplasia, or abnormalities of the subchordal apparatus and papillary muscles. Kutty and colleagues[59] elegantly described abnormally large TCV tethering volumes and greater bending angles of the TCV in those with moderate or severe tricuspid regurgitation in HLHS. Common AV in unbalanced AV septal defect valves also have particular anatomic predisposition toward regurgitation, such as leak through the zone of apposition, prolapse, myxomatous changes, and chordal elongation and/or rupture. Indeed the cumulative incidence of AV valve failure at 25 years for common AV valve was 56% (CI, 46%–67%), for systemic single TCV 46% (CI, 31%–61%), and for a single mitral valve 26% (CI, 21%–30%)[57,58] AV valve regurgitation may lead to increased systemic ventricle end-diastolic pressure, which in turn may cause higher pulmonary vascular resistance and pressure, ultimately precipitating low cardiac output states with accompanying venous hypertension. This hemodynamic cascade may trigger atrial tachyarrhythmia and ventricular dysfunction and may precipitate late Fontan failure in the form of PLE, plastic bronchitis, and other manifestations of lymphatic overload and dysfunction because of the high systemic venous pressures. Mortality rates are also higher once moderate or severe AV valve regurgitation develops.

Surgical strategies aimed at addressing late development or worsening of AV valve regurgitation in Fontan patients are currently challenging to advocate universally because of the suboptimal intermediate and late outcome of such

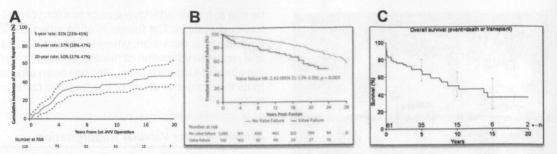

Fig. 19. (A) Cumulative incidence of AV valve failure in Fontan patients. (B) Time-varying covariate Kaplan-Meier curve for estimated freedom from Fontan failure in patients with AV valve failure (*orange line*) and in patients without AV valve failure (*blue line*). (C) Kaplan-Meier survival curve displays the overall transplant-free survival after AV valve surgery after Fontan procedure. With significant AV valve regurgitation, the risk of Fontan failure is increased by more than 2-fold.

intervention. Although operative mortality is low, reoperation for recurrent AV valve regurgitation is common, ranging from 44% to 81%. The higher recurrence rates are mitigated by strategies that entirely exclude the leaking AV valve[60] if there are 2, or if part of a common AV valve, or by use of a mechanical AV valve.[61–63] The decision therefore to intervene on a moderate or severely leaking AV valve in Fontan patients should be taken cautiously, and only when there is a very high likelihood of preventing late recurrence, and when the hemodynamic effects outweigh the surgical risks.

End-Organ Disease and Fontan Surveillance

Long-term cardiac and extracardiac complications have been documented in 60% of Fontan patients at 14 years after Fontan.[64] These late EC complications include Fontan-associated liver disease (FALD), lymphatic dysfunction, subclinical glomerular and tubular dysfunction in at least 10% to 14%,[65] gut dysbiosis[66] with associated bacterial translocation and inflammatory signaling,[67] muscle sarcopenia[68] as well as bone loss, hypothyroidism, glucose intolerance,[69] and structural brain changes accompanying varying degrees of neurodevelopmental challenges (**Table 4**). These EC complications may hail subclinical pathway obstruction atrial arrhythmia, high Fontan pressures, diastolic dysfunction, severe systolic dysfunction, or the presence of AV valve regurgitation. The authors believe, therefore, that disproportionately fast development of end-organ disease should prompt further hemodynamic assessment, including invasive hemodynamic evaluation.

Fontan surveillance is summarized in the recent AHA and Cardiac Society of Australia and New Zealand position statements on the Evaluation and Management of the child and adult with Fontan circulation.[70–73]

General principles of organ surveillance are:

- Adult Fontan patients need to be seen at least annually if they are stable. If hemodynamic or end-organ concerns exist, more frequent evaluation is warranted.
- Patients can be classified into low-, intermediate-, and high-risk groups. This can be because of their hemodynamics, FALD, presence of heart failure, or PLE or plastic bronchitis, or the presence of unstable arrhythmia.
- The presence of early or rapidly progressive end-organ disease should prompt further investigation of the hemodynamics with cardiac MRI ± cardiac catheterization.
- Cardiopulmonary exercise testing with peripheral venous pressure monitoring may be helpful in identifying those with adverse hemodynamics.

See **Table 4** for a summary of the various endo-organ dysfunctions that are seen, their significance, and suggested surveillance thereof.

Therapeutic Options

Surgical management

Fontan patients frequently require surgical intervention after their Fontan surgery. A recent publication from the Australian and New Zealand Fontan registry showed that, in a large cohort of 1428 patients, 435 (30%) underwent at least 1 procedure after their Fontan operation.[1] Most of these patients had late interventions at a median age of 4.2 years after Fontan. Transcatheter fenestration closure and surgical pacemaker-related procedures were the most common procedure. For patients with APFs, conversion to total cavopulmonary connections has been previously discussed. Other common indications for surgery after the Fontan operation include AV valvar

Table 4
End-organ dysfunction in Fontan patients and suggested surveillance

End-Organ	Type of Abnormality	Frequencies of Abnormalities	Significance	Surveillance
Fontan-associated liver disease	Congestion	100%	Low risk	Liver ultrasound ± CT or MRI during adult life, 6 monthly screening if high-risk features • If moderate risk then annually • If low risk consider screening every 2 y Biopsy—as needed
	Fibrosis	>90%	Low risk	
	Cirrhosis	30%	• High risk for operative intervention • Risk for HCC development • Portal hemodynamics • Decompensated cirrhosis	
	Arterialized nodules	33%		CT or MRI (at least dual phase)
	Hepatocellular carcinoma	1–3%		Usually triple phase CT or MRI + targeted biopsy
Renal dysfunction	Glomerular	14% with GFR < 90 mL/min/1.73 m²	Associated with a greater risk of mortality or non-elective hospitalization	Serum creatinine Serum cystatin C Urinary KIM-1 Urinary NAG
	Tubular			
Thyroid dysfunction	Subclinical manifest with high TSH and lowered free T4	24–33%	Correlated with Fontan hemodynamics and may in turn affect cardiovascular functioning through lack of inotropy provided by thyroid hormone	Free T4 TSH
Impaired glucose metabolism	Abnormal fasting glucose	–	Impaired glucose tolerance is associated with greater mortality	Random blood glucose (annually) Oral glucose tolerance test (as needed) Hemoglobin A₁c (every 3 y or as needed)
	Impaired glucose tolerance	34%		
	Diabetes mellitus	4.6%		

(continued on next page)

Table 4
(continued)

End-Organ	Type of Abnormality	Frequencies of Abnormalities	Significance	Surveillance
Muscle loss	Loss of skeletal muscle strength Sarcopenia	Sarcopenia in 10%	Associated with poor exercise performance	Exercise stress testing every 2–3 y
Bone density loss	Loss of bone density in the osteopenic range Secondary hyperparathyroidism 25-Hydroxy vitamin D deficiency	29% — 27%	May be a marker of adverse hemodynamics, such as diastolic dysfunction or significant cyanosis May also be a marker of hypovitaminosis D	Dual energy X-ray absorptiometry scan Ca phosphate, parathyroid hormone
Protein-losing enteropathy	Enteral loss of hepatic lymph effluent, with subsequent hypoproteinemia, nutritional deficiency; immune compromise	9–14%	Associated with marked morbidity, frequent hospitalization, loss of quality of life, eventually leading to death or transplantation, sometimes need for cardiac surgery or cardiac rhythm management	Stool alpha-1-antitrypsin clearance and random levels Radio-labeled albumin excretion from the stool (screening in high-risk populations that manifest clinical symptoms, or that have diminished albumin)
Plastic bronchitis	Airway loss of pulmonary lymphatic effluent, leading to bronchial cast formation, airways obstruction, and symptoms of casting and bronchospasm and airways infection		Marker of significant morbidity and mortality	Screening based on clinical symptomatology and physical findings Bronchoscopy in individuals with a high clinical index of suspicion

Abbreviations: GFR, glomerular filtration rate; HCC, hepatocellular carcinoma; NAG, N-acetyl-β-glucosaminidase; TSH, thyroid stimulating hormone and thyrotropin.

repair/replacement, outflow tract obstruction, or PA reconstruction.

Catheterization-based interventions

Given the vulnerabilities of the Fontan circulation and the challenges with currently available diagnostic tools, routine cardiac catheterizations has been recommended at least once every 10 years in adolescent and adult patients. A particularly useful time to undertake such cardiac catheterization is before transfer to adult care to accurately define the hemodynamic strengths and vulnerabilities of the individual Fontan circulations.[3] However, there is also an important role for catheterization-based interventions that may be triggered by clinical concerns arising from tomographic imaging or from abnormal serum biomarkers. Cardiac magnetic resonance imaging or CT imaging can identify Fontan pathway obstructions that may prompt intervention in the catheterization laboratory. These anatomic lesions can occur anywhere within the venous system, including in the inferior vena cava, Fontan baffle, SVC, cavopulmonary anastomoses, or branch pulmonary arteries. Given the physiologic limitations of a passive circulation and the absence of a subpulmonary ventricle, optimization of the Fontan pathway is critical. A low threshold for balloon dilation or stenting of angiographic narrowings may be considered even if the measured pull back gradient is as low as 1 mm Hg. If left unchecked over years, the cumulative physiologic burden of these lesions can be significant and may accelerate FALD or exercise intolerance.

Cyanosis is another common reason for late reintervention.[4] The causes have already been discussed elsewhere in this article. There are sometimes theoretic benefits for maintaining right-to-left shunts in selected patients with a view to maintaining ventricular preload, decreasing Fontan baffle pressures, and potentially slowing the progression of FALD.

An important emerging role for catheterization-based interventions in Fontan patients is to address lymphatic dysfunction. Inherent in the Fontan circulation is increased systemic venous pressure, which leads to lymphatic congestion and overflow. Increased pressures within the lymphatic system can cause the formation of lymphatic channels that overflow into the gut (PLE), airways (plastic bronchitis), lungs (chylothorax), or the peritoneal cavity (ascites). Initial management should focus on addressing anatomic and reversible hemodynamic issues on the Fontan circulation, followed by various medical therapies.[7] In patients not responsive to medical therapies, fenestration creation in the catheterization laboratory can be helpful.[8] Recently, the group at the Children's Hospital of Philadelphia has shown that catheter-based interventions within the lymphatic system to embolize lymphatic channels can result in sustainable remission of symptoms, especially in plastic bronchitis.[9] This approach may be more effective in patients with

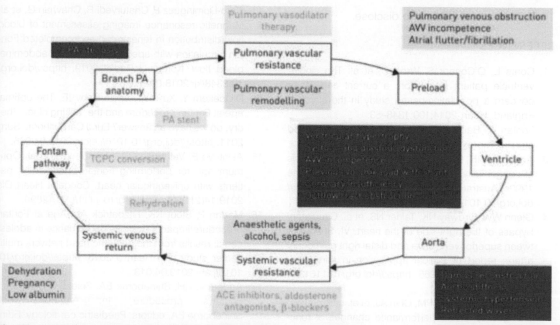

Fig. 20. General considerations and approaches to Fontan management.

plastic bronchitis (compared with PLE[10]) as they have fewer but larger channels more amenable to intervention. There have also been small case series showing that rerouting of the innominate vein to the left atrium (via surgery or transcatheter approach) can also result in remission of symptoms, but at the expense of cyanosis. This is the so-called Hraska procedure.[11,12]

A summary of management approaches can be found in **Fig. 20**.

SUMMARY

In this article the authors have summarized the important anatomic and physiologic substrates for which the Fontan circulation was surgically created. The authors have outlined both normal and abnormal physiologic responses, including exercise performances after the Fontan operation. Having laid the background, the authors then provide contemporary insights into the outcomes with respect to mortality, arrhythmia, end-organ dysfunction, and in the final section provide guidance with respect to treatment strategies. The future direction of the Fontan circulation is at an important juncture. Multiple devices to support the circulation mechanically are under investigation, but probably the most interesting concept is that of combining additional energy to the venous circuit, together with reducing central venous pressures by a modest amount [around 5mm Hg] from baseline.

DISCLOSURE

The authors have nothing to disclose.

REFERENCES

1. Coats L, O'Connor S, Wren C, et al. The single-ventricle patient population: a current and future concern a population-based study in the North of England. Heart 2014;100:1348–53.
2. Fontan F, Baudet E. Surgical repair of tricuspid atresia. Thorax 1971;26:240–8.
3. Anderson RH, Ho SY. Sequential segmental analysis of congenitally malformed hearts: advances for the 1990s. Australas J Card Thorac Surg 1993. https://doi.org/10.1016/1037-2091(93)90074-E.
4. Glenn WW, Ordway NK, Talner NS, et al. Circulatory bypass of the right side of the heart. VI. Shunt between superior vena cava and distal right pulmonary artery; report of clinical application in thirty-eight cases. Circulation 1965. https://doi.org/10.1161/01.CIR.31.2.172.
5. Fogel MA, Weinberg PM, Chin AJ, et al. Late ventricular geometry and performance changes of functional single ventricle throughout staged Fontan reconstruction assessed by magnetic resonance imaging. J Am Coll Cardiol 1996. https://doi.org/10.1016/0735-1097(96)00111-8.
6. Kreutzer GO. Evolutionary process of the Fontan-Kreutzer procedure. Rev Argent Cardiol 2011;79:47–54..
7. Shachar GB, Fuhrman BP, Wang Y, et al. Rest and exercise hemodynamics after the Fontan procedure. Circulation 1982. https://doi.org/10.1161/01.CIR.65.6.1043.
8. Lardo AC, del Nido PJ, Webber SA, et al. Hemodynamic effect of progressive right atrial dilatation in atriopulmonary connections. J Thorac Cardiovasc Surg 1997. https://doi.org/10.1016/S0022-5223(97)70110-7.
9. Migliavacca F, Dubini G, Bove EL, et al. Computational fluid dynamics simulations in realistic 3-D geometries of the total cavopulmonary anastomosis: the influence of the inferior caval anastomosis. J Biomech Eng 2003. https://doi.org/10.1115/1.1632523.
10. Marcelletti C, Corno A, Giannico S, et al. Inferior vena cava-pulmonary artery extracardiac conduit. A new form of right heart bypass. J Thorac Cardiovasc Surg 1990. https://doi.org/10.1016/S0022-5223(19)35562-X.
11. Bridges ND, Lock JE, Castaneda AR. Baffle fenestration with subsequent transcatheter closure. Modification of the Fontan operation for patients at increased risk. Circulation 1990. https://doi.org/10.1161/01.CIR.82.5.1681.
12. Lemler MS, Scott WA, Leonard SR, et al. Fenestration improves clinical outcome of the Fontan procedure: a prospective, randomized study. Circulation 2002;105:207–12.
13. Caro-Dominguez P, Chaturvedi R, Chavhan G, et al. Magnetic resonance imaging assessment of blood flow distribution in fenestrated and completed Fontan circulation with special emphasis on abdominal blood flow. Korean J Radiol 2019. https://doi.org/10.3348/kjr.2018.0921.
14. D'Udekem Y, Xu MY, Konstantinov IE. The optimal age at Fontan procedure and the "ticking clock" theory: do we have an answer? Eur J Cardiothorac Surg 2011. https://doi.org/10.1016/j.ejcts.2010.04.006.
15. Akintoye E, Veldtman GR, Miranda WR, et al. Optimum age for performing Fontan operation in patients with univentricular heart. Congenit Heart Dis 2019;14(2). https://doi.org/10.1111/chd.12690.
16. Madan P, Stout KK, Fitzpatrick AL. Age at Fontan procedure impacts exercise performance in adolescents: results from the pediatric heart network multicenter study. Am Heart J 2013. https://doi.org/10.1016/j.ahj.2013.04.013.
17. Anderson RH, Shineborne EA. Selection criteria for Fontan's procedure. In: Anderson RH, Shineborne EA, editors. Paediatric cardiology. Edinburgh (UK): Churchill Livingstone; 1978. p. 559–66.

18. Malhotra SP, Ivy DD, Mitchell MB, et al. Performance of cavopulmonary palliation at elevated altitude: midterm outcomes and risk factors for failure. Circulation 2008. https://doi.org/10.1161/CIRCULATIONAHA.107.751784.

19. Macé L, Dervanian P, Bourriez a, et al. Changes in venous return parameters associated with univentricular Fontan circulations. Am J Physiol Heart Circ Physiol 2000;279(5):H2335–43. Available at: http://www.ncbi.nlm.nih.gov/pubmed/11045970.

20. Gewillig M, Brown SC, Eyskens B, et al. The Fontan circulation: who controls cardiac output? Interact Cardiovasc Thorac Surg 2010;10:428–33.

21. Pushparajah K, Wong JK, Bellsham-Revell HR, et al. Magnetic resonance imaging catheter stress haemodynamics post-Fontan in hypoplastic left heart syndrome. Eur Heart J Cardiovasc Imaging 2016. https://doi.org/10.1093/ehjci/jev178.

22. Cordina R, O'Meagher S, Gould H, et al. Skeletal muscle abnormalities and exercise capacity in adults with a Fontan circulation. Heart 2013. https://doi.org/10.1136/heartjnl-2013-304249.

23. Ohuchi H, Ono S, Tanabe Y, et al. Long-term serial aerobic exercise capacity and hemodynamic properties in clinically and hemodynamically good, "excellent", Fontan survivors. Circ J 2012;76(1):195–203.

24. Udholm S, Aldweib N, Hjortdal VE, et al. Prognostic power of cardiopulmonary exercise testing in Fontan patients: a systematic review. Open Heart 2018. https://doi.org/10.1136/openhrt-2018-000812.

25. Mair DD, Puga FJ, Danielson GK. The Fontan procedure for tricuspid atresia: early and late results of a 25-year experience with 216 patients. J Am Coll Cardiol 2001. https://doi.org/10.1016/S0735-1097(00)01164-5.

26. Khairy P, Fernandes SM, Mayer JE, et al. Long-term survival, modes of death, and predictors of mortality in patients with Fontan surgery. Circulation 2008;117:85–92.

27. Alsaied T, Bokma JP, Engel ME, et al. Factors associated with long-term mortality after Fontan procedures: a systematic review. Heart 2017;103(2). https://doi.org/10.1136/heartjnl-2016-310108.

28. Poh CL, Zannino D, Weintraub RG, et al. Three decades later: the fate of the population of patients who underwent the atriopulmonary Fontan procedure. Int J Cardiol 2017. https://doi.org/10.1016/j.ijcard.2017.01.057.

29. Ben Ali W, Bouhout I, Khairy P, et al. Extracardiac versus lateral tunnel Fontan: a meta-analysis of long-term results. Ann Thorac Surg 2019. https://doi.org/10.1016/j.athoracsur.2018.08.041.

30. Dori Y, Keller MS, Fogel MA, et al. MRI of lymphatic abnormalities after functional single-ventricle palliation surgery. Am J Roentgenol 2014. https://doi.org/10.2214/AJR.13.11797.

31. Book WM, Gerardin J, Saraf A, et al. Clinical phenotypes of Fontan failure: implications for management. Congenit Heart Dis 2016. https://doi.org/10.1111/chd.12368.

32. Averin K, Hirsch R, Seckeler MD, et al. Diagnosis of occult diastolic dysfunction late after the fontan procedure using a rapid volume expansion technique. Heart 2016;102(14):1109–14.

33. Stout KK, Broberg CS, Book WM, et al. Chronic heart failure in congenital heart disease: a scientific statement from the American Heart Association. Circulation 2016. https://doi.org/10.1161/CIR.0000000000000352.

34. Ostrow AM, Freeze H, Rychik J. Protein-losing enteropathy after Fontan operation: investigations into possible pathophysiologic mechanisms. Ann Thorac Surg 2006;82(2):695–700.

35. Mertens L, Hagler DJ, Sauer U, et al. Protein-losing enteropathy after the Fontan operation: an international multicenter study. J Thorac Cardiovasc Surg 1998. https://doi.org/10.1016/S0022-5223(98)70406-4.

36. Rychik J, Goldberg D, Rand E, et al. End-organ consequences of the Fontan operation: liver fibrosis, protein-losing enteropathy and plastic bronchitis. Cardiol Young 2013;23:830–9.

37. Itkin M, Piccoli DA, Nadolski G, et al. Protein-losing enteropathy in patients with congenital heart disease. J Am Coll Cardiol 2017;69(24):2929–37.

38. Ugaki S, Lord DJE, Sherwood MC, et al. Lymphangiography is a diagnostic and therapeutic intervention for patients with plastic bronchitis after the Fontan operation. J Thorac Cardiovasc Surg 2016;152(2):e47–9.

39. Dori Y, Keller MS, Rychik J, et al. Successful treatment of plastic bronchitis by selective lymphatic embolization in a Fontan patient. Pediatrics 2014. https://doi.org/10.1542/peds.2013-3723.

40. Correa R, Sherwin ED, Kovach J, et al. Mechanism and ablation of arrhythmia following total cavopulmonary connection. Circ Arrhythmia Electrophysiol 2015. https://doi.org/10.1161/CIRCEP.114.001758.

41. Forsdick V, Iyengar AJ, Carins T, et al. Unsatisfactory early and late outcomes after Fontan surgery delayed to adolescence and adulthood. Semin Thorac Cardiovasc Surg 2015. https://doi.org/10.1053/j.semtcvs.2015.05.001.

42. Carins TA, Shi WY, Iyengar AJ, et al. Long-term outcomes after first-onset arrhythmia in Fontan physiology. J Thorac Cardiovasc Surg 2016. https://doi.org/10.1016/j.jtcvs.2016.07.073.

43. Pundi KN, Pundi KN, Johnson JN, et al. Sudden cardiac death and late arrhythmias after the Fontan operation. Congenit Heart Dis 2017. https://doi.org/10.1111/chd.12401.

44. Egbe AC, Connolly HM, McLeod CJ, et al. Thrombotic and embolic complications associated with atrial arrhythmia after Fontan operation: role of prophylactic therapy. J Am Coll Cardiol 2016. https://doi.org/10.1016/j.jacc.2016.06.056.

45. Egbe AC, Connolly HM, Niaz T, et al. Prevalence and outcome of thrombotic and embolic complications in adults after Fontan operation. Am Heart J 2017. https://doi.org/10.1016/j.ahj.2016.09.014.

46. Khairy P, Van Hare GF, Balaji S, et al. PACES/HRS expert consensus statement on the recognition and management of arrhythmias in adult congenital heart disease. Hear Rhythm 2014. https://doi.org/10.1016/j.hrthm.2014.05.009.

47. Yang H, Veldtman GR, Bouma BJ, et al. Non-vitamin K antagonist oral anticoagulants in adults with a Fontan circulation: are they safe. Open Hear 2019;6(1). https://doi.org/10.1136/openhrt-2018-000985.

48. Pujol C, Müssigmann M, Schiele S, et al. Direct oral anticoagulants in adults with congenital heart disease—a single centre study. Int J Cardiol 2020. https://doi.org/10.1016/j.ijcard.2019.09.077.

49. Pujol C, Niesert AC, Engelhardt A, et al. Usefulness of direct oral anticoagulants in adult congenital heart disease. Am J Cardiol 2016. https://doi.org/10.1016/j.amjcard.2015.10.062.

50. Deal BJ, Mavroudis C, Backer CL. Arrhythmia management in the Fontan patient. Pediatr Cardiol 2007; 28:448–56.

51. Deal BJ, Costello JM, Webster G, et al. Intermediate-term outcome of 140 consecutive Fontan conversions with arrhythmia operations. Ann Thorac Surg 2016. https://doi.org/10.1016/j.athoracsur.2015.09.017.

52. Said SM, Burkhart HM, Schaff HV, et al. Fontan conversion: identifying the high-risk patient. Ann Thorac Surg 2014. https://doi.org/10.1016/j.athoracsur.2014.01.083.

53. Masura J, Borodacova L, Tittel P, et al. Percutaneous management of cyanosis in Fontan patients using Amplatzer occluders. Catheter Cardiovasc Interv 2008. https://doi.org/10.1002/ccd.21540.

54. Poterucha JT, Johnson JN, Taggart NW, et al. Embolization of veno-venous collaterals after the Fontan operation is associated with decreased survival. Congenit Heart Dis 2015. https://doi.org/10.1111/chd.12276.

55. Praus A, Fakler U, Balling G, et al. Only hepatic venous blood closes intrapulmonary shunts after cavopulmonary connection. Int J Cardiol 2014; 172(2):477–9.

56. Pike NA, Vricella LA, Feinstein JA, et al. Regression of severe pulmonary arteriovenous malformations after Fontan revision and "hepatic factor" rerouting. Ann Thorac Surg 2004. https://doi.org/10.1016/j.athoracsur.2004.02.003.

57. King G, Gentles TL, Winlaw DS, et al. Common atrioventricular valve failure during single ventricle palliation. Eur J Cardiothorac Surg 2017. https://doi.org/10.1093/ejcts/ezx025.

58. King G, Ayer J, Celermajer D, et al. Atrioventricular valve failure in Fontan palliation. J Am Coll Cardiol 2019. https://doi.org/10.1016/j.jacc.2018.12.025.

59. Kutty S, Colen T, Thompson RB, et al. Tricuspid regurgitation in hypoplastic left heart syndrome mechanistic insights from 3-dimensional echocardiography and relationship with outcomes. Circ Cardiovasc Imaging 2014. https://doi.org/10.1161/CIRCIMAGING.113.001161.

60. King G, Winlaw DS, Alphonso N, et al. Atrioventricular valve closure in Fontan palliation. Eur J Cardiothorac Surg 2019. https://doi.org/10.1093/ejcts/ezz324.

61. Alsaied T, Bokma JP, Engel ME, et al. Predicting long-term mortality after Fontan procedures: a risk score based on 6707 patients from 28 studies. Congenit Heart Dis 2017;12(4). https://doi.org/10.1111/chd.12468.

62. Wong DJ, Iyengar AJ, Wheaton GR, et al. Long-term outcomes after atrioventricular valve operations in patients undergoing single-ventricle palliation. Ann Thorac Surg 2012. https://doi.org/10.1016/j.athoracsur.2012.03.058.

63. Kotani Y, Chetan D, Atlin CR, et al. Longevity and durability of atrioventricular valve repair in single-ventricle patients. Ann Thorac Surg 2012. https://doi.org/10.1016/j.athoracsur.2012.04.048.

64. D'udekem Y, Iyengar AJ, Galati JC, et al. Redefining expectations of long-term survival after the Fontan procedure twenty-five years of follow-up from the entire population of Australia and New Zealand. Circulation 2014. https://doi.org/10.1161/CIRCULATIONAHA.113.007764.

65. Opotowsky AR, Baraona F, Landzberg M, et al. Kidney dysfunction in patients with a single ventricle Fontan circulation. J Am Coll Cardiol 2016. https://doi.org/10.1016/s0735-1097(16)30899-3.

66. Patel JK, Ceylan ET, Bittinger K, et al. Changes in gut microbiome early after Fontan operation. Circulation 2016. Abstract 17908.

67. Sharma R, Bolger AP, Li W, et al. Elevated circulating levels of inflammatory cytokines and bacterial endotoxin in adults with congenital heart disease. Am J Cardiol 2003. https://doi.org/10.1016/S0002-9149(03)00536-8.

68. Possner M, Alsaied T, Siddiqui S, et al. Abdominal skeletal muscle index as a potential novel biomarker in adult Fontan patients. CJC Open 2020;2(2). https://doi.org/10.1016/j.cjco.2019.12.004.

69. Ohuchi H, Miyamoto Y, Yamamoto M, et al. High prevalence of abnormal glucose metabolism in young adult patients with complex congenital heart

disease. Am Heart J 2009. https://doi.org/10.1016/j.ahj.2009.04.021.

70. Rychik J, Atz AM, Celermajer DS, et al. Evaluation and management of the child and adult with Fontan circulation: a scientific statement from the American Heart Association. Circulation 2019;140(6). https://doi.org/10.1161/CIR.0000000000000696.

71. Zentner D, Celermajer DS, Gentles T, et al. Management of people with a Fontan circulation: a Cardiac Society of Australia and New Zealand position statement. Hear Lung Circ 2020. https://doi.org/10.1016/j.hlc.2019.09.010.

72. Gentles TL, Mayer JEJ, Gauvreau K, et al. Fontan operation in five hundred consecutive patients: factors influencing early and late outcome. J Thorac Cardiovasc Surg 1997;114:376–91.

73. Murphy MO, Glatz AC, Goldberg DJ, et al. Management of early Fontan failure: a single-institution experience. Eur J Cardiothorac Surg 2014. https://doi.org/10.1093/ejcts/ezu022.

74. Rathod RH, Prakash A, Kim YY, et al. Cardiac magnetic resonance parameters predict transplantation-free survival in patients with Fontan circulation. Circ Cardiovasc Imaging 2014. https://doi.org/10.1161/CIRCIMAGING.113.001473.

75. Diller G, Giardini A, Dimopoulos K, et al. Predictors of morbidity and mortality in contemporary Fontan patients: results from a multicenter study including cardiopulmonary exercise testing in 321 patients. Eur Heart J 2010;31(24):3073–83.

76. Fernandes SM, Alexander ME, Graham DA, et al. Exercise testing identifies patients at increased risk for morbidity and mortality following Fontan surgery. Congenit Heart Dis 2011;6(4):294–303.

77. Ohuchi H, Negishi J, Noritake K, et al. Prognostic value of exercise variables in 335 patients after the Fontan operation: a 23-year single-center experience of cardiopulmonary exercise testing. Congenit Heart Dis 2015;10(2):105–16.

78. Nathan AS, Loukas B, Moko L, et al. Exercise oscillatory ventilation in patients with Fontan physiology. Circ Heart Fail 2015;8(2):304–11.

79. Egbe AC, Driscoll DJ, Khan AR, et al. Cardiopulmonary exercise test in adults with prior Fontan operation: the prognostic value of serial testing. Int J Cardiol 2017;235:6–10.

80. Atz AM, Zak V, Mahony L, et al. Longitudinal outcomes of patients with single ventricle after the Fontan procedure. J Am Coll Cardiol 2017;69(22):2735–44.

81. Cunningham JW, Nathan AS, Rhodes J, et al. Decline in peak oxygen consumption over time predicts death or transplantation in adults with a Fontan circulation. Am Heart J 2017;189:184–92.

Transcatheter Interventions in Adult Congenital Heart Disease

Jamil A. Aboulhosn, MD[a],*, Ziyad M. Hijazi, MD, MPH[b,c]

KEYWORDS

- Adult congenital heart disease • Transcatheter intervention • Pulmonary valve replacement
- VSD closure • ASD closure • Valvuloplasty

KEY POINTS

- Transcatheter interventions are replacing traditional surgical procedures for many types of native and operated congenital heart disease.
- Transcatheter interventions often require fluoroscopic and echocardiographic guidance.
- Transcatheter pulmonary valve replacement is now considered standard of care in patients with failing bioprosthetic valves and conduits.
- New self-expanding devices are undergoing human trials and will allow for transcatheter valve replacement of patients with large native right ventricular outflow tracts and pulmonary regurgitation.

BACKGROUND

The past 3 decades have witnessed an exponential growth of transcatheter interventions for congenital heart disease (CHD). Nowhere has this been more evident than in the adult CHD population, because survival into adulthood is now the norm for most forms of CHD.[1,2] In 1976 King and Mills published the first report of transcatheter device closure of an atrial septal defect (ASD).[3] Since that time, improvements in device design, catheterization technology, and procedural techniques have brought interventional cardiology to the forefront as a therapeutic intervention that may delay or obviate the need for surgery in CHD. Advances in noninvasive cardiovascular imaging have made diagnostic cardiac catheterization in a shrinking pool of patients. Transthoracic echocardiography with Doppler is now the noninvasive imaging work horse for congenital and structural

cardiology and is cost effective and widely available. Cross-sectional imaging modalities such as computed tomography scans and MRI provide 3-dimensional volumetric data that are invaluable in the assessment of anatomy and function, especially in those with complex anatomy. The combination of echocardiography and cross-sectional imaging provides a powerful noninvasive armamentarium that is capable of accurately assessing most anatomic and physiologic types of CHD thus relegating diagnostic catheterization to a small subset of patients, typically those with single ventricle physiology, pulmonary hypertension, or those in whom noninvasive imaging results in confusing or contradictory findings. Because most hemodynamic determinations can be made by Doppler echocardiography and anatomic determinations can be made by computed tomography scans or MRI, diagnostic catheterizations are

ᵃ Ahmanson/UCLA Adult Congenital Heart Disease Center, Ronald Reagan Medical Center at UCLA, 635 Charles Young Drive South, Los Angeles, CA 90095, USA; ᵇ Sidra Heart Center, Sidra Medicine, Al Gharrafa Street, Ar-Rayyan, Doha, Qatar; ᶜ Weill Cornell Medicine, Cornell University, 525 East 68th Street, New York, NY 10065, USA
* Corresponding author.
E-mail address: jaboulhosn@mednet.ucla.edu

Cardiol Clin 38 (2020) 403–416
https://doi.org/10.1016/j.ccl.2020.04.005
0733-8651/20/© 2020 Elsevier Inc. All rights reserved.

indicated for determination of hemodynamics that cannot be obtained by other modalities. Diagnostic catheterizations continue to be the gold standard for the evaluation of pulmonary pressures, flows, and resistance, especially in single ventricle patients before and after cavopulmonary shunts.

Interventional catheterization can be therapeutic, reparative, or palliative and is becoming an increasingly popular alternative to cardiac surgery. Further, it can be used to complement and enhance surgical results. Interventional catheterization has largely replaced surgery as the treatment of choice for a number of congenital cardiovascular conditions, including ostium secundum ASD, coarctation of the aorta, patent ductus arteriosus, pulmonary artery or valve stenosis, certain types of ventricular septal defects (VSDs), and conduit or bioprosthetic valve dysfunction. Various devices are under clinical trials for the replacement of pulmonic valves in dysfunctional native right ventricular (RV) outflow tracts. These techniques have shown promise and are expected to enter mainstream clinical practice within the next few years. New procedures and devices are continually evolving. This article details a variety of currently available procedures for adult patients with CHD, including the indications for their use, potential risks, and clinical outcomes.

INTERVENTIONS FOR SEMILUNAR VALVE AND VENTRICULAR OUTFLOW TRACT OBSTRUCTIONS
Right Ventricular Outflow Tract Obstruction

Obstruction of the RV outflow tract can occur at multiple levels, namely, subinfundibular, infundibular, valvular, or supravalvular. Although infundibular obstruction can be effectively relieved in younger patients with stenting, subpulmonic stenosis is typically a surgical problem. Although valvar pulmonic stenosis is very amenable to balloon dilation, conduit stenosis, bioprosthetic pulmonary valve dysfunction, and main and branch pulmonary artery stenoses can all benefit from treatment via transcatheter techniques.

PULMONARY VALVE STENOSIS

Balloon valvuloplasty is the treatment of choice for isolated pulmonary valve stenosis if the valve is mobile and doming. The original catheter based technique was initially described by Rubio and Limon-Lason in 1956.[4] The currently used percutaneous static balloon valvuloplasty technique was first reported by Kan and colleagues[5] in

1982. This procedure has proven safe and efficacious over the past 2 decades, making balloon valvuloplasty the treatment of choice for valvular pulmonary stenosis.[6–8] Although the presence of a dysplastic or heavily calcified pulmonary valve (especially with supravalvular narrowing) is associated with less ideal outcomes with this technique,[6] these patients remain as candidates for pulmonary valvuloplasty.

Nearly 15% of patients with pulmonary stenosis have dysplastic valves. These valves can be distinguished from the mobile doming cases by the absence of a pulmonary ejection sound on physical examination or by noninvasive imaging modalities such as echocardiography or MRI.

Infundibular or subinfundibular RV outflow tract obstruction from hypertrophied myocardium is not amenable to balloon angioplasty. Transcatheter stent deployment has shown limited efficacy for relief of muscular subpulmonary stenosis. In some patients with pulmonary valvular and subvalvular obstruction, relief of the valvular stenosis is often accompanied by gradual regression of the subvalvular hypertrophy and a decrease in the degree of obstruction.[9] In the absence of valvar pulmonary stenosis, medical management with beta-blockers can be attempted; however, surgical relief is frequently needed.

Transcatheter balloon valvuloplasty is the treatment of choice in symptomatic patients with isolated mobile pulmonary valve stenosis if the Doppler-estimated peak instantaneous gradient is 36 mm Hg or greater or in asymptomatic patients with more severe stenosis (gradient $\geq$64 mm Hg).[8,10,11] Peak gradients of less than 36 mm Hg typically do not increase with age, and survival is not curtailed; accordingly, there is no indication for intervention.[11] The technique for pulmonary valvuloplasty has changed little since early reports; however, technological advancements resulting in low-profile catheters have decreased the likelihood of vascular entry site injury. The measurement of the pulmonary valve annulus diameter is an important step before proceeding with balloon selection. The desired balloon/annulus ratio is 1.2 to 1.4.[12] Balloon/annulus ratios that exceed 1.5 risk rupturing the pulmonary valve annulus.[13] If the pulmonary annulus is too large for dilatation with a single balloon, 2 balloons can be used. When using 2 balloons, the combined diameters of the 2 balloons ideally should be 1.2 times the optimal diameter of a single balloon.[14] Two balloons have the advantage of less trauma at the venous access site, success with larger diameter pulmonary valves, and potential decompression of the right ventricle during valvuloplasty through gaps between the balloons.

Published reports of short- and long-term outcomes have been favorable.[6,7,15] In a study of 25 consecutive adolescents and adults, Sharieff and colleagues[15] achieved procedural success in 80% with an immediate decrease in peak gradient from a mean of 94 mm Hg to 34 mm Hg. The peak gradient decreased further over 3 years to a mean of 19 mm Hg, mainly owing to regression of infundibular hypertrophy. The VACA registry investigators gathered follow-up data on 533 patients who underwent balloon pulmonary valvuloplasty.[7] Over 8 years of follow-up, 23% of patients had a suboptimal outcome, as judged by either a residual peak systolic gradient of 36 mm Hg or greater or the need for further transcatheter or surgical intervention. Predictors of suboptimal outcome included elevated immediate postprocedure gradient (odds ratio, 1.32 per 10 mm Hg increase), a lower ratio of balloon to annulus diameter, and a dysplastic valve. Restenosis is rare. Pulmonary regurgitation is common and is hemodynamically well-tolerated.[16] Compared with surgical valvotomy, transcatheter balloon valvuloplasty results in lower mortality and morbidity and hence is now considered the standard of care with surgery relegated to those with failed transcatheter interventions or incompatible anatomy.[8,17] Although the residual systolic gradients are higher with balloon valvuloplasty versus surgical valvotomy, there is less regurgitation.

PULMONARY ARTERY STENOSIS

Supravalvular pulmonary artery stenosis may occur in isolation, but is most often associated with other lesions such as tetralogy of Fallot. Branch pulmonary artery stenosis often occurs after surgical shunt placement. Native pulmonary artery stenosis can be found in patients with William's, Noonan's, and Alagille's syndromes, or in patients exposed to rubella infection in utero. The indications for transcatheter or surgical intervention in pulmonary artery stenosis include lesions that result in elevation of RV systolic pressure or those that result in relative underperfusion of a lung segment.[19] Surgical repair of pulmonary artery stenosis is possible, but the results are frequently suboptimal, particularly if the lesions are peripheral. Lock and colleagues[19] first described a percutaneous static balloon angioplasty technique for the treatment of peripheral pulmonary artery stenosis in 1983. An adequate result depends on the use of sufficiently large high-pressure balloons that tear the vascular intima and part of the media, leaving a slim safety margin for this procedure.[20]

Elastic recoil of the angioplastied segment is common with balloon angioplasty alone, prompting the use of stents.[21] The success rate of transcatheter intervention for peripheral pulmonary stenosis is increased from 70% with balloon angioplasty alone to 90% with the use of stents.[20,21] Cutting balloons are more effective than static balloons in relieving peripheral stenoses that cannot be stented.[22] In general, the first and second arcade branches of the pulmonary arteries are usually effectively treated with stents. Diffuse peripheral pulmonary stenosis can be a very difficult problem for which there is no surgical option (short of lung transplantation). Patients with multiple distal stenosis often require multiple balloon dilations. In some patients, thorough and aggressive dilation of these stenoses can decrease the RV pressure; however, care must be taken to avoid rupture of the distal pulmonary vasculature.

PULMONARY VALVE REPLACEMENT

The single most common application of transcatheter valve replacement in adult CHD is in prosthetic pulmonary valve dysfunction, RV to pulmonary artery conduit failure or the dysfunctional RV outflow tract. The vast majority of adult patients with CHD requiring transcatheter pulmonary valve replacement (TCPVR) are those with repaired tetralogy of Fallot. Other etiologies include congenital pulmonary valve stenosis that has been surgically intervened upon with resultant pulmonary regurgitation, those with repaired truncus arteriosus with subsequently dysfunctional RV to pulmonary artery conduits, and those with congenital aortic valve pathology that have undergone the Ross operation and subsequently developed conduit dysfunction. Among those with tetralogy of Fallot, surgical intervention in infancy is typically performed to patch the VSD and to relieve RV outflow tract obstruction. In those with pulmonary atresia, placement of a RV to pulmonary artery conduit is typical, whereas among those with pulmonary valve stenosis and hypoplastic annulus, surgical relief of the obstruction is often achieved by dividing the annulus of the pulmonary valve and patch augmentation of the RV outflow tract. In past decades, transannular patch augmentation was widely used and therefore this surgical variant is commonly encountered in the adult CHD population, resulting in predominant pulmonary regurgitation and large and often aneurysmal RV outflow tracts. In contrast, patients who have undergone surgical conduit placement (typically using a valved aortic or pulmonic homograft) present with predominant conduit stenosis or mixed stenosis and regurgitation. Adult patients with CHD born with pulmonary atresia have typically undergone multiple surgical procedures for the placement or replacement of conduits and many have eventually undergone bioprosthetic pulmonary valve replacement. The number of surgical procedures performed correlates with an increase in arrhythmia risk and risk of heart failure.[23] Although the indications and timing of PVR, be it surgical or transcatheter, remain controversial, it is widely accepted that those with severe stenosis and exercise limitation will benefit with subsequent improvement in exercise capacity.[8,24] In adult patients with CHD with predominant pulmonary regurgitation, the 2018 American College of Cardiology/American Heart Association adult CHD guidelines recommend consideration of valve replacement in symptomatic patients or those with evidence of RV or left ventricular systolic dysfunction, severe RV enlargement with an indexed RV end-diastolic volume of greater than 160 mL/m^2, or an indexed RV end-systolic volume of greater than 80 mL/m^2 and those with decreases in exercise capacity.[8]

Homograft conduits, either aortic or pulmonary, have been used extensively since the 1960s and are often present in adult patients with CHD. Progressive dysfunction occurs in the majority of homografts and most require replacement within 15 years from implantation, sooner if implanted in

a young child[25] (**Fig. 1**). Heavily calcified aortic homografts are prone to dissection and rupture if aggressively dilated with high-pressure balloons or to beyond their original implantation size and therefore covered stent platforms are often used to decrease the risk of uncontained rupture. Pulmonary homografts typically are not as extensively calcified, but do have a tendency to dilate with resultant regurgitation. Pulmonary homografts can often be dilated to a slightly larger diameter than the original implant diameter if deemed imperative. Infective endocarditis is a serious concern and may have occurred in up to 10% of patients with dysfunctional homografts being considered for intervention; a prior history of endocarditis, immunocompromise, and residual stenosis after TCPVR are risk factor for endocarditis after TCPVR.[26–29] Surgical placement of stented bioprosthetic valves is widely used in adult patients with CHD with dysfunctional conduits and native RV outflow tracts. As with conduits, bioprosthetic valves have a finite life span and the majority require replacement within 15 years of implantation. A dysfunctional bioprosthetic valve provides an ideal landing zone for TCPVR, often referred to as a valve in valve procedure and is associated with excellent outcomes[30,31] (**Fig. 2**). Balloon-expandable transcatheter valves are now widely used to replace dysfunctional atrioventricular bioprosthesis with high success rates and minimal complications (**Fig. 3**). In the presence of

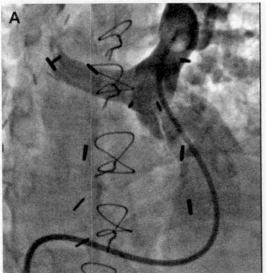 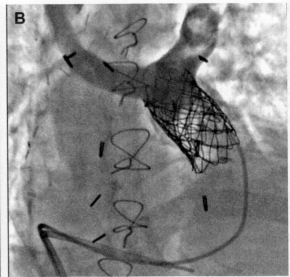

Fig. 1. A 28-year old patient with pulmonary atresia and major aortopulmonary collateral arteries status post bilateral unifocalization and RV to pulmonary artery aortic homograft with progressive stenosis and regurgitation. (*A*) Left pulmonary artery angiogram demonstrating severe pulmonary regurgitation with flow reversal to the right ventricle. (*B*) Status post covered stent placement followed by Melody valve placement with resolution of pulmonary regurgitation.

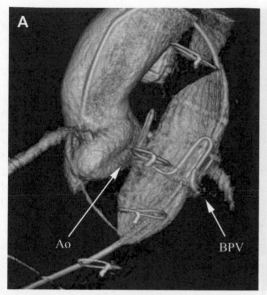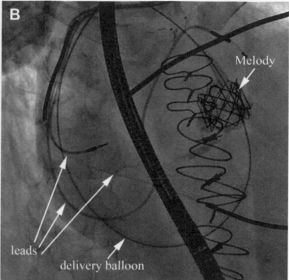

Fig. 2. (*A*) Three-dimensional (3D) rotational aortic angiography with 3D reconstruction during high pressure balloon dilation of a bioprosthetic pulmonary valve (BPV). Note the distortion of the aortic root (Ao). (*B*) Fluoroscopic image post Melody valve placement from a jugular venous approach in a 68 year old man with repaired tetralogy of Fallot, interrupted inferior vena cava, advanced left ventricular failure with biventricular resynchronization and multiple intracardiac leads.

undersized bioprosthetic valves that were placed in childhood, a valve in valve procedure can still be performed by increasing the size of the bioprosthetic valve with the use of high pressure balloons to fracture the valve ring.[32]

In the current era of TCPVR, the most widely used valves in adult CHD in the United States are the Melody valve (Medtronic Minneapolis, MN) and Edwards Sapien Valve (Edwards Lifesciences, Irvine, CA). The Melody valve is a bovine jugular vein cuff and valve sewn onto a platinum iridium stent frame. The valve sizes range from 18 to 22 mm but the valve functions well with a greater range of implant diameters (12–24 mm). The Edwards Sapien valve is now in its third generation; the first generation is no longer available commercially. The second-generation Sapien XT is approved by the US Food and Drug Administration for use in dysfunctional conduits and a prospective trial was just concluded assessing the Sapien S3 in both conduits and bioprosthetic valves (COMPASSION S3 Clinical Trial NCT02744677). Both the XT and S3 are made of bovine pericardial tissue hand sewn onto a cobalt chromium stent platform with the addition of an expanded polytetrafluoroethylene cuff or skirt on the S3 model around the base. The Sapien valves range in size from 20 to 29 mm and are deployed through an expandable sheath design. The larger diameter of the Sapien valves allow for the treatment of conduits, bioprosthesis, and native RV

outflow tracts that exceed 24 mm in diameter and therefore cannot be treated with the Melody valve. Both valve platforms are associated with excellent short- and intermediate-term outcomes.[27,33–35] Stent fracture has been noted to be a problem with the Melody valve, especially when prestenting is not performed within conduits or native RV outflow tracts, prestenting does not seem to be necessary in bioprosthetic valves given the presence of a metallic or plastic ring within which the stent platform can be protected from compressive forces.[36] The Sapien valve's cobalt chromium stent frame is significantly more durable, able to withstand high compressive forces, and not prone to fracture; therefore, prestenting before Sapien valve implantation does not seem to be necessary.[37,38] It is imperative to evaluate for coronary arterial compression before valve implantation because coronary compression can occur in approximately 6% of patients.[39] High-risk substrates for coronary artery compression include those with anomalous coronary arterial anatomy and patients with surgically reimplanted coronary arteries.

The treatment of large diameter (>30 mm) native RV outflow tracts is especially challenging, given that the largest commercially available balloon expandable TCPVR platforms are the 29-mm Sapien XT or Sapien 3 valves. The 29-mm Sapien 3 valve can be expanded beyond its nominal diameter by overinflation, with additional volume with

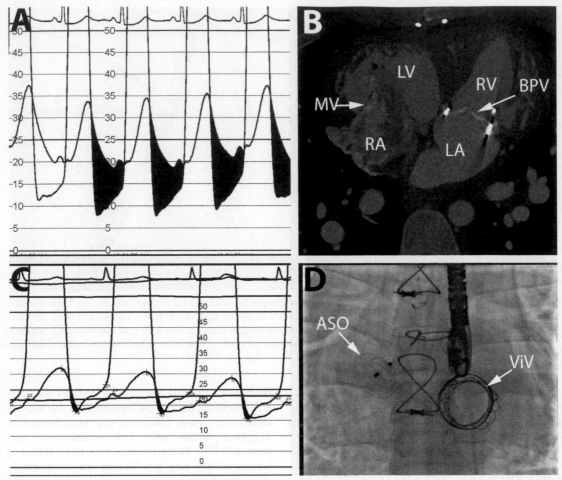

Fig. 3. A 33-year-old with congenitally corrected transposition of the great arteries status post surgical left atrioventricular valve replacement with a bioprosthetic bovine valve (BPV) that has become severely stenotic. (*A*) Simultaneous left atrial (LA) and RV pressures with a mean diastolic gradient of 9 mm Hg. (*B*) Electrocardiogram-gated computed tomography angiogram demonstrating decreased opening of a thickened and partially calcified BPV. In contrast, note the wide opening of the mitral valve between the right atrium (RA) and the subpulmonic left ventricle. (*C*) After trans-septal transcatheter placement of a 29-mm Sapien 3, there is no longer a resting mean diastolic gradient across the valve. (*D*) Fluoroscopic en-face view of the Sapien 3 valve within the dysfunctional BPV (valve in valve procedure [ViV]). The large fenestration created within the atrial septum by passage of a 26F sheath was closed with an Amplatzer septal occluder (ASO). MV, mitral valve.

an eventual maximal outer diameter of 31 mm. Hybrid surgical plication of the pulmonary artery can be considered via a sternotomy or thoracotomy to establish a landing zone for TCPVR.[40] The Venus P Valve (Venus Medtech, Hangzhuo, China) and the Harmony valve (Medtronic), are self-expanding covered hourglass-shaped RV outflow tract reducer platforms with the valve in the central waist, both valves are currently in clinical trials. Edwards Life Sciences has developed a self-expanding RV outflow tract reducer that does not house a valve platform, the Alterra adaptive RV outflow tract reducer. The Sapien 3 29 mm valve is subsequently implanted (during same procedure or during a separate procedure) within the Alterra

RV outflow tract reducer. This system is currently in clinical trial testing (**Fig. 4**).

Coarctation of the Aorta

Both native and recurrent coarctations of the aorta in adult patients with CHD are usually discrete narrowings beyond the subclavian artery; however, more diffuse forms of the disease may also be encountered, including the presence of a hypoplastic arch or a gothic angulation of the arch. A significant coarctation is defined as having a resting peak to peak gradient of 20 mm Hg or greater.[41] However, significant arterial collaterals may result in unimpressive gradients in those

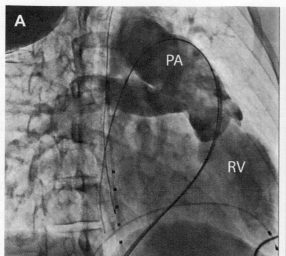
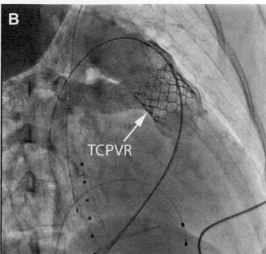

Fig. 4. (A) Severe pulmonary regurgitation in a patient with native RV outflow tract. Note the reflux of contrast from the pulmonary artery to the right ventricle (RV). (B) After placement of the Alterra adaptive stent with subsequent TCPVR with a 29-mm Sapien 3.

with significant aortic narrowing, additionally, those with poor ventricular systolic function may have lower gradients.

Transcatheter balloon angioplasty of aortic coarctation was initially performed in 1982 by Singer and colleagues.[42] This treatment has been applied to discrete native and recurrent narrowing of the descending aorta with a high immediate success rate; however, aortic wall complications occurred in 23% of patients and reobstruction occurred in 19%.[43–46] An alternative treatment option is stent implantation, first

reported by Suarez de Lezo and colleagues[47] in 1995. Open and closed cell design stents and covered stent platforms are now widely used in preference to balloon angioplasty alone (**Fig. 5**). The immediate results are excellent with a low risk of complications (<5%) and a low risk of aortic wall injury (3.1%), the intermediate reobstruction rate is 15%; however, the majority of these are mild restenosis.[43] Intermediate results demonstrate the 3-year freedom from reintervention ranges from 73% to 88% and the rate of aneurysm formation is relatively low.[48,49] The availability of

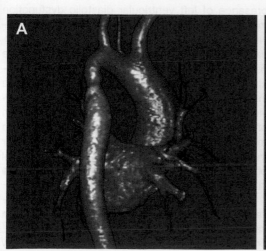
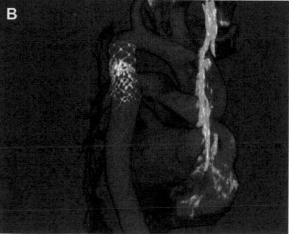

Fig. 5. (A) MRI angiography with 3-dimensional volume rendering, right posterior projection, demonstrating severe recurrent coarctation in a patient that had undergone surgical end-to-end repair in infancy. (B) Computed tomography angiography, similar projection, after covered Cheatham platinum stent placement and EV-3 Mega LD open cell uncovered stent placement with complete resolution of aortic narrowing.

covered balloon and self-expanding stent platforms may further improve the safety profile of stents and allow for exclusion of aneurysms.[50]

OCCLUSION DEVICES
Patent Ductus Arteriosus

The ductus arteriosus, a communication between the aorta and pulmonary artery, may persist in a wide variety of sizes and forms.[51] PDA closure is indicated in patients with left-to-right shunting who are symptomatic of heart failure or asymptomatic patients with left heart enlargement.[41,52] In adults (and children) with PDA, the outcomes after closure have been very good, including in select patients with moderately increased pulmonary artery pressure and resistance.[53] The Eisenmenger syndrome remains a contraindication to closure. Some authors have advocated the use of temporary balloon occlusion to demonstrate the hemodynamic tolerability of duct closure.[54] Reactivity of the pulmonary vascular bed to pulmonary vasodilating agents and/or a decrease in pulmonary artery pressure and resistance with test balloon occlusion portend a positive outcome with device occlusion. Indications for closure of a small PDA without significant shunting are not well-established and the closure of the silent ductus remains a source of debate. Endarteritis is a rare complication in the current era, but has been reported.[55,56] The closure of all PDAs can be accomplished via catheterization with minimal morbidity and a high rate of success.[57] Currently available devices include coils which are used for closure of small sized PDAs and multiple occlusion devices, including the Amplatzer duct occlude (approved in the United States), Occlutech PDA device, and a variety of Chinese Amplatzer like devices not approved in the United States[58–62] (see **Fig. 7**). The Nit-Occlud device (pfm Medical, Cologne, Germany) is a coil-type device with a controlled delivery system that is the successor to the hourglass-shaped nitinol coil.

Patients with medial aortic wall abnormalities, as in Marfan syndrome and older patients with calcified PDA, should be approached cautiously. PDA occlusion may be performed with aortic covered stent placement.[63] Patients with PDA and pulmonary hypertension but acceptable pulmonary vascular resistance (<6 Woods units) can be closed using an Amplatzer Muscular VSD device to decrease risk of device embolization.

Atrial Septal Defects

ASD is one of the most commonly encountered congenital heart malformations in the adult. The treatment of secundum type ASD has changed drastically over the last 2 decades. Surgical closure had been the preferred treatment since the inception of cardiopulmonary bypass. Although the operative outcomes are excellent, surgical closure carries the risk of complications.[64] Transcatheter device closure has now supplanted surgery as the standard therapy for most secundum ASDs. Accurate defect sizing, determination of adequate rims, and the exclusion of associated cardiac anomalies are the cornerstones to successful percutaneous defect closure.[65] Transthoracic and transesophageal echocardiography are widely used to screen defects for closure and rule out partial anomalous pulmonary venous connections.[66–68] Intracardiac echocardiography has also been advocated as a method for both selection of septal occluder size and for guidance during transcatheter closure.[69,70]

Survival into adulthood is the rule; however, life expectancy is not normal in the patient with an unrepaired defect, with mortality increasing by 6% per year after age 40.[71,72] Progressive dyspnea on exertion and palpitations frequently present in adulthood owing to progressive right heart dilation and dysfunction, pulmonary hypertension, tricuspid regurgitation, and atrial arrhythmias. The degree of left-to-right shunt increases with age as left ventricular compliance decreases and systemic arterial resistance increases. Indications for ASD closure include the presence of significant shunting ad defined by calculating a Qp:Qs of 1.5:1.0 or greater and/or the presence of right heart enlargement on transthoracic echocardiography in the presence of normal or low pulmonary vascular resistance.[41] Defect closure in older adults seems to be beneficial; however, the presence of left ventricular diastolic dysfunction may result in increased left atrial pressure after device closure of ASD. Therefore, careful hemodynamic assessment of the left atrial pressure before closure and during temporary balloon occlusion of the defect is of paramount importance in such patients. The use of fenestrated ASD devices may help in such patients.[73] The exclusion of patients with severe pulmonary hypertension may be obviated by pulmonary artery vasodilator therapy that may decrease pulmonary arterial pressure and resistance, permitting shunt closure in these patients.[74,75]

Advancements in device design and catheterization technology have led to the availability of a variety of transcatheter occlusion devices.[76,77] Transcatheter device closure compares favorably with surgical closure in terms of efficacy and is associated with shorter hospital stays and fewer postprocedural complications.[78] Although the details of the procedure vary depending on the

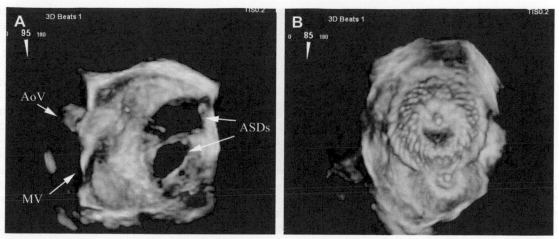

Fig. 6. (*A*) Three-dimensional transesophageal echocardiogram, left atrial view demonstrating 2 large ostium secundum type ASDs, the aortic valve (AoV) and the mitral valve (MV) are labeled for orientation. (*B*) After closure with 2 Amplatzer septal occlude devices (ASD).

device used, in general the procedure is performed under fluoroscopic and transesophageal or intracardiac echocardiographic guidance. Published results vary with each device, but in general, complete closure is achieved in 60% to 90% of cases within hours of deployment, with 80% to 100% closure over 1 year of follow-up.[79] The Amplatzer septal occluder (AGA Medical, Plymouth, MN) remains the most widely used ASD closure device in the United States (**Fig. 6**). The long-term outcomes of device closure using the Amplatzer septal occluder are excellent.[80] Amplatzer septal occluders ranging from 4 to 38 mm have been approved by the US Food and Drug Administration; a 40-mm device is available outside the United States and has been successfully used

but there is an increased risk of device embolization.[81] All device types risk rare short-term complications of embolization, thrombus formation, aortic root perforation, pericardial effusion, and dysrhythmias. A variety of devices from W. L. Gore & Associates (Flagstaff, AZ), including the Helex septal occluder, the Cardioform septal occluder, and most recently the Gore Cardioform ASD occluder, can be used for effective ASD closure.[82] Sporadic cases of late erosions have been reported with both the Amplatzer and Gore devices.[83,84] Patients who had received Amplatzer septal occluders with perforation were more likely to have a deficient anterior–superior rim and had received larger device to unstretched defect diameter.[84]

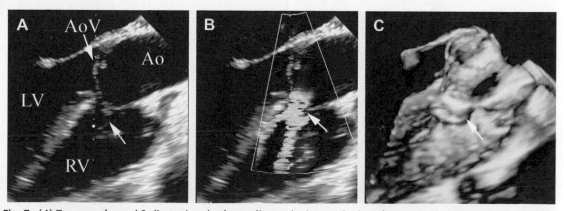

Fig. 7. (*A*) Transesophageal 2-dimensional echocardiography long axis view demonstrating a communication between the aorta (Ao) and the right ventricle (RV) (*white arrow*) above the aortic valve (AoV) via a prolapsing aortic root sinus. (*B*) Color Doppler image demonstrating flow from the Ao to the RV via the ruptured right coronary sinus. (*C*) Three-dimensional transesophageal echocardiography after device closure of the ruptured sinus of Valsalva with an Amplatzer muscular VSD device (*white arrow*).

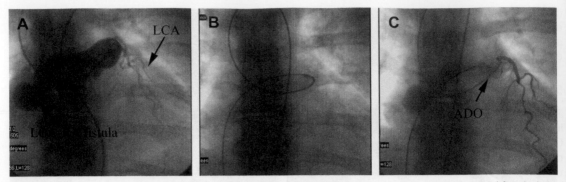

Fig. 8. (*A*) Coronary angiography demonstrating a severely dilated left coronary artery to right atrial fistula (LCA-RA fistula). There are small branches of the LCA emerging from the fistula. (*B*) A wire rail is created from the femoral artery to the femoral vein allowing for advancement of a sheath from the right atrial into the fistula. (*C*) Placement of an Amplatzer duct occluder (ADO) into the fistula.

Ventricular Septal Defects

Although transcatheter device closure of ASD is widely accepted and now considered standard of care (discussed elsewhere in this article), closure of a VSD presents certain challenges that have required careful device modification. These challenges include the variable thickness of the ventricular septum, the variable location of many VSDs, the high pressures in the ventricles, and the close proximity of the aortic valve and conduction tissue to the membranous septum. VSD closure devices must avoid interference with valve function and the conduction system, and they must not produce arrhythmias, hemolysis, or device migration.[18]

The Amplatzer muscular VSD occluder (Abbott Laboratories, Chicago, IL) is in many ways similar to the Amplatzer ASD occlusion device; a Dacron polyester patch placed inside 2 nitinol disks connected by a waist. The Amplatzer muscular VSD occluder has demonstrated safety and efficacy in the closure of congenital and acquired (eg, after a myocardial infarction) muscular VSDs.[85–88] Other Amplatzer occlusion devices are also used for VSD closure, closure of ruptured sinus of Valsalva aneurysms (see **Fig. 6**) and other high-flow communications (**Fig. 7**), including the Amplatzer Duct Occluder, the vascular plugs, and the Amplatzer septal occluder. Closure of perimembranous VSDs is feasible but the development of conduction abnormalities is a major concern[89]

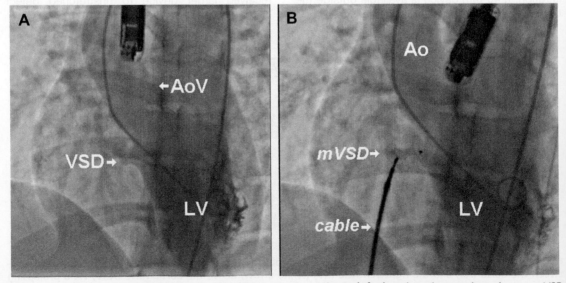

Fig. 9. (*A*) Left ventricular (LV) angiography demonstrating right to left shunting via a perimembranous VSD below the level of the aortic valve (AoV). (*B*) LVA angiography after muscular VSD device (mVSD) placement. The device is still attached to the delivery cable.

(Figs. 8 and 9). Closure of membranous VSDs associated with aneurysms of the ventricular septum is feasible and safe with a low risk of conduction system abnormalities.[90]

SUMMARY

Transcatheter interventions have become an indispensable tool in the treatment of adults with CHD. From closure of intracardiac and extracardiac communications to replacement of dysfunctional valves, the growing armamentarium of transcatheter tools is supplanting traditional surgical approaches. The next decade promises exponential advances in valve replacement and repair techniques, further refinement of stent and occlusion device technology, and an expanding role for transcatheter treatment of adults with CHD.

DISCLOSURE

Dr Aboulhosn is a consultant and proctor for Edwards Lifesciences, a consultant for Medtronic Inc and Abbott Pharmaceuticals. Dr Hijazi is a consultant for Occlutech and Numed, he is a speaker for Venus and Medtech.

REFERENCES

1. Moons P, Bovijn L, Budts W, et al. Temporal trends in survival to adulthood among patients born with congenital heart disease from 1970 to 1992 in Belgium. Circulation 2010;122:2264–72.
2. Gilboa SM, Salemi JL, Nembhard WN, et al. Mortality resulting from congenital heart disease among children and adults in the United States, 1999 to 2006. Circulation 2010;122:2254–63.
3. King TD, Thompson SL, Steiner C, et al. Secundum atrial septal defect. Nonoperative closure during cardiac catheterization. JAMA 1976;235:2506–9.
4. Rubio V, Limon-Lason R. Treatment of pulmonary valvular stenosis and tricuspid stenosis using a modified catheter. Arch Inst Cordiol Mexico 1952; 23:183–92.
5. Kan JS, White RI Jr, Mitchell SE, et al. Percutaneous balloon valvuloplasty: a new method for treating congenital pulmonary valve stenosis. N Engl J Med 1982;307:540–2.
6. Stanger P, Cassidy SC, Girod DA, et al. Balloon pulmonary valvuloplasty: results of the valvuloplasty and angioplasty of congenital anomalies registry. Am J Cardiol 1990;65:775–83.
7. McCrindle BW. Independent predictors of long-term results after balloon pulmonary valvuloplasty. Valvuloplasty and Angioplasty of Congenital Anomalies (VACA) Registry investigators. Circulation 1994;89: 1751–9.
8. Stout KK, Daniels CJ, Aboulhosn JA, et al. 2018 AHA/ACC guideline for the management of adults with congenital heart disease: a report of the American College of Cardiology/American Heart Association task force on clinical practice guidelines. J Am Coll Cardiol 2019;73:e81–192.
9. Fawzy ME, Galal O, Dunn B, et al. Regression of infundibular pulmonary stenosis after successful balloon pulmonary valvuloplasty in adults. Cathet Cardiovasc Diagn 1990;21:77–81.
10. Allen HD, Beekman RH 3rd, Garson A Jr, et al. Pediatric therapeutic cardiac catheterization: a statement for healthcare professionals from the Council on cardiovascular disease in the young, American Heart Association. Circulation 1998;97:609–25.
11. Hayes CJ, Gersony WM, Driscoll DJ, et al. Second natural history study of congenital heart defects. Results of treatment of patients with pulmonary valvar stenosis. Circulation 1993;87:I28–37.
12. Rao PS. Transcatheter treatment of pulmonary outflow tract obstruction: a review. Prog Cardiovasc Dis 1992;35:119–58.
13. Ring JC, Kulik TJ, Burke BA, et al. Morphologic changes induced by dilation of the pulmonary valve anulus with overlarge balloons in normal newborn lambs. Am J Cardiol 1985;55:210–4.
14. Butto F, Amplatz K, Bass JL. Geometry of the proximal pulmonary trunk during dilation with two balloons. Am J Cardiol 1986;58:380–1.
15. Sharieff S, Shah-e-Zaman K, Faruqui AM. Short- and intermediate-term follow-up results of percutaneous transluminal balloon valvuloplasty in adolescents and young adults with congenital pulmonary valve stenosis. J Invasive Cardiol 2003;15:484–7.
16. Rao PS, Galal O, Patnana M, et al. Results of three to 10 year follow up of balloon dilatation of the pulmonary valve. Heart 1998;80:591–5.
17. O'Connor BK, Beekman RH, Lindauer A, et al. Intermediate-term outcome after pulmonary balloon valvuloplasty: comparison with a matched surgical control group. J Am Coll Cardiol 1992;20:169–73.
18. Schneider DJ, Levi DS, Serwacki MJ, et al. Overview of interventional pediatric cardiology in 2004. Minerva Pediatr 2004;56:1–28.
19. Lock JE, Castaneda-Zuniga WR, Fuhrman BP, et al. Balloon dilation angioplasty of hypoplastic and stenotic pulmonary arteries. Circulation 1983;67:962–7.
20. Nakanishi T, Tobita K, Sasaki M, et al. Intravascular ultrasound imaging before and after balloon angioplasty for pulmonary artery stenosis. Catheter Cardiovasc Interv 1999;46:68–78.
21. Nakanishi T. Balloon dilatation and stent implantation for vascular stenosis. Pediatr Int 2001;43:548–52.
22. Magee AG, Wax D, Saiki Y, et al. Experimental branch pulmonary artery stenosis angioplasty using a novel cutting balloon. Can J Cardiol 1998;14: 1037–41.

23. Khairy P, Aboulhosn J, Gurvitz MZ, et al. Arrhythmia burden in adults with surgically repaired tetralogy of Fallot: a multi-institutional study. Circulation 2010; 122:868–75.

24. Lurz P, Nordmeyer J, Giardini A, et al. Early versus late functional outcome after successful percutaneous pulmonary valve implantation: are the acute effects of altered right ventricular loading all we can expect? J Am Coll Cardiol 2011;57:724–31.

25. Kaza AK, Lim HG, Dibardino DJ, et al. Long-term results of right ventricular outflow tract reconstruction in neonatal cardiac surgery: options and outcomes. J Thorac Cardiovasc Surg 2009;138:911–6.

26. Lluri G, Levi DS, Miller E, et al. Incidence and outcome of infective endocarditis following percutaneous versus surgical pulmonary valve replacement. Catheter Cardiovasc Interv 2018;91:277–84.

27. McElhinney DB, Benson LN, Eicken A, et al. Infective endocarditis after transcatheter pulmonary valve replacement using the Melody valve: combined results of 3 prospective North American and European studies. Circ Cardiovasc Interv 2013;6:292–300.

28. Sadeghi S, Wadia S, Lluri G, et al. Risk factors for infective endocarditis following transcatheter pulmonary valve replacement in patients with congenital heart disease. Catheter Cardiovasc Interv 2019;94: 625–35.

29. McElhinney DB, Sondergaard L, Armstrong AK, et al. Endocarditis after transcatheter pulmonary valve replacement. J Am Coll Cardiol 2018;72:2717–28.

30. Gillespie MJ, Rome JJ, Levi DS, et al. Melody valve implant within failed bioprosthetic valves in the pulmonary position: a multicenter experience. Circ Cardiovasc Interv 2012;5:862–70.

31. Finch W, Levi DS, Salem M, et al. Transcatheter melody valve placement in large diameter bioprostheses and conduits: what is the optimal "Landing zone"? Catheter Cardiovasc Interv 2015; 86:E217–23.

32. Shahanavaz S, Asnes JD, Grohmann J, et al. Intentional fracture of bioprosthetic valve frames in patients undergoing valve-in-valve transcatheter pulmonary valve replacement. Circ Cardiovasc Interv 2018;11:e006453.

33. Kenny D, Rhodes JF, Fleming GA, et al. 3-year outcomes of the Edwards SAPIEN transcatheter heart valve for conduit failure in the pulmonary position from the COMPASSION multicenter clinical trial. JACC Cardiovasc Interv 2018;11:1920–9.

34. Cheatham JP, Hellenbrand WE, Zahn EM, et al. Clinical and hemodynamic outcomes up to 7 years after transcatheter pulmonary valve replacement in the US melody valve investigational device exemption trial. Circulation 2015;131:1960–70.

35. Sinha S, Aboulhosn J, Asnes J, et al. Initial results from the off-label use of the SAPIEN S3 valve for percutaneous transcatheter pulmonary valve replacement: a multi-institutional experience. Catheter Cardiovasc Interv 2019;93:455–63.

36. McElhinney DB, Cheatham JP, Jones TK, et al. Stent fracture, valve dysfunction, and right ventricular outflow tract reintervention after transcatheter pulmonary valve implantation: patient-related and procedural risk factors in the US Melody Valve Trial. Circ Cardiovasc Interv 2011;4:602–14.

37. Ghobrial J, Levi DS, Aboulhosn J. Native right ventricular outflow tract transcatheter pulmonary valve replacement without pre-stenting. JACC Cardiovasc Interv 2018;11:e41–4.

38. Morgan GJ, Sadeghi S, Salem MM, et al. SAPIEN valve for percutaneous transcatheter pulmonary valve replacement without "pre-stenting": a multi-institutional experience. Catheter Cardiovasc Interv 2019;93:324–9.

39. Morray BH, McElhinney DB, Cheatham JP, et al. Risk of coronary artery compression among patients referred for transcatheter pulmonary valve implantation: a multicenter experience. Circ Cardiovasc Interv 2013;6:535–42.

40. Suleiman T, Kavinsky CJ, Skerritt C, et al. Recent development in pulmonary valve replacement after tetralogy of Fallot repair: the emergence of hybrid approaches. Front Surg 2015;2:22.

41. Stout KK, Daniels CJ, Aboulhosn JA, et al. 2018 AHA/ACC guideline for the management of adults with congenital heart disease: executive summary: a report of the American College of Cardiology/ American Heart Association Task Force on clinical practice guidelines. J Am Coll Cardiol 2019;73: 1494–563.

42. Singer MI, Rowen M, Dorsey TJ. Transluminal aortic balloon angioplasty for coarctation of the aorta in the newborn. Am Heart J 1982;103:131–2.

43. Forbes TJ, Kim DW, Du W, et al. Comparison of surgical, stent, and balloon angioplasty treatment of native coarctation of the aorta: an observational study by the CCISC (Congenital Cardiovascular Interventional Study Consortium). J Am Coll Cardiol 2011;58:2664–74.

44. Lock JE, Bass JL, Amplatz K, et al. Balloon dilation angioplasty of aortic coarctations in infants and children. Circulation 1983;68:109–16.

45. Kan JS, White RI Jr, Mitchell SE, et al. Treatment of restenosis of coarctation by percutaneous transluminal angioplasty. Circulation 1983;68:1087–94.

46. McCrindle BW, Jones TK, Morrow WR, et al. Acute results of balloon angioplasty of native coarctation versus recurrent aortic obstruction are equivalent. Valvuloplasty and Angioplasty of Congenital Anomalies (VACA) Registry Investigators. J Am Coll Cardiol 1996;28:1810–7.

47. Suarez de Lezo J, Pan M, Romero M, et al. Balloon-expandable stent repair of severe coarctation of aorta. Am Heart J 1995;129:1002–8.

48. Fletcher SE, Nihill MR, Grifka RG, et al. Balloon angioplasty of native coarctation of the aorta: midterm follow-up and prognostic factors. J Am Coll Cardiol 1995;25:730–4.

49. Ovaert C, McCrindle BW, Nykanen D, et al. Balloon angioplasty of native coarctation: clinical outcomes and predictors of success. J Am Coll Cardiol 2000; 35:988–96.

50. Taggart NW, Minahan M, Cabalka AK, et al. Immediate outcomes of covered stent placement for treatment or prevention of aortic wall injury associated with coarctation of the aorta (COAST II). JACC Cardiovasc Interv 2016;9:484–93.

51. Krichenko A, Benson LN, Burrows P, et al. Angiographic classification of the isolated, persistently patent ductus arteriosus and implications for percutaneous catheter occlusion. Am J Cardiol 1989;63: 877–80.

52. Fisher RG, Moodie DS, Sterba R, et al. Patent ductus arteriosus in adults–long-term follow-up: nonsurgical versus surgical treatment. J Am Coll Cardiol 1986;8: 280–4.

53. Pas D, Missault L, Hollanders G, et al. Persistent ductus arteriosus in the adult: clinical features and experience with percutaneous closure. Acta Cardiol 2002;57:275–8.

54. Roy A, Juneja R, Saxena A. Use of Amplatzer duct occluder to close severely hypertensive ducts: utility of transient balloon occlusion. Indian Heart J 2005; 57:332–6.

55. Balzer DT, Spray TL, McMullin D, et al. Endarteritis associated with a clinically silent patent ductus arteriosus. Am Heart J 1993;125:1192–3.

56. Parthenakis H, Kanakaraki MK, Vardas PE. Images in cardiology: silent patent ductus arteriosus endarteritis. Heart 2000;84:619.

57. Schneider DJ, Moore JW. Patent ductus arteriosus. Circulation 2006;114:1873–82.

58. Moore JW, Khan M. Gianturco coil occlusion of patent ductus arteriosus. Curr Interv Cardiol Rep 2001; 3:80–5.

59. Pass RH, Hijazi Z, Hsu DT, et al. Multicenter USA Amplatzer patent ductus arteriosus occlusion device trial: initial and one-year results. J Am Coll Cardiol 2004;44:513–9.

60. Masura J, Tittel P, Gavora P, et al. Long-term outcome of transcatheter patent ductus arteriosus closure using Amplatzer duct occluders. Am Heart J 2006;151. 755.e7- 755.e10.

61. Eicken A, Balling G, Gildein HP, et al. Transcatheter closure of a non-restrictive patent ductus arteriosus with an Amplatzer muscular ventricular septal defect occluder. Int J Cardiol 2006;117(1):e40–2.

62. Spies C, Ujivari F, Schrader R. Transcatheter closure of a 22 mm patent ductus arteriosus with an Amplatzer atrial septal occluder. Catheter Cardiovasc Interv 2005;64:352–5.

63. Sadiq M, Malick NH, Qureshi SA. Simultaneous treatment of native coarctation of the aorta combined with patent ductus arteriosus using a covered stent. Catheter Cardiovasc Interv 2003;59:387–90.

64. Du ZD, Hijazi ZM, Kleinman CS, et al. Comparison between transcatheter and surgical closure of secundum atrial septal defect in children and adults: results of a multicenter nonrandomized trial. J Am Coll Cardiol 2002;39:1836–44.

65. Varma C, Benson LN, Silversides C, et al. Outcomes and alternative techniques for device closure of the large secundum atrial septal defect. Catheter Cardiovasc Interv 2004;61:131–9.

66. Cooke JC, Gelman JS, Harper RW. Echocardiologists' role in the deployment of the Amplatzer atrial septal occluder device in adults. J Am Soc Echocardiogr 2001;14:588–94.

67. Magni G, Hijazi ZM, Pandian NG, et al. Two- and three-dimensional transesophageal echocardiography in patient selection and assessment of atrial septal defect closure by the new DAS-Angel Wings device: initial clinical experience. Circulation 1997; 96:1722–8.

68. Carcagni A, Presbitero P. Transcatheter closure of secundum atrial septal defects with the Amplatzer occluder in adult patients. Ital Heart J 2002;3:182–7.

69. Butera G, Chessa M, Bossone E, et al. Transcatheter closure of atrial septal defect under combined transesophageal and intracardiac echocardiography. Echocardiography 2003;20:389–90.

70. Zanchetta M, Rigatelli G, Pedon L, et al. Transcatheter atrial septal defect closure assisted by intracardiac echocardiography: 3-year follow-up. J Interv Cardiol 2004;17:95–8.

71. Perloff JK. Ostium secundum atrial septal defect–survival for 87 and 94 years. Am J Cardiol 1984; 53:388–9.

72. Campbell M. Natural history of atrial septal defect. Br Heart J 1970;32:820–6.

73. Abdelkarim A, Levi DS, Tran B, et al. Fenestrated Transcatheter ASD closure in adults with diastolic dysfunction and/or pulmonary hypertension: case series and review of the literature. Congenit Heart Dis 2016;11:663–71.

74. Schwerzmann M, Zafar M, McLaughlin PR, et al. Atrial septal defect closure in a patient with "irreversible" pulmonary hypertensive arteriopathy. Int J Cardiol 2006;110:104–7.

75. Bradley EA, Ammash N, Martinez SC, et al. Treat-to-close": non-repairable ASD-PAH in the adult: results from the North American ASD-PAH (NAAP) multicenter registry. Int J Cardiol 2019;291:127–33.

76. Banerjee A, Bengur AR, Li JS, et al. Echocardiographic characteristics of successful deployment of the Das AngelWings atrial septal defect closure device: initial multicenter experience in the United States. Am J Cardiol 1999;83:1236–41.

77. Walsh KP, Tofeig M, Kitchiner DJ, et al. Comparison of the Sideris and Amplatzer septal occlusion devices. Am J Cardiol 1999;83:933–6.

78. Du ZD, Koenig P, Cao QL, et al. Comparison of transcatheter closure of secundum atrial septal defect using the Amplatzer septal occluder associated with deficient versus sufficient rims. Am J Cardiol 2002;90:865–9.

79. Rao PS. Comparative summary of atrial septal defect occlusion devices. Philadelphia: Lippincott, Williams & Wilkins; 2003.

80. Masura J, Gavora P, Podnar T. Long-term outcome of transcatheter secundum-type atrial septal defect closure using Amplatzer septal occluders. J Am Coll Cardiol 2005;45:505–7.

81. Lopez K, Dalvi BV, Balzer D, et al. Transcatheter closure of large secundum atrial septal defects using the 40 mm Amplatzer septal occluder: results of an international registry. Catheter Cardiovasc Interv 2005;66:580–4.

82. de Hemptinne Q, Horlick EM, Osten MD, et al. Initial clinical experience with the GORE((R)) CARDIO-FORM ASD occluder for transcatheter atrial septal defect closure. Catheter Cardiovasc Interv 2017; 90:495–503.

83. Kumar P, Orford JL, Tobis JM. Two cases of pericardial tamponade due to nitinol wire fracture of a gore septal occluder. Catheter Cardiovasc Interv 2019. https://doi.org/10.1002/ccd.28596.

84. Amin Z, Hijazi ZM, Bass JL, et al. Erosion of Amplatzer septal occluder device after closure of secundum atrial septal defects: review of registry of complications and recommendations to minimize future risk. Catheter Cardiovasc Interv 2004;63: 496–502.

85. Chessa M, Carminati M, Cao QL, et al. Transcatheter closure of congenital and acquired muscular ventricular septal defects using the Amplatzer device. J Invasive Cardiol 2002;14:322–7.

86. Thanopoulos BD, Karanassios E, Tsaousis G, et al. Catheter closure of congenital/acquired muscular VSDs and perimembranous VSDs using the Amplatzer devices. J Interv Cardiol 2003;16:399–407.

87. Holzer R, Balzer D, Cao QL, et al. Device closure of muscular ventricular septal defects using the Amplatzer muscular ventricular septal defect occluder: immediate and mid-term results of a U.S. registry. J Am Coll Cardiol 2004;43:1257–63.

88. Holzer R, Balzer D, Amin Z, et al. Transcatheter closure of postinfarction ventricular septal defects using the new Amplatzer muscular VSD occluder: results of a U.S. Registry. Catheter Cardiovasc Interv 2004;61:196–201.

89. Holzer R, de Giovanni J, Walsh KP, et al. Transcatheter closure of perimembranous ventricular septal defects using the Amplatzer membranous VSD occluder: immediate and midterm results of an international registry. Catheter Cardiovasc Interv 2006;68: 620–8.

90. Pedra CA, Pedra SR, Esteves CA, et al. Percutaneous closure of perimembranous ventricular septal defects with the Amplatzer device: technical and morphological considerations. Catheter Cardiovasc Interv 2004;61:403–10.

Adults with Congenital Heart Disease and Arrhythmia Management

Jeremy P. Moore, MD, MS[a,b,*], Paul Khairy, MD, PhD[c,d]

KEYWORDS

- Adult congenital heart disease • Intra-atrial reentrant tachycardia • Ventricular tachycardia
- Catheter ablation • Sinus node dysfunction • Sudden cardiac death • Pacemaker
- Implantable cardioverter-defibrillator

KEY POINTS

- Atrial tachyarrhythmias are the most common rhythm disturbances in adult congenital heart disease (ACHD) and are characterized by a gradual transition from intra-atrial reentrant tachycardia to atrial fibrillation over the lifetime of the individual.
- Ventricular tachyarrhythmia and sudden cardiac death occur up to 100 times more frequently among ACHD than acquired heart disease.
- Cardiac resynchronization is an important adjunctive therapy for select ACHD patients with heart failure and electrical dyssynchrony.
- There have been major advances in rhythm management for ACHD in recent years, stemming from a combination of technologic and technical innovations.

 Video content accompanies this article at http://www.cardiology.theclinics.com.

OVERVIEW

A rapid expansion of the population of adults with congenital heart disease (ACHD) and arrhythmia has given rise to the specialty of ACHD electrophysiology. ACHD patients experience rhythm abnormalities that are often poorly tolerated and require advanced medical or interventional therapies. Common examples are the bradyarrhythmias of sinus node dysfunction and atrioventricular (AV) block, the tachyarrhythmias of intra-atrial reentrant tachycardia, atrial fibrillation, and ventricular tachycardia (VT), and pathologic electrical delay resulting in "ventricular dyssynchrony" (**Fig. 1**). In addition, primary prevention of sudden cardiac death is indicated in many situations. This article reviews the pathophysiology, clinical characteristics, and treatment strategies for these commonly encountered arrhythmias among ACHD.

SINUS NODE DYSFUNCTION

Sinus node dysfunction (SND) is prevalent in ACHD, primarily because of the cumulative effects of atrial distention and fibrosis from abnormal hemodynamics and direct surgical trauma to the sinoatrial nodal complex or its vascular supply. Patients at particular risk include those who have undergone the Mustard or Senning operation[1,2] and cavopulmonary shunts. SND after the Mustard operation, for instance, has been reported to be as great as 50% at

[a] Ahmanson-UCLA/Adult Congenital Heart Disease Center, Los Angeles, CA, USA; [b] Department of Pediatrics, UCLA Medical Center, Los Angeles, CA, USA; [c] Electrophysiology Service and Adult Congenital Heart Disease Center; [d] Department of Medicine, Montreal Heart Institute, Université de Montreal, 5000 Bélanger Street, Montreal, Quebec H1T 1C8, Canada
* Corresponding author. 100 Medical Plaza Drive, Suite 770, Los Angeles, CA 90095.
E-mail address: jpmoore@mednet.ucla.edu

Cardiol Clin 38 (2020) 417–434
https://doi.org/10.1016/j.ccl.2020.04.006
0733-8651/20/Published by Elsevier Inc.

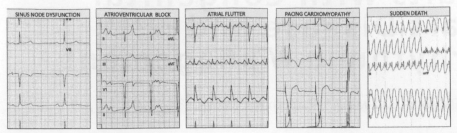

| SINUS NODE DYSFUNCTION | ATRIOVENTRICULAR BLOCK | ATRIAL FLUTTER | PACING CARDIOMYOPATHY | SUDDEN DEATH |

Fig. 1. Summary of the major forms of rhythm disturbance among patients with adult congenital heart disease.

20 years after surgery.[2] Both the lateral tunnel and extracardiac total cavopulmonary connection (TCPC) operations are associated with an approximately 15% risk of SND at 10 years after surgery.[3] Maintenance of sinus rhythm is important for optimal Fontan physiology,[4] and SND has been implicated in manifestations of Fontan failure (eg, plastic bronchitis or protein-losing enteropathy) that may be reversible with restoration of atrial-based rhythm.[5]

Indications for pacing in the setting of SND are firstly symptom based, but may also be guided by significant bradycardia.[6] Transvenous pacing is usual for patients who are remote from surgery unless there are unacceptable impediments to this approach (eg, limited access to the atrial myocardium or residual intracardiac shunt).[7] Many perceived barriers can be overcome by innovative techniques. For instance, transhepatic-transbaffle approaches have been described, and transvenous atrial pacing after extracardiac Fontan operation is technically feasible by transpulmonary puncture.[8,9] (**Fig. 2**). Long-term outcomes of these unconventional strategies remain to be determined, particularly with regard to complications such as bleeding, lead migration, and hepatic function (with transhepatic approaches), and concerns regarding lead extractions in the event of infection. Surgical pacing is typically used if there is known SND at the time of operation or when converting an older style of Fontan to TCPC.[10]

ATRIOVENTRICULAR BLOCK

AV block may occur either spontaneously or as an iatrogenic sequela of operative repair for ACHD. Spontaneous AV block is notably seen in congenitally corrected transposition of the great arteries (CCTGA), where superior displacement of the AV node results in a long and tenuous nonbranching conducting bundle.[11,12] The annual incidence of spontaneous AV block in CCTGA is reported to be approximately 2%.[13] Other important congenital defects associated with spontaneous

AV block include AV septal defects and atrial septal defects.[14] Surgical iatrogenic AV block has become less common with advanced surgical techniques, but can occur when suture lines are placed in the vicinity of the AV conduction system.

More recently, leadless cardiac pacing has emerged as an option to avoid problems associated with conventional pacing. These include intravascular infection, lead fracture, and venous thrombosis. Among ACHD, additional concerns include preservation of AV valve function and thromboembolic risk (**Fig. 3**).[15] Importantly, current leadless pacing systems are capable of pacing and sensing only the ventricular myocardium

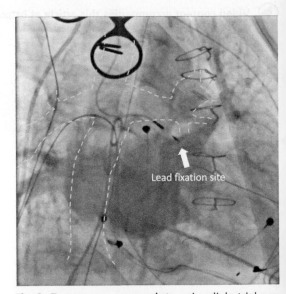

Fig. 2. Transvenous approach to epicardial atrial pacing for an extracardiac Fontan patient. Dotted white lines represent the course of the Fontan pathway. The pacing lead has been placed from the right subclavian vein, through the Glenn anastomosis, and into the pulmonary artery. Puncture into the extracardiac space was performed and the lead affixed to the atrial epi-myocardium. This approach can be used for patients in whom a surgical thoracotomy is undesirable.

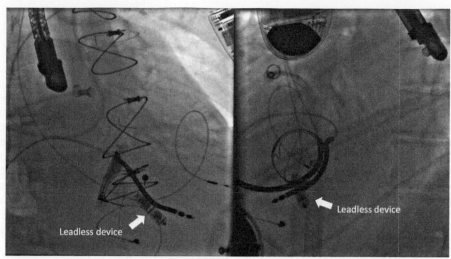

Fig. 3. Placement of a leadless cardiac pacemaker from the femoral approach in a patient with permanent atrial fibrillation and atrioventricular block after tricuspid valve replacement. The prior ICD lead had failed after being entrapped during the valve surgery, leaving the patient with a slow ventricular escape rhythm. The leadless pacemaker was implanted to avoid future disruption of tricuspid valve function.

and are therefore limited in their application. Future technology intends to identify atrial contraction from intracardiac accelerometer waveforms, permitting maintenance of AV synchrony and expanding the currently limited leadless pacemaker implant indications.[16]

CARDIAC RESYNCHRONIZATION THERAPY

Spontaneous or pacing-induced electrical delay develops frequently among patients with congenital heart disease (CHD). Abnormal electrical excitation can result in inefficient myocardial energetics, with early contraction and simultaneous systolic stretch of opposing ventricular walls. For acquired heart disease, cardiac resynchronization therapy (CRT) has been shown to promote reverse ventricular remodeling, improve quality of life, and decrease mortality.[17]

Among patients with ACHD and a systemic left ventricle, there is evidence that CRT is beneficial for both spontaneous or pacing-induced types of left ventricular (LV) electromechanical delay,[18] but there are fewer data for other forms of CHD. In a limited fashion, CRT has also been evaluated in the context of failure of the subpulmonary right ventricle, the systemic right ventricle, and the single ventricle.

Subpulmonary Right Ventricle

Subpulmonary right ventricular (RV) dysfunction is not uncommon among patients with tetralogy of Fallot and related variants, where right bundle branch block can contribute to ventricular dyssynchrony, often in combination with hemodynamic derangements of the pulmonary or tricuspid valve(s). Initially, pacing studies were limited to acute improvement in RV systolic function in the catheterization laboratory or in the postoperative setting.[19,20] More recently, long-term improvement in New York Heart Association class and objective measures of aerobic capacity have been demonstrated,[21] along with indices of RV remodeling.[22] In general, strategies involve lead fixation at the site of latest RV endocardial activation to achieve fusion with intrinsic AV conduction. Currently CRT for the subpulmonary right ventricle carries a class IIb indication based on limited data.[6]

Systemic Right Ventricle

A significant proportion of patients with d-transposition of the great arteries (DTGA) after the Senning or Mustard operation or unrepaired or physiologically repaired CCTGA carry a CRT indication based on current guidelines.[23] The feasibility and potential benefits of CRT for the systemic right ventricle were initially demonstrated for CCTGA patients undergoing concomitant surgery,[24] and since then various multicenter[18,25,26] and single-center studies have shown potential benefit. Although most have reported a favorable response, a notable minority have reported either very poor response[26] or even clinical deterioration.[27] Accordingly, there remains uncertainty as to the role of CRT for the systemic right ventricle, and this topic has been identified as a high-impact research question in recent ACHD clinical practice guidelines.[28]

An important consideration for systemic RV resynchronization is the route of implantation. For patients with CCTGA, the cardiac veins are anomalous in ~20% of patients, with ectopic location, duplication, and atresia reported.[29] Despite this, successful cannulation and CRT lead placement via a posteroseptal coronary sinus ostium can be achieved in most patients, with alternative cannulation techniques for the remainder (Fig. 4).[30] In rare CCTGA and most Mustard or Senning patients, epicardial lead placement may be required and can be approached via lateral thoracotomy or lower midline sternotomy, respectively.[31]

Single Ventricle

Electrical dyssynchrony, especially resulting from permanent ventricular pacing, has been shown to be associated with progressive AV valve regurgitation, ventricular systolic dysfunction, and reduced transplant-free survival among patients with single-ventricle anatomy.[32,33] Echocardiographic characterization of mechanical contraction in the form of classic-pattern dyssynchrony may be useful for a subset of patients who are most likely to respond favorably to CRT.[34] Although both multisite pacing[35] and single ventricular apical pacing[32]

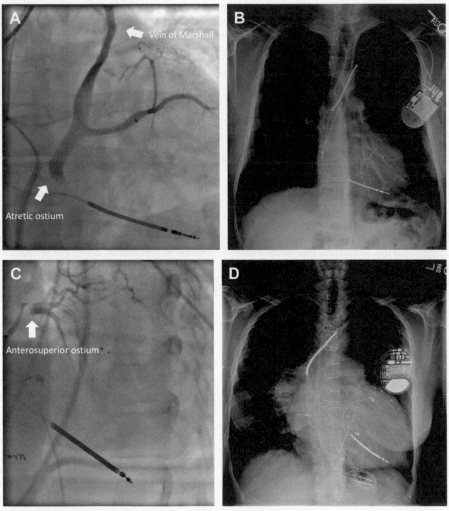

Fig. 4. Transvenous cardiac resynchronization therapy lead placement for patients with CCTGA with absent or diminutive posteroseptal coronary sinus ostia (CSO). (*A, B*) Intraprocedural lead placement and postoperative radiograph for a patient with atresia of the posterior CSO. A lead was placed through a persistent vein of Marshall that drained the coronary venous circulation. (*C, D*) Identical views of a patient with a diminutive conventional posterior CSO with lead placement through a large vein at the base of the right atrial appendage.

have been proposed as strategies to improve long-term clinical outcomes, data are lacking, and the optimal approach to resynchronization for the single-ventricle patient remains unknown.

CONDUCTION SYSTEM PACING

Recently, direct His-bundle pacing has been shown to be a physiologic alternative to CRT in acquired heart disease. This approach circumvents many of the challenges encountered in conventional CRT that include inadequate coronary venous tributaries, elevated ventricular pacing threshold, phrenic nerve capture, and lead dislodgment, among others. His-bundle pacing may be particularly useful for ACHD patients with, or at high risk for, pacing-induced cardiomyopathy, especially when combined with challenging coronary sinus anatomy such as CCTGA (**Fig. 5**).[30] To date, only isolated case reports demonstrate the feasibility of His-bundle pacing for CCTGA[36–38] and further data are needed before there is widespread endorsement of this approach. This issue was the topic of a recent multicenter investigation conducted by the joint Pediatric and Congenital Electrophysiology Society and International Society of Adult Congenital Heart Disease Electrophysiology Research Collaboration.[39]

SUPRAVENTRICULAR TACHYCARDIA
Intra-Atrial Reentrant Tachycardia

Intra-atrial reentrant tachycardia (IART) is the most common tachyarrhythmia observed among patients with ACHD, with a cumulative incidence approaching 50% by the age of 65 years.[40] The development of IART is associated with multiple adverse clinical outcomes including stroke, heart failure, and all-cause mortality.[40,41] Of patients developing IART, those with DTGA and Mustard or Senning baffles, pulmonary hypertension, valvular heart disease, and single-ventricle anatomy face the highest mortality risk.[41,42]

In many cases, IART is the cumulative effect of diffuse injury to the atrial myocardium and maturation of surgical barriers, both highly prevalent in ACHD.[43] Importantly, long-term antiarrhythmic drug therapy for maintenance of sinus rhythm and ventricular rate control for IART are generally considered only moderately effective strategies in ACHD. Instead, 3 principal management strategies are useful for maintenance of sinus rhythm.

Catheter ablation
D-transposition of the great arteries after the Mustard or Senning operation IART in the setting of DTGA after the Mustard or Senning operation is frequently associated with a relatively slow atrial rate owing to extensive areas of diseased myocardium and robust AV node conduction. This can result in 1:1 atrial-ventricular conduction, and together with an inherently compromised systemic right ventricle may be associated with degeneration to malignant ventricular arrhythmia.[42] IART circuits for these patients are usually biatrial or situated within the morphologic right atrium, which is separated from the venous circulation by a

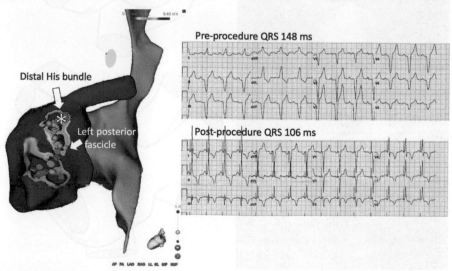

Distal His bundle

Left posterior fascicle

Pre-procedure QRS 148 ms

Post-procedure QRS 106 ms

Fig. 5. A patient with CCTGA and heart block who developed pacing-induced cardiomyopathy after conventional dual-chamber pacemaker placement. The morphologic left conduction system was mapped and a lead was affixed to the distal His bundle (*asterisk*). The QRS duration decreased following this procedure, and the heart failure resolved.

surgical baffle. This chamber can therefore be approached by direct baffle puncture or by a retrograde course.[44,45]

Most frequently, IART circuits develop around the tricuspid valve annulus.[46] Additional reentrant circuits have been shown to depend on the underlying surgical anatomy. After the Mustard operation, for instance, reentry around a morphologic right atrial free wall atriotomy or patch is common, whereas reentry around the right pulmonary veins and the nearby surgical counterincision is observed after the Senning operation (**Fig. 6**, Video 1).[47–49] The mapping procedure entails thorough evaluation of the entire morphologic right atrium to target all reentry circuits and reduce the risk for possible recurrent tachycardia. Ultrahigh-density mapping may play a role in more precise circuit delineation so that these substrates may be comprehensively targeted.[50] Other substrates that are often observed include focal atrial tachycardias and AV nodal reentry tachycardia.[47,51] Tachycardia recurrence after IART ablation is reportedly 30%,[46,47] but a more contemporary study involving comprehensive circuit delineation using high-density mapping is lacking.

Fontan operation The modified atriopulmonary Fontan operation is associated with massive right atrial enlargement owing to long-standing venous hypertension. The incidence of IART after this surgery has been estimated to be 50% at 20 postoperative years. Surgical placement of the atrial baffle, the anastomosis from the morphologic right atrium to the pulmonary artery, and the atriotomy incision may also serve as electrical barriers for reentry (**Fig. 7**, Video 2).[43,52] Moreover, reentry around the systemic AV annulus and a dilated inferior vena cava may also occur, resulting in multiple potential circuits in any given individual.[53,54] Evaluation for periannular reentry usually requires baffle puncture when present.[45] Extreme atrial muscle hypertrophy after the atriopulmonary Fontan operation[55] can challenge the

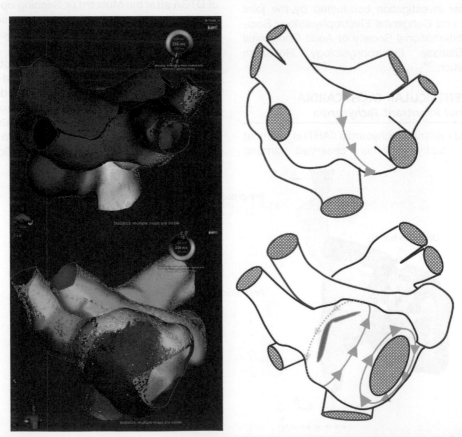

Fig. 6. Demonstration of intra-atrial reentry circuits after Senning operation. The leftward panels demonstrate ultrahigh-density activation mapping and the rightward panels a schematic view. There are simultaneous or "dual-loop" wavefronts around the right pulmonary veins and nearby surgical incision as well as the tricuspid valve annulus.

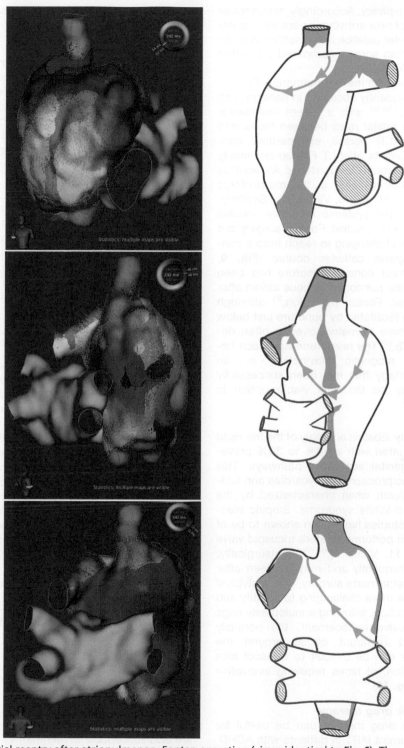

Fig. 7. Intra-atrial reentry after atriopulmonary Fontan operation (views identical to **Fig. 6**). The patient had previously undergone catheter ablation of periannular, septal, and caval circuits. There was a residual wavefront using scar on the posterior wall of the massively dilated morphologic right atrium that passed between the superior vena cava and atriopulmonary anastomosis.

limits of lesion delivery. Accordingly, recurrences and the onset of new arrhythmias are more common after catheter ablation in the setting of atriopulmonary Fontan surgery compared with other forms of ACHD.

In comparison with the atriopulmonary Fontan, IART is less frequently observed in patients with TCPC surgery,[3,56,57] with a recent multicenter study showing similar rates between those with lateral tunnel (LT) versus extracardiac conduits.[58] IART circuits after LT Fontan commonly involve reentry around the systemic AV annulus as well as atriotomy scar in the morphologic right atrial free wall (**Fig. 8**, Video 3).[59] Similarly, circuits around the systemic AV valve annulus are seen after extracardiac Fontan surgery but are much more challenging to reach from a conventional prograde catheter course (**Fig. 9**, Video 4).[60] Direct conduit puncture has been used to reach the pulmonary venous atrium after the extracardiac Fontan operation,[61] although access can be facilitated by puncture just below the conduit where cavoatrial overlap often develops (**Fig. 10**).[62] The retrograde approach using remote magnetic navigation is an alternative strategy that has been successfully used and may be the only viable option in some cases.[63]

Ebstein anomaly Ebstein anomaly of the tricuspid valve is associated with a 20% to 30% prevalence of congenital accessory pathways. This can result in reciprocating tachycardias and sudden cardiac death when characterized by the Wolff-Parkinson-White syndrome. Empiric electrophysiology studies have been shown to be of high yield when performed before tricuspid valve surgery (**Fig. 11**, Video 5).[64,65] Postsurgically, IART occurs frequently and may be seen after modified right atrial maze surgery, where atypical circuits may be more challenging to identify and ablate.[66] In addition, following annuloplasty rings or tricuspid valve replacement, the normally straightforward reentrant circuit around the tricuspid valve can be difficult to transect with catheter ablation, at times requiring innovative techniques (**Fig. 12**).[67]

Antiarrhythmic drug therapy

Antiarrhythmic drug therapy can be useful for control of recurrent IART in patients with ACHD. The most successful for maintenance of sinus rhythm are those with class III properties, owing to their efficacy for the prevention of reentry.[68–70] Catheter ablation is generally preferable to long-term antiarrhythmic drug therapy in patients with ACHD given their potential proarrhythmic side effects, limited effectiveness, and end-organ toxicities.[6]

Antitachycardia pacing

Antitachycardia pacing can result in acute termination of IART through antidromic penetration into the tachycardia circuit, thereby abolishing electrical propagation through wavefront collision. Although initial case reports were concerning for acceleration of the tachycardia and degeneration to malignant ventricular arrhythmia,[71] recent single-center studies have suggested both safety and efficacy of this approach for patients with ACHD.[72,73]

Of the available therapeutic strategies, catheter ablation has realized the most dramatic improvements over the past several decades. Although no randomized trials exist or are likely to take place, early and aggressive catheter ablation therapy is likely to be the optimal approach for most patients with ACHD at experienced centers.

ATRIAL FIBRILLATION

Atrial fibrillation (AF) has been increasingly recognized as being of major importance for the aging ACHD population, with estimates that are 20 times higher than the age-matched population.[74] AF surpasses IART as the predominant atrial tachyarrhythmia after 50 years of age with progression to more persistent forms with time.[75] ACHD at high risk include single ventricle, left-sided obstructive lesions, and palliated CHD.[76] To date, catheter ablation as a definitive therapy for AF using radiofrequency or cryothermal energy is effective but suboptimal, with recurrences reported between 40% and 50% after 1 year at experienced centers.[77–79]

ARRHYTHMIA/SUDDEN CARDIAC DEATH
Ventricular Tachycardia

Sustained monomorphic VT can develop in the setting of various CHD lesions and may result in hemodynamic instability or sudden cardiac death (SCD). Although tetralogy of Fallot is best characterized, VT after multiple forms of ACHD has been described. The VT mechanism after surgical repair is most often reentry (70%–80%).[80,81] Interestingly, unoperated patients with Ebstein anomaly are also susceptible to reentrant VT using intrinsic scar within the atrialized portion of the right ventricle.[82]

After tetralogy of Fallot surgery, postoperative scar predisposes to reentrant VT through a limited number of anatomic isthmuses.[83,84] Conduction slowing has been shown to be a

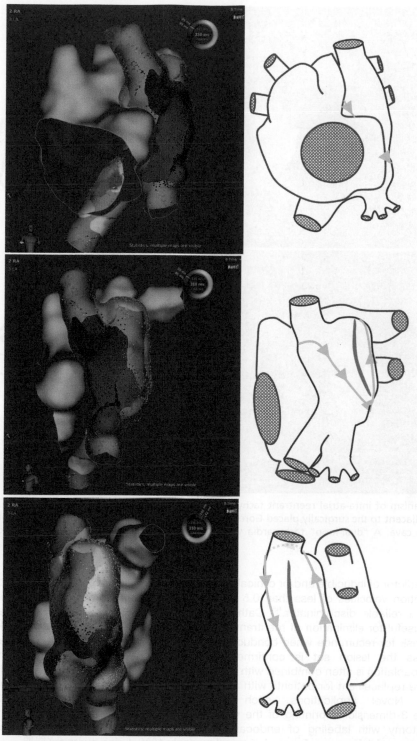

Fig. 8. Intra-atrial reentry after lateral tunnel Fontan in situs inversus. A wavefront using both portions of the morphologic right atrium is depicted. Catheter ablation at a narrow channel between an atriotomy and the inferior vena cava eliminated the tachycardia.

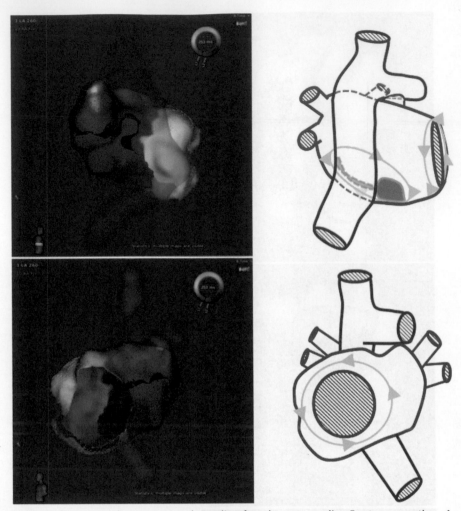

Fig. 9. Mechanism of intra-atrial reentrant tachycardia after the extracardiac Fontan operation. An atriotomy was found adjacent to the surgically placed GoreTex tube that extended down to the remnant of the oversewn inferior vena cava. A "dual-loop" tachycardia was active around the free wall atriotomy and the tricuspid annulus.

powerful predictor of inducible and/or clinical VT, with conduction velocities of less than 0.5 m/s serving as a reliable discriminator.[85] Catheter ablation is useful for elimination of reentrant VT with a low risk for recurrence when conduction block across the lesion set is confirmed.[86] Surgical cryoablation is often combined with pulmonary valve replacement for patients with clinical VT.[87] Novel applications, such as preoperative 3-dimensional printing of the ventricular anatomy with labeling of endocardial scar, may be useful for more focused surgical VT ablation (**Fig. 13**).

Sudden Cardiac Death

Mortality in CHD has experienced a shift from childhood to adulthood over the past several decades,[88] of which SCD is a major contributor. SCD is the mode of death in approximately 20% to 30% of ACHD mortalities, surpassed only by heart failure.[89–93] The overall risk of SCD in ACHD is between 25 and 100 times higher than that of the general population of comparable age.[94] This risk is progressive with time and is strongly associated with congenital lesion complexity.[92] The mechanism of SCD is VT/ventricular fibrillation in 80% of ACHD patients with approximately 70% of events occurring at rest (only 10% during exercise).[90,95]

Factors that have been associated with SCD among ACHD patients include increased QRS duration and fragmentation, conduction disturbances and delayed repolarization, pulmonary hypertension, supraventricular tachycardia, and

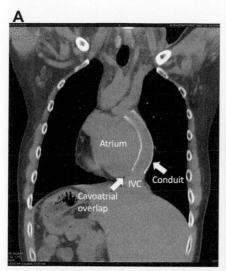 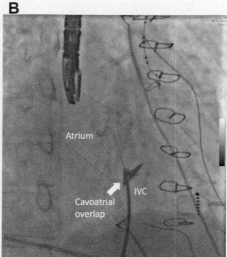

Fig. 10. Transcaval puncture for access to the pulmonary venous atrium after extracardiac Fontan for recurrent intra-atrial reentrant tachycardia. (*A*) Preoperative computed tomography angiogram demonstrating a region of overlap between the inferior vena cava and the pulmonary venous atrium. (*B*) Fluoroscopy demonstrates contrast in the region of overlap. Contrast is injected through the needle tip into the pulmonary venous atrium before the sheath and dilator are advanced.

impaired ventricular systolic function.[89,95,96] In particular, progression of QRS duration, QT dispersion, and ventricular dysfunction are highly predictive of SCD events.[97] Nonsustained VT (NSVT) has not been shown to be predictive of SCD for the general ACHD population, in contradistinction to its predictive value for tetralogy of Fallot.[95,98,99]

The ACHD lesions at greatest risk for SCD include those with a systemic right ventricle, single ventricle, or cyanotic forms CHD that include Eisenmenger syndrome[91,94,100,101] and tetralogy of Fallot. More recently, postoperative Ebstein anomaly has been reported to be associated with a relatively high risk for SCD based on the experience of a single center that included nearly 1000 patients.[102] With the exception of tetralogy of Fallot, clinical risk scores for these lesions are limited.

Sudden death in tetralogy of Fallot was recognized as a consequence of ventricular arrhythmia as early as the mid 1970s. Many predictors have been identified over the last several decades. These have included QRS duration, surgical technique and timing, indices of RV and LV systolic function, degree and complexity of ventricular rhythms as recorded by Holter monitoring, and, more recently, RV mass z score and LV ejection fraction.[103] Importantly, NSVT and increased LV end-diastolic pressure have been shown to be strong predictors of appropriate ICD shocks in a large population of patients with tetralogy of

Fallot[99] and can be used in the calculation of baseline SCD risk. A Bayesian approach to risk stratification for primary-prevention ICD placement has been suggested for the tetralogy of Fallot population, for whom programmed ventricular stimulation is useful when the pretest probability of SCD lies between 1% and 11.5%.[104]

At present, expert consensus guidelines have been endorsed in the form of a joint statement from the Pediatric and Congenital Electrophysiology and Heart Rhythm Societies in 2014,[6] which were largely adopted by the European Society of Cardiology.[105] These guidelines provide a primary-prevention approach to the ACHD patient at risk for SCD, providing evidence-based recommendations for ICD placement. Unfortunately, current risk-stratification schemes are limited to a small subset of patients at elevated SCD risk.[106] An ongoing prospective study is under way to validate a proposed risk-stratification score that is based on clinical factors identified from the CONCOR registry among a diverse group of ACHD patients.[107]

Implantable Cardioverter-Defibrillators

To date, the only treatment strategy that has been shown to effectively prevent SCD in ACHD population remains the implantable cardioverter-defibrillator (ICD). In general, ACHD patients experience a relatively high proportion of both appropriate and inappropriate ICD shocks in

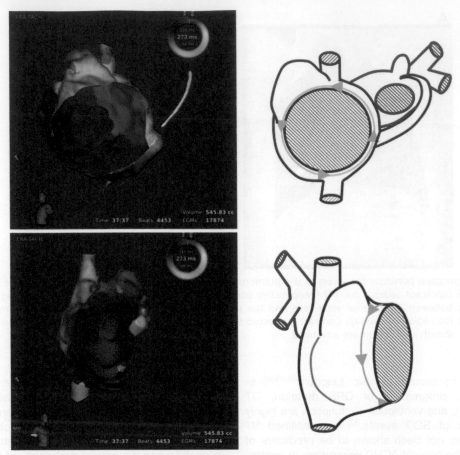

Fig. 11. Preoperative mapping of intra-atrial reentry before surgical valve repair in a patient with Ebstein anomaly. Massive right atrial enlargement is present with perpetuation of counterclockwise reentry around the tricuspid annulus owing to long conduction course rather than discrete slowing.

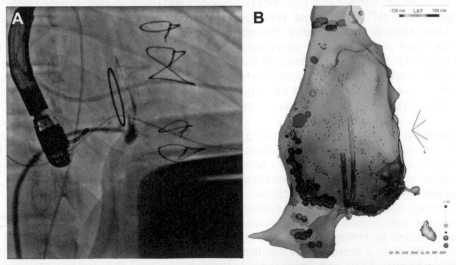

Fig. 12. Subvalvular catheter ablation for a patient with Ebstein anomaly who had previously undergone surgical tricuspid valve replacement. Recurrent intra-atrial reentrant tachycardia that was resistant to catheter ablation in the region of the tricuspid valve. (*A*) Needle puncture below the prosthetic valve. (*B*) Location of successful subvalvular catheter ablation on the 3-dimensional electroanatomic map.

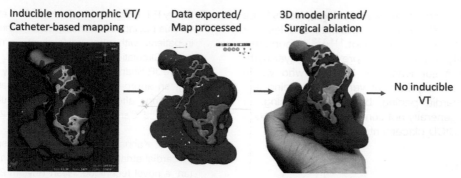

Inducible monomorphic VT/
Catheter-based mapping

Data exported/
Map processed

3D model printed/
Surgical ablation

No inducible
VT

Fig. 13. Example of 3-dimensional (3D) printing for operative planning of tetralogy of Fallot. The procedural 3D map of a patient with clinical sustained monomorphic ventricular tachycardia (VT) with pulmonary valve dysfunction is shown. The 3D print was created to assist with concomitant surgical cryoablation of the RV free wall, after which VT was no longer inducible.

comparison with patients with acquired forms of heart disease.[108] Conventional ICD placement involves a subcutaneous or submuscular pulse generator with intravascular leads for both detection of ventricular arrhythmia and delivery of high-voltage defibrillation shocks. Such ICD therapies are highly effective for termination of malignant ventricular arrhythmia in this population.

Importantly, transvenous ICD placement may not be possible for many forms of ACHD owing to unique anatomic constraints. Examples include superior baffle occlusion after the Mustard operation for DTGA, prior TCPC Fontan surgery, and significant right-to-left intracardiac shunting as observed in the Eisenmenger syndrome. For such patients, the subcutaneous ICD (SICD) may serve as an alternative option (**Fig. 14**).[109,110] The

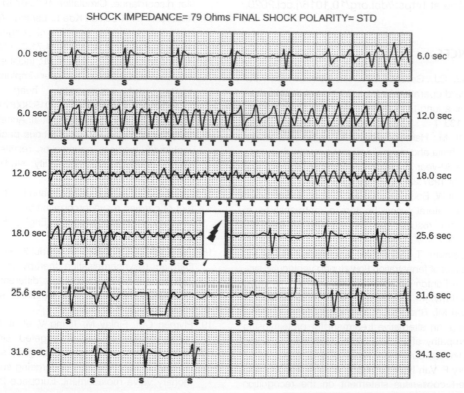

SHOCK IMPEDANCE= 79 Ohms FINAL SHOCK POLARITY= STD

Fig. 14. Appropriate subcutaneous implantable cardioverter-defibrillator (SICD) shock in Eisenmenger syndrome. This patient had demonstrated recurrent episodes of both atrial and ventricular arrhythmia by an implantable loop recorder, prompting SICD placement. The successful shock occurred approximately 1 year after implantation.

preprocedure mandatory screening appears to be most favorable for Fontan patients and less for those with tetralogy of Fallot.[111,112] Importantly, the inability of the SICD to prevent bradyarrhythmia is a major limitation. Patients who would benefit from any form of ventricular pacing (eg, antitachycardia pacing, bradycardia pacing, or CRT) are generally not considered suitable candidates for SICD placement.

SUMMARY

Arrhythmia concerns abound in ACHD. Advances in technology and techniques have improved the therapeutic approaches available for this challenging population. As the congenital population continues to age, increased arrhythmia and ongoing advances in the specialty are to be expected.

DISCLOSURE

The author has nothing to disclose.

SUPPLEMENTARY DATA

Supplementary data related to this article can be found online at https://doi.org/10.1016/j.ccl.2020.04.006.

REFERENCES

1. Hayes CJ, Gersony WM. Arrhythmias after the mustard operation for transposition of the great arteries: a long-term study. J Am Coll Cardiol 1986; 7(1):133–7.
2. Gelatt M, Hamilton RM, McCrindle BW, et al. Arrhythmia and mortality after the mustard procedure: a 30-year single-center experience. J Am Coll Cardiol 1997;29(1):194–201.
3. Ben Ali W, Bouhout I, Khairy P, et al. Extracardiac versus lateral tunnel Fontan: a meta-analysis of long-term results. Ann Thorac Surg 2019;107(3): 837–43.
4. Hasselman T, Schneider D, Madan N, et al. Reversal of fenestration flow during ventricular systole in Fontan patients in junctional or ventricular paced rhythm. Pediatr Cardiol 2005;26(5):638–41.
5. Cohen MI, Rhodes LA, Wernovsky G, et al. Atrial pacing: an alternative treatment for protein-losing enteropathy after the Fontan operation. J Thorac Cardiovasc Surg 2001;121(3):582–3.
6. Khairy P, Van Hare GF, Balaji S, et al. PACES/HRS expert consensus statement on the recognition and management of arrhythmias in adult congenital heart disease: executive summary. Heart Rhythm 2014;11(10):e81–101.

7. Khairy P, Landzberg MJ, Gatzoulis MA, et al. Transvenous pacing leads and systemic thromboemboli in patients with intracardiac shunts: a multicenter study. Circulation 2006;113(20):2391–7.
8. Moore JP, Shannon KM. Transpulmonary atrial pacing: an approach to transvenous pacemaker implantation after extracardiac conduit Fontan surgery. J Cardiovasc Electrophysiol 2014;25(9): 1028–31.
9. Hoyt W, Kannankeril PJ, Fish FA. Transpulmonary epicardial atrial pacing after the extracardiac Fontan: a novel technique. Heart Rhythm 2018;15(5): S103.
10. Mavroudis C, Deal BJ, Backer CL, et al. J. Maxwell Chamberlain Memorial Paper for congenital heart surgery. 111 Fontan conversions with arrhythmia surgery: surgical lessons and outcomes. Ann Thorac Surg 2007;84(5):1457–65 [discussion: 1465–6].
11. Anderson RH, Arnold R, Wilkinson JL. The conducting system in congenitally corrected transposition. Lancet 1973;1(7815):1286–8.
12. Anderson RH, Becker AE, Arnold R, et al. The conducting tissues in congenitally corrected transposition. Circulation 1974;50(5):911–23.
13. Huhta JC, Maloney JD, Ritter DG, et al. Complete atrioventricular block in patients with atrioventricular discordance. Circulation 1983;67(6):1374–7.
14. Andersen TA, Troelsen Kde L, Larsen LA. Of mice and men: molecular genetics of congenital heart disease. Cell Mol Life Sci 2014;71(8):1327–52.
15. Russell MR, Galloti R, Moore JP. Initial experience with transcatheter pacemaker implantation for adults with congenital heart disease. J Cardiovasc Electrophysiol 2019;30(8):1362–6.
16. Chinitz L, Ritter P, Khelae SK, et al. Accelerometer-based atrioventricular synchronous pacing with a ventricular leadless pacemaker: results from the Micra atrioventricular feasibility studies. Heart Rhythm 2018;15(9):1363–71.
17. Cleland JG, Daubert JC, Erdmann E, et al. The effect of cardiac resynchronization on morbidity and mortality in heart failure. N Engl J Med 2005; 352(15):1539–49.
18. Janousek J, Gebauer RA, Abdul-Khaliq H, et al. Cardiac resynchronisation therapy in paediatric and congenital heart disease: differential effects in various anatomical and functional substrates. Heart 2009;95(14):1165–71.
19. Plymen CM, Finlay M, Tsang V, et al. Haemodynamic consequences of targeted single- and dual-site right ventricular pacing in adults with congenital heart disease undergoing surgical pulmonary valve replacement. Europace 2015;17(2): 274–80.
20. Stephenson EA, Cecchin F, Alexander ME, et al. Relation of right ventricular pacing in tetralogy of

Fallot to electrical resynchronization. Am J Cardiol 2004;93(11):1449–52. A1412.

21. Kubus P, Materna O, Tax P, et al. Successful permanent resynchronization for failing right ventricle after repair of tetralogy of Fallot. Circulation 2014; 130(22):e186–90.

22. Janousek J, Kovanda J, Lozek M, et al. Pulmonary right ventricular resynchronization in congenital heart disease: acute improvement in right ventricular mechanics and contraction efficiency. Circ Cardiovasc Imaging 2017;10(9) [pii:e006424].

23. Diller GP, Okonko D, Uebing A, et al. Cardiac resynchronization therapy for adult congenital heart disease patients with a systemic right ventricle: analysis of feasibility and review of early experience. Europace 2006;8(4):267–72.

24. Janousek J, Tomek V, Chaloupecky VA, et al. Cardiac resynchronization therapy: a novel adjunct to the treatment and prevention of systemic right ventricular failure. J Am Coll Cardiol 2004;44(9): 1927–31.

25. Dubin AM, Janousek J, Rhee E, et al. Resynchronization therapy in pediatric and congenital heart disease patients: an international multicenter study. J Am Coll Cardiol 2005;46(12):2277–83.

26. Cecchin F, Frangini PA, Brown DW, et al. Cardiac resynchronization therapy (and multisite pacing) in pediatrics and congenital heart disease: five years experience in a single institution. J Cardiovasc Electrophysiol 2009;20(1):58–65.

27. Kiesewetter C, Michael K, Morgan J, et al. Left ventricular dysfunction after cardiac resynchronization therapy in congenital heart disease patients with a failing systemic right ventricle. Pacing Clin Electrophysiol 2008;31(2):159–62.

28. Stout KK, Daniels CJ, Aboulhosn JA, et al. 2018 AHA/ACC guideline for the management of adults with congenital heart disease: executive summary: a report of the American College of Cardiology/ American Heart Association Task Force on clinical practice guidelines. Circulation 2019;139(14): e637–97.

29. Bottega NA, Kapa S, Edwards WD, et al. The cardiac veins in congenitally corrected transposition of the great arteries: delivery options for cardiac devices. Heart Rhythm 2009;6(10):1450–6.

30. Moore JP, Cho D, Lin JP, et al. Implantation techniques and outcomes after cardiac resynchronization therapy for congenitally corrected transposition of the great arteries. Heart Rhythm 2018;15(12):1808–15.

31. Moore JP, Gallotti RG, Shannon KM, et al. A minimally invasive hybrid approach for cardiac resynchronization of the systemic right ventricle. Pacing Clin Electrophysiol 2019;42(2):171–7.

32. Kodama Y, Kuraoka A, Ishikawa Y, et al. Outcome of patients with functional single ventricular heart after pacemaker implantation: what makes it poor, and what can we do? Heart Rhythm 2019;16(12): 1870–4.

33. Bulic A, Zimmerman FJ, Ceresnak SR, et al. Ventricular pacing in single ventricles-A bad combination. Heart Rhythm 2017;14(6):853–7.

34. Rosner A, Khalapyan T, Dalen H, et al. Classic-pattern dyssynchrony in adolescents and adults with a Fontan circulation. J Am Soc Echocardiogr 2018;31(2):211–9.

35. O'Leary ET, Gauvreau K, Alexander ME, et al. Dual-site ventricular pacing in patients with fontan physiology and heart block: does it mitigate the detrimental effects of single-site ventricular pacing? JACC Clin Electrophysiol 2018;4(10):1289–97.

36. Kean AC, Kay WA, Patel JK, et al. Permanent nonselective His bundle pacing in an adult with L-transposition of the great arteries and complete AV block. Pacing Clin Electrophysiol 2017;40(11): 1313–7.

37. Mahata I, Macicek SL, Morin DP. Direct His bundle pacing using retrograde mapping in complete heart block and L-transposition of the great arteries. HeartRhythm Case Rep 2019;5(6):291–3.

38. Vijayaraman P, Mascarenhas V. Three-dimensional mapping guided permanent His bundle pacing in a patient with corrected transposition of great arteries. HeartRhythm Case Rep 2019;5(12):600–2.

39. Moore JP, Gallotti R, Shannon KM, et al. Permanent conduction system pacing for congenitally corrected transposition of the great arteries: A Pediatric and Congenital Electrophysiology Society (PACES)/International Society for Adult Congenital Heart Disease (ISACHD) Collaborative Study. Heart Rhythm 2020. [Epub ahead of print].

40. Bouchardy J, Therrien J, Pilote L, et al. Atrial arrhythmias in adults with congenital heart disease. Circulation 2009;120(17):1679–86.

41. Yap SC, Harris L, Chauhan VS, et al. Identifying high risk in adults with congenital heart disease and atrial arrhythmias. Am J Cardiol 2011;108(5): 723–8.

42. Khairy P. Sudden cardiac death in transposition of the great arteries with a Mustard or Senning baffle: the myocardial ischemia hypothesis. Curr Opin Cardiol 2017;32(1):101–7.

43. Collins KK, Love BA, Walsh EP, et al. Location of acutely successful radiofrequency catheter ablation of intraatrial reentrant tachycardia in patients with congenital heart disease. Am J Cardiol 2000; 86(9):969–74.

44. El-Said HG, Ing FF, Grifka RG, et al. 18-year experience with transseptal procedures through baffles, conduits, and other intra-atrial patches. Catheter Cardiovasc Interv 2000;50(4):434–9.

45. Correa R, Walsh EP, Alexander ME, et al. Transbaffle mapping and ablation for atrial tachycardias

after Mustard, Senning, or Fontan operations. J Am Heart Assoc 2013;2(5):e000325.

46. Wu J, Deisenhofer I, Ammar S, et al. Acute and long-term outcome after catheter ablation of supraventricular tachycardia in patients after the Mustard or Senning operation for D-transposition of the great arteries. Europace 2013;15(6):886–91.

47. Gallotti RG, Madnawat H, Shannon KM, et al. Mechanisms and predictors of recurrent tachycardia after catheter ablation for d-transposition of the great arteries after the Mustard or Senning operation. Heart Rhythm 2017;14(3):350–6.

48. Zrenner B, Dong J, Schreieck J, et al. Delineation of intra-atrial reentrant tachycardia circuits after mustard operation for transposition of the great arteries using biatrial electroanatomic mapping and entrainment mapping. J Cardiovasc Electrophysiol 2003;14(12):1302–10.

49. Sardana R, Chauhan VS, Downar E. Unusual intraatrial reentry following the Mustard procedure defined by multisite magnetic electroanatomic mapping. Pacing Clin Electrophysiol 2003;26(4 Pt 1):902–5.

50. Moore JP, Buch E, Gallotti RG, et al. Ultrahigh-density mapping supplemented with global chamber activation identifies noncavotricuspid-dependent intra-atrial re-entry conduction isthmuses in adult congenital heart disease. J Cardiovasc Electrophysiol 2019;30(12):2797–805.

51. Kanter RJ, Papagiannis J, Carboni MP, et al. Radiofrequency catheter ablation of supraventricular tachycardia substrates after Mustard and Senning operations for d-transposition of the great arteries. J Am Coll Cardiol 2000;35(2):428–41.

52. Anne W, van Rensburg H, Adams J, et al. Ablation of post-surgical intra-atrial reentrant tachycardia. Predilection target sites and mapping approach. Eur Heart J 2002;23(20):1609–16.

53. Mandapati R, Walsh EP, Triedman JK. Pericaval and periannular intra-atrial reentrant tachycardias in patients with congenital heart disease. J Cardiovasc Electrophysiol 2003;14(2):119–25.

54. Moore BM, Anderson R, Nisbet AM, et al. Ablation of atrial arrhythmias after the atriopulmonary fontan procedure: mechanisms of arrhythmia and outcomes. JACC Clin Electrophysiol 2018;4(10):1338–46.

55. Wolf CM, Seslar SP, den Boer K, et al. Atrial remodeling after the Fontan operation. Am J Cardiol 2009;104(12):1737–42.

56. Stephenson EA, Lu M, Berul CI, et al. Arrhythmias in a contemporary fontan cohort: prevalence and clinical associations in a multicenter cross-sectional study. J Am Coll Cardiol 2010;56(11):890–6.

57. d'Udekem Y, Iyengar AJ, Galati JC, et al. Redefining expectations of long-term survival after the Fontan procedure: twenty-five years of follow-up from the entire population of Australia and New Zealand. Circulation 2014;130(11 Suppl 1):S32–8.

58. Deshaies C, Hamilton RM, Shohoudi A, et al. Thromboembolic risk after atriopulmonary, lateral tunnel, and extracardiac conduit Fontan surgery. J Am Coll Cardiol 2019;74(8):1071–81.

59. El Yaman MM, Asirvatham SJ, Kapa S, et al. Methods to access the surgically excluded cavotricuspid isthmus for complete ablation of typical atrial flutter in patients with congenital heart defects. Heart Rhythm 2009;6(7):949–56.

60. Moore JP, Shannon KM, Fish FA, et al. Catheter ablation of supraventricular tachyarrhythmia after extracardiac Fontan surgery. Heart Rhythm 2016;13(9):1891–7.

61. Dave AS, Aboulhosn J, Child JS, et al. Transconduit puncture for catheter ablation of atrial tachycardia in a patient with extracardiac Fontan palliation. Heart Rhythm 2010;7(3):413–6.

62. Moore JP, Hendrickson B, Brunengraber DZ, et al. Transcaval puncture for access to the pulmonary venous atrium after the extracardiac total cavopulmonary connection operation. Circ Arrhythm Electrophysiol 2015;8(4):824–8.

63. Bessiere F, Mongeon FP, Therrien J, et al. Magnetic-guided catheter ablation of twin AV nodal reentrant tachycardia in a patient with left atrial isomerism, interrupted inferior vena cava, and Kawashima-Fontan procedure. Clin Case Rep 2017;5(12):2105–10.

64. Shivapour JK, Sherwin ED, Alexander ME, et al. Utility of preoperative electrophysiologic studies in patients with Ebstein's anomaly undergoing the Cone procedure. Heart Rhythm 2014;11(2):182–6.

65. Huang CJ, Chiu IS, Lin FY, et al. Role of electrophysiological studies and arrhythmia intervention in repairing Ebstein's anomaly. Thorac Cardiovasc Surg 2000;48(6):347–50.

66. Hassan A, Tan NY, Aung H, et al. Outcomes of atrial arrhythmia radiofrequency catheter ablation in patients with Ebstein's anomaly. Europace 2018;20(3):535–40.

67. Moore JP, Gallotti RG, Chiriac A, et al. Catheter ablation of supraventricular tachycardia after tricuspid valve surgery in patients with congenital heart disease: a multicenter comparative study. Heart Rhythm 2020;17(1):58–65.

68. Koyak Z, Kroon B, de Groot JR, et al. Efficacy of antiarrhythmic drugs in adults with congenital heart disease and supraventricular tachycardias. Am J Cardiol 2013;112(9):1461–7.

69. Banchs JE, Baquero GA, Nickolaus MJ, et al. Clinical efficacy of dofetilide for the treatment of atrial tachyarrhythmias in adults with congenital heart disease. Congenit Heart Dis 2014;9(3):221–7.

70. El-Assaad I, Al-Kindi SG, Abraham J, et al. Use of dofetilide in adult patients with atrial arrhythmias and congenital heart disease: a PACES collaborative study. Heart Rhythm 2016;13(10):2034–9.

71. Rhodes LA, Walsh EP, Gamble WJ, et al. Benefits and potential risks of atrial antitachycardia pacing after repair of congenital heart disease. Pacing Clin Electrophysiol 1995;18(5 Pt 1):1005–16.

72. Kamp AN, LaPage MJ, Serwer GA, et al. Antitachycardia pacemakers in congenital heart disease. Congenit Heart Dis 2015;10(2):180–4.

73. Kramer CC, Maldonado JR, Olson MD, et al. Safety and efficacy of atrial antitachycardia pacing in congenital heart disease. Heart Rhythm 2018; 15(4):543–7.

74. Mandalenakis Z, Rosengren A, Lappas G, et al. Atrial fibrillation burden in young patients with congenital heart disease. Circulation 2018;137(9): 928–37.

75. Labombarda F, Hamilton R, Shohoudi A, et al. Increasing prevalence of atrial fibrillation and permanent atrial arrhythmias in congenital heart disease. J Am Coll Cardiol 2017;70(7):857–65.

76. Kirsh JA, Walsh EP, Triedman JK. Prevalence of and risk factors for atrial fibrillation and intra-atrial reentrant tachycardia among patients with congenital heart disease. Am J Cardiol 2002;90(3):338–40.

77. Liang JJ, Frankel DS, Parikh V, et al. Safety and outcomes of catheter ablation for atrial fibrillation in adults with congenital heart disease: a multicenter registry study. Heart Rhythm 2019;16(6):846–52.

78. Sohns C, Nurnberg JH, Hebe J, et al. Catheter ablation for atrial fibrillation in adults with congenital heart disease: lessons learned from more than 10 years following a sequential ablation approach. JACC Clin Electrophysiol 2018;4(6):733–43.

79. Abadir S, Waldmann V, Dyrda K, et al. Feasibility and safety of cryoballoon ablation for atrial fibrillation in patients with congenital heart disease. World J Cardiol 2019;11(5):149–58.

80. van Zyl M, Kapa S, Padmanabhan D, et al. Mechanism and outcomes of catheter ablation for ventricular tachycardia in adults with repaired congenital heart disease. Heart Rhythm 2016; 13(7):1449–54.

81. Yang J, Brunnquell M, Liang JJ, et al. Long term follow-up after ventricular tachycardia ablation in patients with congenital heart disease. J Cardiovasc Electrophysiol 2019;30(9):1560–8.

82. Moore JP, Shannon KM, Gallotti RG, et al. Catheter ablation of ventricular arrhythmia for Ebstein's anomaly in unoperated and post-surgical patients. JACC Clin Electrophysiol 2018;4(10):1300–7.

83. Moore JP, Seki A, Shannon KM, et al. Characterization of anatomic ventricular tachycardia isthmus pathology after surgical repair of tetralogy of Fallot. Circ Arrhythm Electrophysiol 2013;6(5):905–11.

84. Zeppenfeld K, Schalij MJ, Bartelings MM, et al. Catheter ablation of ventricular tachycardia after repair of congenital heart disease: electroanatomic identification of the critical right ventricular isthmus. Circulation 2007;116(20):2241–52.

85. Kapel GF, Sacher F, Dekkers OM, et al. Arrhythmogenic anatomical isthmuses identified by electroanatomical mapping are the substrate for ventricular tachycardia in repaired tetralogy of Fallot. Eur Heart J 2017;38(4):268–76.

86. Kapel GF, Reichlin T, Wijnmaalen AP, et al. Re-entry using anatomically determined isthmuses: a curable ventricular tachycardia in repaired congenital heart disease. Circ Arrhythm Electrophysiol 2015;8(1):102–9.

87. Sandhu A, Ruckdeschel E, Sauer WH, et al. Perioperative electrophysiology study in patients with tetralogy of Fallot undergoing pulmonary valve replacement will identify those at high risk of subsequent ventricular tachycardia. Heart Rhythm 2018;15(5):679–85.

88. Khairy P, Ionescu-Ittu R, Mackie AS, et al. Changing mortality in congenital heart disease. J Am Coll Cardiol 2010;56(14):1149–57.

89. Verheugt CL, Uiterwaal CS, van der Velde ET, et al. Mortality in adult congenital heart disease. Eur Heart J 2010;31(10):1220–9.

90. Zomer AC, Vaartjes I, Uiterwaal CS, et al. Circumstances of death in adult congenital heart disease. Int J Cardiol 2012;154(2):168–72.

91. Engelings CC, Helm PC, Abdul-Khaliq H, et al. Cause of death in adults with congenital heart disease—an analysis of the German National Register for Congenital Heart Defects. Int J Cardiol 2016; 211:31–6.

92. Diller GP, Kempny A, Alonso-Gonzalez R, et al. Survival prospects and circumstances of death in contemporary adult congenital heart disease patients under follow-up at a large tertiary centre. Circulation 2015;132(22):2118–25.

93. Videbaek J, Laursen HB, Olsen M, et al. Long-term nationwide follow-up study of simple congenital heart disease diagnosed in otherwise healthy children. Circulation 2016;133(5):474–83.

94. Silka MJ, Hardy BG, Menashe VD, et al. A population-based prospective evaluation of risk of sudden cardiac death after operation for common congenital heart defects. J Am Coll Cardiol 1998;32(1):245–51.

95. Koyak Z, Harris L, de Groot JR, et al. Sudden cardiac death in adult congenital heart disease. Circulation 2012;126(16):1944–54.

96. Vehmeijer JT, Koyak Z, Bokma JP, et al. Sudden cardiac death in adults with congenital heart disease: does QRS-complex fragmentation discriminate in structurally abnormal hearts? Europace 2018;20(F11):f122–8.

97. Koyak Z, de Groot JR, Bouma BJ, et al. Sudden cardiac death in adult congenital heart disease: can the unpredictable be foreseen? Europace 2017;19(3):401–6.

98. Teuwen CP, Ramdjan TT, Gotte M, et al. Non-sustained ventricular tachycardia in patients with congenital heart disease: an important sign? Int J Cardiol 2016;206:158–63.

99. Khairy P, Harris L, Landzberg MJ, et al. Implantable cardioverter-defibrillators in tetralogy of Fallot. Circulation 2008;117(3):363–70.

100. Gallego P, Gonzalez AE, Sanchez-Recalde A, et al. Incidence and predictors of sudden cardiac arrest in adults with congenital heart defects repaired before adult life. Am J Cardiol 2012;110(1):109–17.

101. Greutmann M, Tobler D, Kovacs AH, et al. Increasing mortality burden among adults with complex congenital heart disease. Congenit Heart Dis 2015;10(2):117–27.

102. Attenhofer Jost CH, Tan NY, Hassan A, et al. Sudden death in patients with Ebstein anomaly. Eur Heart J 2018;39(21):1970–1977a.

103. Valente AM, Gauvreau K, Assenza GE, et al. Contemporary predictors of death and sustained ventricular tachycardia in patients with repaired tetralogy of Fallot enrolled in the INDICATOR cohort. Heart 2014;100(3):247–53.

104. Khairy P. Programmed ventricular stimulation for risk stratification in patients with tetralogy of Fallot: a Bayesian perspective. Nat Clin Pract Cardiovasc Med 2007;4(6):292–3.

105. Priori SG, Blomstrom-Lundqvist C, Mazzanti A, et al. 2015 ESC guidelines for the management of patients with ventricular arrhythmias and the prevention of sudden cardiac death: the Task Force for the management of patients with ventricular arrhythmias and the prevention of sudden cardiac death of the European Society of Cardiology (ESC). Endorsed by: Association for European Paediatric and Congenital Cardiology (AEPC). Eur Heart J 2015;36(41):2793–867.

106. Vehmeijer JT, Koyak Z, Budts W, et al. Prevention of sudden cardiac death in adults with congenital heart disease: do the guidelines fall short? Circ Arrhythm Electrophysiol 2017;10(7).

107. Vehmeijer JT, Koyak Z, Zwinderman AH, et al. PREVENTION-ACHD: PRospEctiVE study on implaNTable cardioverter-defibrillator therapy and suddeN cardiac death in Adults with Congenital Heart Disease; rationale and design. Neth Heart J 2019;27(10):474–9.

108. Vehmeijer JT, Brouwer TF, Limpens J, et al. Implantable cardioverter-defibrillators in adults with congenital heart disease: a systematic review and meta-analysis. Eur Heart J 2016;37(18):1439–48.

109. Moore JP, Mondesert B, Lloyd MS, et al. Clinical experience with the subcutaneous implantable cardioverter-defibrillator in adults with congenital heart disease. Circ Arrhythm Electrophysiol 2016; 9(9). https://doi.org/10.1161/CIRCEP.116.004338.

110. Ferrero P, Ali H, Barman P, et al. Entirely subcutaneous defibrillator and complex congenital heart disease: data on long-term clinical follow-up. World J Cardiol 2017;9(6):547–52.

111. Alonso P, Osca J, Rueda J, et al. Conventional and right-sided screening for subcutaneous ICD in a population with congenital heart disease at high risk of sudden cardiac death. Ann Noninvasive Electrocardiol 2017;22(6). https://doi.org/10.1111/anec.12461.

112. Garside H, Leyva F, Hudsmith L, et al. Eligibility for subcutaneous implantable cardioverter defibrillators in the adult congenital heart disease population. Pacing Clin Electrophysiol 2019;42(1):65–70.

Surgery for Adult Congenital Heart Disease

Tracy Geoffrion, MD, MPH[a],*, Stephanie Fuller, MD, MS[a,b]

KEYWORDS

- Surgery • ACHD • Fontan • Transplant • Congenital

KEY POINTS

- Describe the primary lesions found in adults with congenital heart disease requiring surgical intervention in adulthood.
- Review adult congenital heart disease diagnosis and treatment relating to surgery.
- Summarize surgical therapies used for adults with congenital cardiac disease.

INTRODUCTION

Technical and medical improvements for congenital cardiac disease in children have resulted in an increasing population of patients who survive into adulthood. Many of these patients are subject to progression of their native palliated disease or suffer from sequelae of their childhood repair and require repeat surgical intervention. In 2018, the American College of Cardiology/American Heart Association updated their published guidelines regarding the surgical management of adult congenital heart disease (ACHD).[1] An overview of surgical techniques, surgical decision-making strategies, and controversies in care when operating on the patient with ACHD is detailed here.

BASICS OF ADULT CONGENITAL CARDIAC SURGERY

There is no consensus as to the best location in which adult congenital cardiac operations should be performed. However, there are many who promote using adult hospital resources for these patients given their comorbid conditions.[2] Each facility (adult vs pediatric) has unique benefits for this patient population, including the availability of adult specialists, adult-sized equipment, psychosocial support, and cardiologists and surgeons

well-versed in congenital heart disease lesions.[2] The Adult Congenital Heart Association has delineated comprehensive program features and services that constitute excellence in care of this unique population.[3]

Regardless of location, appropriate personnel are heavily emphasized. There are data supporting improved surgical outcomes when procedures are performed by surgeons specifically trained in congenital cardiac surgery.[4]

Preoperative Evaluation

Preoperatively, patients should receive a thorough evaluation by a multidisciplinary team that specializes in ACHD. In addition, adult specialists should be consulted as needed to address acquired health issues as a part of preoperative clearance, such as renal insufficiency, hepatopathy, and restrictive lung disease. Once a surgical plan is developed, medical optimization should be performed before undertaking surgical intervention. In some cases, this goal requires inpatient admission for medical management and a comprehensive dental evaluation. Significant consideration should be given to those patients with known or suspected commonly associated genetic syndromes such as trisomy 21 and DiGeorge syndrome, because they may pose unique issues for

[a] The Division of Cardiothoracic Surgery, Children's Hospital of Philadelphia, 3401 Civic Center Boulevard, Philadelphia, PA 19104, USA; [b] Division of Cardiothoracic Surgery, Children's Hospital of Philadelphia, The Perelman School of Medicine, University of Pennsylvania, 3401 Civic Center Boulevard, Philadelphia, PA 19104, USA
* Corresponding author.
E-mail address: Geoffriont@email.chop.edu

Cardiol Clin 38 (2020) 435–443
https://doi.org/10.1016/j.ccl.2020.04.013
0733-8651/20/© 2020 Elsevier Inc. All rights reserved.

perioperative care. Preoperative assessment by anesthesiologists should include a detailed history of prior anesthetic exposures, airway concern, and cervical spine issues when immobilized and positioned for surgery.

Multimodal imaging should be performed to clearly evaluate the current anatomy. This imaging includes chest radiography, transthoracic echocardiography, and cardiac catheterization with evaluation of left and right heart pressures and coronary anatomy. Additionally, cardiac MRI can be very useful in evaluating patients for complex repairs. Emerging modalities such as 3-dimensional echocardiography of computed tomography scans are advocated as well. Most surgeons request computed tomography with scans or without angiography and/or vascular ultrasound examinations of the neck and groin to determine the potential for injury on reoperative sternotomy and evaluate prospective sites of vascular access. In the operating room, all patients should undergo a preoperative transesophageal echocardiogram, ideally performed by a cardiologist who specializes in ACHD.

Reoperative surgery

Although there are many technical considerations in the conduct of ACHD operations, for most of these patients this operation is not their first. The reoperative sternotomy carries an increased risk at baseline secondary to the formation of scar tissue in the mediastinum. Many remotely placed patches and baffles become calcified, creating a hostile operative environment for safe mediastinal reentry, dissection, and cannulation to cardiopulmonary bypass. Additionally, reoperative patients have atypical anatomy that may be unfamiliar to the operating surgeon. Frequently, it is challenging to identify and access the necessary structures, further increasing the risk of injury to the heart, great vessels, and lungs during redo sternotomy, chest opening, and dissection.

Cannulation for cardiopulmonary bypass in the patient with ACHD varies by operative procedure with the intent of providing optimal exposure and safety.[5] The most commonly used strategies are ascending aorta and right atrial, ascending aorta and bicaval, femoral artery and femoral vein, right axillary artery, and femoral vein or right atria. In addition, partial bypass or left sided bypass may be used in unique instances. Aortoatrial cannulation is typically used for closed cardiac and great vessel operations. Aortobicaval cannulation is the most commonly used procedure for congenital cardiac surgery because it provides exposure of the intracardiac structures and is particularly

protective when atrial or ventricular shunting lesions exist. In situations where the process of entering the chest is likely to be difficult or risky, femoral bypass can be initiated before sternotomy to support the patient should a major structure be entered. When the ascending aorta is unable to be cannulated for anatomic or technical reasons, the axillary artery may be used for antegrade arterial bypass inflow. The femoral vein, right atrium, or vena cavae can then be used for venous cannulation. Alternative arterial access via the innominate or carotid arteries can also be used if needed.[6] Hence, it is always necessary to document the patency of peripheral vessels given that these patients often have multiple surgeries, catheterizations, and central access, all of which may lead to occlusion of these vessels. It is always necessary to proceed safely and ensure the availability of appropriately typed and crossed blood products. Peripheral cannulae must always be readily available on in reoperative sternotomy in case of mediastinal injury. In the cases of catastrophic injury upon sternal reentry, surgeons should be prepared to initiate deep hypothermic circulatory arrest for cerebral protection during low flow states to repair the most serious of injuries, such as those to the ascending aorta, aortic arch, and innominate vein.

Multiple strategies are used for myocardial protection during the operative procedure. Primarily, the heart should be nondistended on cardiopulmonary bypass. Many procedures that are exclusively right sided (ie, pulmonary valve replacement) may be performed with the support of cardiopulmonary bypass without cardiac arrest, given confirmation that there are no intracardiac communications at the atrial or ventricular levels. For those cases requiring cardiac standstill, the goal is to achieve both electrical and mechanical arrest of the myocardium. Multiple commercially available cardioplegia solutions are available and used. They are all isotonic and hyperkalemic to induce a polarized cardiac arrest. Again, it is important to note that some procedures require the use of deep hypothermic circulatory arrest. Thus, effective and safe cooling and rewarming strategies must be used together with a cardiopulmonary bypass plan that allows for increased duration of bypass to allow for temperature regulation.

The decision to proceed with surgery is not always straightforward. Certain anatomic or physiologic findings have proven to be relatively prohibitive. These include anatomic risks of reentry into the chest cavity, both venovenous and arterial collateral burden in the mediastinum and pleural cavities, the risk of bleeding during or after surgery, and the severity of ventricular dysfunction such that there is concern about the ability to wean from cardiopulmonary bypass. Recent guidelines have established that, for shunt lesions, in patients with severe pulmonary artery hypertension (greater than 2/3 systemic) or a net right-to-left shunt, surgery is contraindicated.[1] Additionally, severe comorbid conditions or profound frailty can make recovery from any operation challenging. These considerations illustrate the benefit of a multidisciplinary approach to the treatment of these complex patients. Although a number of previous sternotomies is often cited as a concern for sternal reentry, there is no prescribed number of previous sternotomies at which sternal reentry alone becomes prohibitive. These factors should be carefully considered in deciding whether an operation will improve the quality or length of a patient's life.

SHUNTING LESIONS
Atrial Septal Defect and Partial Anomalous Pulmonary Venous Return

Although commonly performed as de novo procedures in adults, these may also be reoperative owing to residual shunts. The repair of an atrial septal defect (ASD) and partial anomalous pulmonary venous return is most commonly performed through a median sternotomy, although alternative access sites include a right minithoracotomy or robotic-assisted surgery through the right chest. Small defects can be closed primarily, but the larger defects typically require patch closure using either autologous pericardium, bovine pericardium, or homograft. The repair of partial anomalous pulmonary venous return with sinus venosus ASD requires using the patch to direct anomalous flow into the left atrium. If there is no associated ASD, one must be created such that the veins can be tunneled to the left atrium without obstruction. For cases in which the right pulmonary veins are high on the superior vena cava and a baffle cannot be created to redirect flow, the Warden procedure is used. This procedure involves the division of the superior vena cava just above the highest anomalous pulmonary vein and anastomosis to the right atrial appendage. The orifice of the superior vena cava is then baffled to the right atrial appendage, which has been cleared of any trabeculations. Anomalous left-sided veins can be rerouted to the left atrium by connecting the draining vertical vein to the left atrial appendage either directly or with the use of a polytetrafluoroethylene graft. The risks of closure of an ASD or partial anomalous pulmonary venous return include residual ASD, pleural effusions, heart block, air embolism, atrial dysrhythmias, pulmonary venous obstruction, and superior vena cava obstruction.[7]

Ventricular Septal Defect

Isolated ventricular septal defects (VSDs) are rare in adults, but may present as a small restrictive VSD detected in a patient who has been lost to follow-up, develops infective endocarditis, or meets surgical indications as an adult. The surgical approach to the lesion is based on the specific type of defect. The transatrial approach uses a right atriotomy to access conoventricular, canal-type, and some muscular defects through the tricuspid valve. Other methods include access through a right ventriculotomy or through the pulmonary valve for conoseptal hypoplasia defects. Small VSDs can be closed primarily with pledgetted sutures, but larger defects should be closed with a patch of Dacron, Gore-Tex, or glutaraldehyde treated pericardium. The specific risks associated relate to the surrounding structures including the conduction system, aortic valve, tricuspid valve, or pulmonary valve.

Atrioventricular Septal Defect

An atrioventricular septal defect may present across the spectrum from incomplete atrioventricular canals to complete. Although it is unlikely that a patient with a complete canal will undergo their first surgical intervention as an adult, the less severe forms of disease are often seen de novo in adulthood. More commonly, previously repaired atrioventricular septal defect lesions can develop complications or disease progression in adulthood. Most commonly, this involves residual intracardiac atrial or ventricular shunting lesions, atrioventricular valve regurgitation often owing to a residual cleft, atrioventricular valve stenosis, or the development of left ventricular outflow tract obstruction. Surgical techniques are tailored to the specific lesions such as closure of residual ASD or VSD lesions as described elsewhere in this article, valve repair or potentially replacement, and resection of subaortic obstruction. The risks of these operations can include any of those mentioned previously for ASD or VSD. If valve repair or replacement are performed, these patients can also be at risk for valve stenosis, prosthetic valve infection or thrombosis, patient–prosthesis mismatch, and complications associated with systemic anticoagulation for mechanical valves.

Patent Ductus Arteriosus

Closure of a patent ductus arteriosus during adult-hood can be complicated. Historically, these patients were managed surgically. The duct was ligated and potentially divided or patch closed through a pulmonary arteriotomy via sternotomy or thoracotomy, with or without the use of cardio-pulmonary bypass.[8] However, minimally invasive and catheter-based techniques are now often being used.[9] Contraindications to these techniques include wide and short ducts, or chests that are otherwise inaccessible via video-assisted thora-coscopic surgery owing to scarring or pleural disease. Additionally, patent ductus arteriosus associated with aneurysms may not be closeable with these methods.[10] Last, those with extensive calcification also pose a high risk for surgical ligation.

LEFT-SIDED OBSTRUCTIVE LESIONS
Congenital Mitral Stenosis

Current American Heart Association guidelines for isolated mitral stenosis support percutaneous balloon valvotomy as first-line procedural therapy for mitral stenosis with appropriate valve morphology as assessed by the Wilkins score. For those who are not candidates for balloon val-vuloplasty, mitral valve surgery with repair or replacement is indicated.[10] The mitral valve can be accessed directly into the left atrium via the interatrial groove or through the atrial septum. Minimally invasive techniques such as right mini-thoracotomy port access and robotic mitral surgery are increasingly popular and have been shown to have equivalent outcomes.[11] Repair techniques for mitral stenosis vary based on the etiology and are limited. These include commis-surotomy, chordal splitting, leaflet augmentation with patch material, and papillary muscle division. When valve replacement is required, a mechanical, or bioprosthetic prosthesis can be used. The primary risks associated with surgery include heart block, circumflex coronary injury, coronary sinus injury, and perivalvular leak or dehiscence.

Subaortic Stenosis

Surgery for subaortic stenosis is typically performed with aortic and right atrial cannulation and cardioplegic arrest. The lesions creating the stenosis are a fibrous membrane below the valve and/or septal hypertrophy. The subaortic membrane is approached through a transverse incision in the ascending aorta, just above the valve. The fibromuscular ring is visualized through the aortic valve and excised in its entirety. The

risks include damage to aortic valve leaflets, resulting in valve insufficiency, injury to conduction tissue causing heart block, and injury to the anterior leaflet of the mitral valve.[7] A myectomy is performed for hypertrophy of the ventricular septum. Transaortic exposure is typically used and the hypertrophied septum is sharply excised from just below the valve toward the apex. In addition to these risks, there is the additional risk of iatrogenic VSD from excess septal muscle excision. Diffuse tunnel-like subvalvar obstruction of the left ventricular outflow tract may require augmentation with more complex aortico-ventriculoplasty operations potentially in combination with aortic valve replacement.[12] For example, the modified Konno procedure involves complete resection of the subaortic ventricular septum through an incision in the right ventricle. The defect or newly created VSD is then closed with a patch.[5] Often, the right ventricle requires a patch enlargement at the incision site as well. This technique has additional risk of damage to the pulmonary and tricuspid valves during the enlargement of the ventricular septum.

Aortic Stenosis

Adult congenital aortic stenosis can be related to calcific or degenerative disease of otherwise normal valves or be secondary to a bicuspid valve. Surgery for aortic stenosis is often direct aortic valve replacement with bioprosthetic or mechanical valve. Some centers employ mini-mally invasive access through a right minithora-cotomy or hemisternotomy for valve replacement. Risks specific to surgical valve replacement include heart block, damage to or occlusion of the coronary arteries, injury to the anterior leaflet of the mitral valve, paravalvular leak, and patient–prosthesis mismatch. In cases where the aortic annulus is too small to fit an adequately sized prosthesis, the aortic root must also be enlarged. There are several aortic annular enlargement techniques used. In addition, assuming there is a normal pulmonic valve, the Ross procedure can be used in adult patients requiring a valve replacement. The Ross procedure involves an autologous root replacement from the pulmonary outflow and requires the use of a homograft to replace the right ventricular outflow tract (RVOT), thus creating both neo-aortic and neopulmonic replacements. Patients often require revision of the homograft. The auto-graft in the aortic position may be prone to dilation or neoaortic valve regurgitation. There are increasing data to support the use of transcath-eter aortic valve replacement for bicuspid aortic valve stenosis.[12–14] However, caution should be used in young patients because there are no long-term data regarding durability and complications.

Supravalvular Aortic Stenosis

Repair of supravalvular aortic stenosis involves patch enlargement of aorta at the level of the sinotubular junction.[15] Additional options in the adult population include aortic root and/or ascending aortic replacement. The integrity of the aortic valve determines whether a concomitant valve replacement is indicated. If the coronary ostia are involved in the stenosis, the patient may require ostioplasty or ostial reimplantation. If this is not feasible and the patient has concern for ischemic events, coronary bypass may be necessary. During patch aortoplasty of the aortic root, there is an inherent risk to the aortic valve leaflets or otherwise normal coronary ostia.

Coarctation of the Aorta

Transcatheter balloon dilation and stenting is commonly used to treat coarctation in the adult.[16] If unsuccessful, surgical repair of coarctation is similar other open surgical intervention on the descending thoracic aorta. This intervention is typically performed through a left posterolateral thoracotomy. An end-to-end anastomosis is used if technically feasible; otherwise, a Dacron interposition graft is placed.[17] Often left heart bypass can be used to support the distal circulation while the aorta is clamped. The primary risks are neurologic, the most severe being spinal ischemia and ensuing paralysis.

Cor Triatriatum Sinister

Surgical repair for cor triatriatum involves excision of the membrane that divides the left atrium. This procedure is performed on bypass with bicaval cannulation. The membrane is accessed through the atrium or the interatrial septum[7] and the specific technical risk is damage to the mitral valve, resulting in mitral regurgitation. Confirmation that all 4 pulmonary veins return normally to the left atrium is necessary.

RIGHT-SIDED LESIONS
Pulmonary Valve Disease

In adults with moderate or severe pulmonary stenosis, balloon valvuloplasty has shown to be an efficacious first-line therapy with good short- and long-term results.[18] For those who fail percutaneous intervention or are not candidates for catheter-based interventions, surgical pulmonary valve repair or replacement is indicated. Pulmonary valve replacement in adults is most often a reoperation after childhood RVOT reconstruction. Bioprosthetic valves are commonly used with an extension of pericardium or graft material onto the proximal portion of the RVOT to prevent mechanical distortion.[5] Alternatively, for patients with a severely dilated RVOT, plication of the RVOT is advocated. If there are no residual intracardiac defects, the operation can be performed safely on cardiopulmonary bypass with the heart warm and beating.

Branch Pulmonary Artery Stenosis

Branch pulmonary artery stenosis frequently accompanies valve disease and can sometimes be alleviated with percutaneous balloon dilation and ensuing stent placement. If that is unsuccessful or if the patient is undergoing another procedure, they can be augmented surgically with a patch. These patches are typically bovine pericardium, autologous pericardium, synthetic pericardium, or homograft.

Tetralogy of Fallot

Patients with repaired tetralogy of Fallot often require reintervention on the RVOT in adulthood. Pulmonary regurgitation, stenosis, or a combination of both are the most commonly seen morphologies and the type of adult intervention required depends on the type of repair that was performed previously.[19] Isolated pulmonary valve disease can be repaired as described elsewhere in this article. RVOT reconstruction with a right ventricle-to-pulmonary artery conduit in childhood carries the risk of developing valve incompetence or conduit obstruction. Catheter-based intervention of conduits with stenting or placement of a transcatheter valve inside previously placed conduits is used,[20,21] but surgical replacement of the pathway is often warranted. This procedure is performed with cardiopulmonary bypass and the previously implanted conduit is removed from the pulmonary artery and right ventricular surface. Patch augmentation or repair of the pulmonary artery is often needed to reconstruct an appropriately sized confluent pulmonary artery bifurcation on which to attach the distal end of the new conduit. Removal of the old conduit from the ventricle is performed with focus on damaging as little native right ventricular myocardium as possible. Options for conduit include homograft and the Hancock Dacron conduit with a porcine bioprosthetic valve.[22] The proximal anastomosis is often augmented with a patch of homograft or Gore-Tex to avoid distortion. Additionally, annular dilation often causes some degree of tricuspid regurgitation in adults with repaired tetralogy of Fallot. This finding is often addressed at the time of conduit exchange or valve replacement and the technical details are discussed in the section on Ebstein's Anomaly and Tricuspid Valve Regurgitation. The addition of arrhythmia surgery can also be used for patients with atrial arrhythmias. Other lesions seen in adults with repaired tetralogy of Fallot that could require operations include branch pulmonary artery stenosis, residual VSD, and RVOT aneurysm.

Ebstein's Anomaly and Tricuspid Valve Regurgitation

Regurgitation of a dysplastic and regurgitant tricuspid valve can be surgically treated with valve repair (annular reduction, leaflet resection, or repair in the cases of perforation) or replacement. For Ebstein's anomaly, there are multiple repair techniques. These included the Hardy, Danielson, Carpentier, and Cone techniques, which involve plication of the atrialized right ventricle, reconstruction of the valve to address the downward displacement of the septal leaflets with potential rotation of the anterior and posterior leaflets, reduction of the right atrium, and closure (total or subtotal) of any atrial communications.[23] Additionally, replacement can be considered if there is not a viable reconstructive option. Although mechanical valves provide superior durability, they are not used frequently in the tricuspid position owing to thrombosis. Porcine bioprosthetic valves have demonstrated a survival advantage in some series.[24]

There is a risk of right heart failure after tricuspid repair after these operations and some surgeons support leaving or creating a small atrial-level communication to unload the right ventricle. If right heart failure is profound and refractory, a bidirectional cavopulmonary anastomosis can be added, creating a functional 1.5 ventricle repair. Hence, all these patients should undergo thorough cardiac catheterization with calculation of pulmonary vascular resistance before surgery. This process can provide better tolerance of residual tricuspid dysfunction, right ventricular dysfunction, and decreased operative mortality.[25] Additional risks of tricuspid valve surgery include damage to the conduction system or coronary arteries and thromboembolism. Atrial tachyarrhythmias are also commonly found in this population either before or after surgery and some investigators advocate a full electrophysiologic assessment in the preoperative period.[25]

OTHER LESIONS
Repaired Transposition of the Great Arteries

Patients with ventricular arterial discordance who underwent repair of transposition in infancy with either atrial or arterial switch operations can often develop sequelae in adulthood and require surveillance. For those patients who underwent atrial switch, they carry a significant risk of systemic atrioventricular (tricuspid) valve regurgitation, right ventricular systolic failure, baffle obstruction or baffle leak, and atrial arrhythmias. Many of these patients require pacemakers, which lead to baffle obstruction.[26–28] Patients with history of arterial switch operations are at risk of coronary artery stenosis, neoaortic root dilation with valve regurgitation, pulmonary artery stenosis, and RVOT obstruction.[29] These complications can often be managed percutaneously in some cases, but may require tricuspid valve repair or replacement, coronary artery bypass, or aortic valve or root replacement.[30] For those patients with atrial switch who develop systemic ventricular failure, orthotopic heart transplantation is recommended.

Coronary Anomalies

The most common coronary anomalies discovered in adulthood are anomalous aortic origin of the coronary artery. Owing to the abnormal take off of these coronaries, patients may present with coronary ischemia. Anomalous aortic origin of the left coronary should be repaired, whereas the right-sided coronary lesions should be repaired when evidence of ischemia exists. The coronary unroofing procedure maintains the same location of the coronary, but allows for relief to the intimal obstruction of the coronary along the intramural path along the aorta. In adults, ischemia from other congenital coronary pathologies such as anomalous coronary artery from the pulmonary artery and ostial stenosis are rare. These pathologies can be addressed with coronary reimplantation, ostial patch, coronary unroofing, or coronary artery bypass grafting depending on the anatomy of the lesions.

Fontan Physiology

Fontan physiology predisposes adult patients to both cardiac and noncardiac complications. They are at risk for developing protein losing enteropathy, plastic bronchitis, Fontan-associated liver disease and various forms of cardiac failure. Surgical strategies that have been used to improve symptoms of these conditions include Fontan conversion to extracardiac Fontan, cardiac pacing, Fontan fenestration, thoracic duct ligation, surgical rerouting of the innominate vein to the left atrium, and heart or combined heart–liver transplantation. The use of mechanical circulatory support in this population is controversial and there is not currently a device approved specifically for Fontan circulation.[31,32] However, promising case reports and single center data supports the use of ventricular assist devices for isolated ventricular failure and total artificial heart devices for Fontan failure.[33]

Acquired Disease in Congenital Patients

As patients with congenital cardiac disease become adults, they are susceptible to the same acquired diseases as those in the general population. Specific acquired pathologies in the ACHD population include degenerative valve disease, arrhythmias, great vessel and aortic root aneurysms, coronary atherosclerosis, and endocarditis. For some of these conditions, indications for surgery are not always clear and extrapolated from the general population. Thus, the traditionally accepted guidelines for patients without ACHD should be used as a guide.

Ascending Aorta and Aortic Root Pathology

The American Heart Association guidelines for the diagnosis, surveillance, and management of aortic root and ascending aorta pathology focus on the size of ascending or arch pathology, the presence of symptoms, and aortic valve competence.[34] These guidelines should be used to aid in decision making on the timing of surgical intervention for patients with ACHD with similar pathology. Exceptions include for those patients with known genetic syndromes and connective tissue disorders such as Turners disease or Marfan syndrome, patients with conotruncal defects who have a predisposition to aortopathy such as tetralogy of Fallot and truncus arteriosus, and those with a reconstructed neoaorta such as those patients with a Norwood or who have undergone the arterial switch and have a neoaortic root. The surgical management of these disease processes varies widely by centers, but includes replacement of the aortic valve and replacement of the aortic root with or without the aortic valve, ascending aorta, and/or aortic arch. When possible, valve-sparing procedures are preferred. These operations can be performed with a variety of different cannulation and myocardial protection strategies based on the location of the disease and the operative procedure planned.

Coronary Artery Atherosclerosis

Coronary artery bypass can be used in patients with ACHD who have reversible ischemia related to coronary artery atherosclerosis. Accepted indications for bypass for patients without ACHD should be followed. These cases can be challenging owing to variations in coronary anatomy and prior operative intervention.

MECHANICAL SUPPORT AND TRANSPLANTATION

Mechanical circulatory support is becoming more commonly used in adult patients with congenital heart disease to support the left ventricle, right ventricle, or both. Implantable devices can be used in patients with low output heart failure as bridge to recovery, destination therapy, or bridge to transplantation.[35] All devices require anticoagulation. Technical considerations in patients with ACHD include the size of the ventricular cavity, access to the necessary structures for cannula implantation in the reoperative setting, associated comorbid conditions (renal or hepatic failure, elevated pulmonary venous pressures), the presence of semilunar valve regurgitation, and the presence of intracardiac shunts. In the Fontan population, atrial device positioning with excision of the atrioventricular valve has been reported with success.[36]

Extracorporeal membrane oxygenation is widely used in the ACHD population. Venovenous or venoarterial circuits can be used depending on the underlying pathology.[37] Often, the cannulation strategies must be adjusted given anomalies of systemic venous drainage. Some options include central cannulation of the aorta and atrium, femoral vein and femoral artery, axillary artery and femoral vein, or femoral artery and internal jugular artery. Although the carotid artery is frequently used in pediatric cannulation for extracorporeal membrane oxygenation, it is not typically used for adults. For those patients requiring long term support, cannulation style should support ambulation and recovery.

For patients with ACHD with severe refractory heart failure and no other surgical options, orthotopic heart transplantation may be indicated.[38] Transplantation in the ACHD population is often higher risk than patients without ACHD because they have undergone multiple prior operations and could have developed aortopulmonary and venovenous collaterals that increase the risk of massive bleeding during repeat operations. Additionally, these patients often require more thoughtful approaches to the operation owing to anatomic variations, venous drainage, and great vessel anatomy.[39,40] In patients who have been on a single ventricle pathway, the elevated venous pressures lead to liver dysfunction or failure that also affects coagulation. In some instances, combined heart and liver transplantation is being used.[31] The problem of increased pulmonary vascular resistance from longstanding heart failure also poses additional questions regarding the decision to transplant. In fact, combined heart and lung transplantation may be feasible. Overall, the outcomes for thoracic transplantation in patients with ACHD have been favorable with a median survival of 15 years for patients with ACHD.[41] Given the high risk, it is important to select carefully those patients with ACHD who will benefit from transplantation.

SUMMARY

There are an increasing number of patients with congenital cardiac disease surviving into adulthood. The complex anatomy and physiology pose unique challenges to surgeons from both a technical and perioperative management standpoint. The management of these patients should be performed by a specialized multidisciplinary team in an experienced center.

DISCLOSURE

The authors have nothing to disclose.

REFERENCES

1. Stout KK, Daniels CJ, Aboulhosn JA, et al. 2018 AHA/ACC guideline for the management of adults with congenital heart disease: executive summary: a report of the American College of Cardiology/American Heart Association Task Force on Clinical Practice Guidelines. Circulation 2019;139(14): e637–97.
2. Kogon BE, Plattner C, Leong T, et al. Adult congenital heart surgery: adult or pediatric facility? Adult or pediatric surgeon? Ann Thorac Surg 2009;87: 833–40.
3. ACHA ACHD PROGRAM CRITERIA. Adult congenital heart association. Available at: https://www.achaheart.org/provider-support/accreditation-program/accreditation-program-documents/. Accessed February 28, 2020.
4. Karamlou T, Diggs BS, Person T, et al. National practice patterns for management of adult congenital heart disease. operation by pediatric heart surgeons decreases in-hospital death. Circulation 2008;118: 2345–52.
5. Kaiser L, Kron IL, Spray TL, editors. Mastery of cardiothoracic surgery. Philadelphia: Lippincott Williams & Wilkins; 2013.
6. Brown ML, Dearani JA, Burkhart HM. The adult with congenital heart disease: medical and surgical

considerations for management. Curr Opin Pediatr 2009;21(5):561–4.
7. Khonsari S, Sintek C. Cardiac surgery: safeguards and pitfalls in operative technique. Phildelphia: Lippincott Williams & Wilkins; 2008.
8. Djukanovic BP, Micovic S, Stojanovic I, et al. The current role of surgery in treating adult patients with patent ductus arteriosus. Congenit Heart Dis 2014;9(5):433–7.
9. Jacobs JP, Giroud JM, Quintessenza JA, et al. The modern approach to patent ductus arteriosus treatment: complementary roles of video-assisted thoracoscopic surgery and interventional cardiology coil occlusion. Ann Thorac Surg 2003;76:1421–8.
10. Nishimura RA, Otto CM, Bonow RO, et al. 2014 AHA/ACC guideline for the management of patients with valvular heart disease: a report of the American College of cardiology/American Heart Association Task Force on practice guidelines. J Am Coll Cardiol 2014;63(22):e57–185.
11. Dogan S, Aybek T, Risteski PS, et al. Minimally invasive port access versus conventional mitral valve surgery: prospective randomized study. Ann Thorac Surg 2005;79(2):492–8.
12. Silversides CK, Kiess M, Beauchesne L, et al. Canadian Cardiovascular Society 2009 Consensus Conference on the management of adults with congenital heart disease: outflow tract obstruction, coarctation of the aorta, tetralogy of Fallot, Ebstein anomaly and Marfan's syndrome. Can J Cardiol 2010;26(3):e80–97.
13. Sridhara S, Gavhane PU, Pandya B, et al. Meta-analysis comparing safety and outcomes after transcatheter aortic valve replacement in bicuspid aortic stenosis. Circulation 2019;140(Suppl_1): A13208.
14. Makkar RR. Outcomes of transcatheter aortic valve replacement with balloon expandable SAPIEN 3 valve in bicuspid aortic stenosis: an analysis of the STS/ACC TVT registry. Oral Presentation at the American College of Cardiology Annual Meeting 2019. New Orleans, Louisiana. Available at: http://www.clinicaltrialresults.org–www.clinicaltrialresults.org/Slides/ACC2019/Makkar_STSTVT.pdf.
15. Coskun TS, Coskun OK, El Arousy M, et al. Surgical repair of congenital supravalvular aortic stenosis in adult. ASAIO J 2007;53(6):e5–6.
16. Carr JA. The results of catheter-based therapy compared with surgical repair of adult aortic coarctation. J Am Coll Cardiol 2006;47(6):1101–7.
17. Bouchart F, Dubar A, Tabley A, et al. Coarctation of the aorta in adults: surgical results and long-term follow-up. Ann Thorac Surg 2000;70(5):1483–8.
18. Stanger P, Cassidy SC, Girod DA, et al. Balloon pulmonary valvuloplasty: results of the valvuloplasty and angioplasty of congenital anomalies registry. Am J Cardiol 1990;65(11):775–83.

19. Tretter JT, Morello M, Chaudhry A, et al. The management of tetralogy of Fallot after corrective surgery. Cardiovasc J S Afr 2018;15(1):6–15.

20. Peng LF, McElhinney DB, Nugent A, et al. Endovascular stenting of obstructed right ventricle-to-pulmonary artery conduits. Circulation 2006;113:2598–605.

21. Ong K, Boone R, Gao M, et al. Right ventricle to pulmonary artery conduit reoperations in patients with tetralogy of Fallot or pulmonary atresia associated with ventricular septal defect. Am J Cardiol 2013;111(11):1638–43.

22. Burri M, Lange R. Surgical treatment of Ebstein's anomaly. Thorac Cardiovasc Surg 2017;65(8):639–48.

23. Brown ML, Dearani JA, Danielson GK, et al. Comparison of the outcome of porcine bioprosthetic versus mechanical prosthetic replacement of the tricuspid valve in the Ebstein anomaly. Am J Cardiol 2009;103(4):555–61.

24. Chauvaud S, Fuzellier JF, Berrebi A, et al. Bi-directional cavopulmonary shunt associated with ventriculo and valvuloplasty in Ebstein's anomaly: benefits in high risk patients. Eur J Cardiothorac Surg 1998;13(05):514–9.

25. Dearani JA, Mora BN, Nelson TJ, et al. Ebstein anomaly review: what's now, what's next? Expert Rev Cardiovasc Ther 2015;13(10):1101–9.

26. Tobler D, Williams WG, Jegatheeswaran A, et al. Cardiac outcomes in young adult survivors of the arterial switch operation for transposition of the great arteries. J Am Coll Cardiol 2010;56(1):58–64.

27. Love BA, Mehta D, Fuster VF. Evaluation and management of the adult patient with transposition of the great arteries following atrial-level (Senning or Mustard) repair. Nat Clin Pract Cardiovasc Med 2008;5(8):454–67.

28. Dobson R, Danton M, Nicola W, et al. The natural and unnatural history of the systemic right ventricle in adult survivors. J Thorac Cardiovasc Surg 2013;145(6):1493–503.

29. Kempny A, Wustmann K, Borgia F, et al. Outcome in adult patients after arterial switch operation for transposition of the great arteries. Int J Cardiol 2013;167(6):2588–93.

30. Haeffele C, Lui GK. Dextro-transposition of the great arteries: long-term sequelae of atrial and arterial switch. Cardiol Clin 2015;33(4):543–58.

31. Reardon LC, DePasquale EC, Tarabay J, et al. Heart and heart–liver transplantation in adults with failing Fontan physiology. Clin Transplant 2018;32(8):e13329.

32. Rychik J, Atz AM, Celermajer DS, et al. Evaluation and management of the child and adult with Fontan circulation: a scientific statement from the American heart association. Circulation 2019;140(6):e234–84.

33. Woods RK, Ghanayem NS, Mitchell ME, et al. Mechanical circulatory support of the Fontan patient. In Seminars in Thoracic and Cardiovascular Surgery: Pediatric Cardiac Surgery Annual 2017 Jan 1 (Vol. 20, pp. 20-27). WB Saunders.

34. Hiratzka LF, Bakris GL, Beckman JA, et al. 2010 ACCF/AHA/AATS/ACR/ASA/SCA/SCAI/SIR/STS/SVM guidelines for the diagnosis and management of patients with thoracic aortic disease. J Am Coll Cardiol 2010;55(14):e27–129.

35. Steiner JM, Krieger EV, Stout KK, et al. Durable mechanical circulatory support in teenagers and adults with congenital heart disease: a systematic review. Int J Cardiol 2017;245:135–40.

36. Mascio CE. Unique cannulation technique and atrioventricular valve excision for HeartWare HVAD in the small Fontan patient. Oper Tech Thorac Cardiovasc Surg 2016;21(4):322–9.

37. Derk G, Laks H, Biniwale R, et al. Novel techniques of mechanical circulatory support for the right heart and Fontan circulation. Int J Cardiol 2014;176(3):828–32.

38. Ross HJ, Law Y, Book WM, et al. Transplantation and mechanical circulatory support in congenital heart disease: a scientific statement from the American Heart Association. Circulation 2016;133(8):802–20.

39. Gupta D, Reid J, Moguillansky D, et al. Heart transplantation for adult congenital heart disease: overview and special considerations. Cardiovasc Innov Appl 2018;3(1):73–84.

40. Fynn-Thompson F. Heart transplantation in adults with congenital heart disease. Methodist DeBakey Cardiovasc J 2019;15(2):145.

41. Khush KK, Cherikh WS, Chambers DC, et al. The International thoracic Organ transplant registry of the International Society for heart and lung transplantation: thirty-fifth adult heart transplantation report—2018; focus theme: multiorgan transplantation. J Heart Lung Transplant 2018;37(10):1155–68.

Congenital Heart Disease and Pulmonary Hypertension

Andrew Constantine, MBBS, MA[a,b],
Konstantinos Dimopoulos, MD, MSc, PhD[a,b],*,
Alexander R. Opotowsky, MD, MPH, MMSc[c]

KEYWORDS

- Pulmonary hypertension • Adult congenital heart disease • Precapillary • Postcapillary
- Echocardiography • Cardiac catheterization • Eisenmenger syndrome

KEY POINTS

- Pulmonary hypertension is common in adults living with congenital heart disease.
- Thoughtful diagnosis and classification are required for appropriate management.
- Extensive expertise and a high index of suspicion allow timely and accurate diagnosis.

INTRODUCTION

Pulmonary hypertension (PH) affects 5% to 10% of patients with congenital heart disease (CHD) and is associated with significant exercise limitation and increased morbidity and mortality.[1–4] The presence of PH also carries significant implications with regard to pregnancy and surgical procedures, both cardiac and noncardiac, affecting perioperative risk. PH, thus, needs to be identified early in all adults with CHD (ACHD) and managed appropriately to avoid pitfalls and optimize outcome. However, the diagnosis and management can be intricate. This review provides a general guide on how to diagnose and manage the ACHD patient with suspected PH of various types.

APPROACH TO THE ADULT CONGENITAL HEART DISEASE PATIENT WITH SUSPECTED PULMONARY HYPERTENSION
Clinical History

The symptoms of PH are notoriously nonspecific, especially in the context of patients with CHD, who may experience symptoms caused by residual hemodynamic lesions, arrhythmias, heart failure, or extracardiac features of a coexistent syndrome. Exertional dyspnea is common and can be graded using the Borg dyspnea scale (eg, assessed before and after a 6-minute walk test). Fatigue is commonly an associated feature in PH. Effort-induced syncope in adults with PH and CHD may occur because of their inability to augment their cardiac output appropriately in

a Adult Congenital Heart Centre & The National Centre for Pulmonary Hypertension, Royal Brompton Hospital, Royal Brompton & Harefield NHS Foundation Trust, Sydney Street, London SW3 6NP, UK; b The National Heart and Lung Institute, Imperial College London, Guy Scadding Building, Cale Street, London SW3 6LY, UK; c Department of Pediatrics, The Heart Institute, Cincinnati Children's Hospital, University of Cincinnati College of Medicine, Cincinnati, OH 45229, USA
* Corresponding author. Adult Congenital Heart Centre & The National Centre for Pulmonary Hypertension, Royal Brompton Hospital, Royal Brompton & Harefield NHS Foundation Trust, Sydney Street, London SW3 6NP, UK.
E-mail address: k.dimopoulos02@gmail.com

Cardiol Clin 38 (2020) 445–456
https://doi.org/10.1016/j.ccl.2020.04.008

response to the demand imposed by exercise or exertion and/or severe hypoxia, and is associated with increased mortality. Chest pain is not uncommon and can be ischemic in nature, the result of increased metabolic demands of the hypertrophied right ventricle, reduced right ventricular (RV) diastolic coronary perfusion, hypoxemia, or compression of the left main stem by a dilated main pulmonary artery (PA).[5] Noncardiac chest pain can arise from pulmonary embolism (eg, embolization of in situ PA thrombi in Eisenmenger patients), PA dissection, or rupture. Hemoptysis is also common and can be massive and life-threatening.

Components of the clinical history may raise suspicion for PH, especially the type of underlying CHD, timing and type of repair, and coexistent genetic syndromes, which may increase the risk of PH by various mechanisms. For example, patients with Down syndrome are prone to develop pulmonary vascular disease early in life in the presence of CHD but can also develop PH because of bronchopulmonary dysplasia, obstructive sleep apnea, and other reasons.

History of associated thromboembolism, respiratory disease, HIV infection, or portal hypertension should also not be ignored.

Further evidence is gathered from the physical examination (**Table 1**) and routine tests, including electrocardiography, chest radiography, exercise testing, and echocardiography.

Echocardiography

Echocardiography is an essential tool in the assessment and follow-up of patients with CHD. Imaging should be performed in an accredited unit using a protocolized approach that includes screening for PH. Clinical and echocardiographic suspicion of PH should be confirmed by cardiac catheterization (**Fig. 1**). Standard echocardiographic criteria for PH, as recommended by international PH guidelines, do apply to many, but not all, CHD patients with biventricular circulation. For example, peak tricuspid regurgitation (TR) flow velocity and other supporting signs related to the ventricles, pulmonary artery, or inferior vena cava and the right atrium can help estimate

Table 1	
Examination findings in pulmonary hypertension associated with congenital heart disease	
Inspection	Clubbing of toes and/or fingers
	Abnormalities of facies, stature, or extremities (genetic syndrome)
	Skin discoloration (cyanosis, pallor, jaundice)
	Petechiae or purpura
	Tortuous retinal vessels (on fundoscopy)
	Raised jugular venous pulse
	Respiratory rate and use of accessory muscles
	Previous surgical scars
	Peripheral edema
Palpation/Percussion	Right ventricular heave
	Left parasternal tap
	Hepatomegaly
	Ascites
	Pitting edema
Auscultation	Eisenmenger
	• Loud pulmonary component of S2
	• Single or narrowly split S2
	• Ejection click at upper left parasternal border
	• Early diastolic decrescendo murmur of high-pressure pulmonary regurgitation (Graham Steell)
	• High-pitched tricuspid regurgitation murmur
	• 3rd and 4th heart sounds
	In PAH-CHD with systemic-to-pulmonary shunts
	• VSD: holosystolic murmur in 4th intercostal space at the left parasternal border
	• Post-tricuspid shunt with Qp:Qs >2: mid-diastolic flow murmur across the MV

Abbreviations: MV, mitral valve; PAH-CHD, pulmonary arterial hypertension associated with congenital heart disease; Qp:Qs, ratio of pulmonary to systemic flow; S2, second heart sound; VSD, ventricular septal defect.

Table 2
Assumptions of the recommended pulmonary artery systolic pressure calculation from peak tricuspid regurgitation velocity and examples of congenital heart defects in which these assumptions do not hold[8]

Assumption About "Normal" Physiology	Situation Where Assumption Violated
RV directly communicates with the PA	Unrepaired pulmonary atresia
RV does not directly communicate with the aorta/systemic circulation	Univentricular circulation Nonrestrictive VSD ccTGA and post-atrial switch for TGA
Absence of obstruction between the proximal RV and distal pulmonary arterioles	Double-chambered RV RV outflow tract obstruction/subpulmonary stenosis Valvular pulmonary stenosis Supravalvular pulmonary stenosis Branch PA stenosis
RA pressure can be estimated using IVC size and collapsibility with respiration	Torrential TR IVC not directly communicating with RA (eg, TCPC) Mechanical ventilation

Abbreviations: (cc)TGA, (congenitally corrected) transposition of the great arteries; IVC, inferior vena cava; PA, pulmonary artery; RA, right atrium; RV, right ventricle; TCPC, total cavopulmonary connection; TR, tricuspid regurgitation; VSD, ventricular septal defect.

the probability of PH.[6,7] However, a fundamental understanding of each patient's anatomy and physiology is critical because standard criteria do not apply and can mislead in subsets of patients with not only complex CHD but also simple forms of CHD. In pulmonary stenosis, the gradient across the right ventricular outflow tract or pulmonary valve contributes to the TR velocity, and must be accounted for in the estimation of PA systolic pressure. In more complex CHD, TR velocity may have no relation to PA pressure (**Table 2**) and alternative signs should be sought.[8]

Cardiac Catheterization

Right heart catheterization remains the only method for confirming a true diagnosis of PH, distinguishing between precapillary and postcapillary hemodynamics, assessing the severity of PH, and performing vasoreactivity challenge. Meticulous attention to detail and an in-depth knowledge of underlying cardiac anatomy are required to access the heart and pulmonary arteries and thus gather and interpret clinically useful information. Cardiac catheterization should, therefore, be undertaken at a specialist center combining ACHD and PH expertise.

Precapillary PH is characterized by the presence of a mean PA pressure (mPAP) $\geq$25 mm Hg, a pulmonary artery wedge pressure (PAWP) $\leq$15 mm Hg, and pulmonary vascular resistance (PVR) $\geq$3WU.[6] By contrast, postcapillary PH is defined

by mPAP $\geq$25 mm Hg and PAWP greater than 15 mm Hg, and can be isolated or combined, based on a PVR of less than or $\geq$3 WU (Wood units) or a diastolic pressure gradient (diastolic PA pressure − PAWP) of less than or $\geq$7 mm Hg, respectively. Recent data from normal subjects, showing that an mPAP greater than 20 mm Hg represents two standard deviations above the mean normal mPAP, have led to the adoption of this cutoff in the new hemodynamic definition of PH in the 6th World Symposium proceedings (**Fig. 2**).[9] Although this new definition is based on scientific data rather than an arbitrary limit, one must acknowledge that no specific evidence about this exists for CHD, and the 25-mm Hg cutoff has appeared ubiquitously in PH research. When PAWP cannot be accurately measured, the left ventricular (LV) end-diastolic pressure should be used to estimate left atrial pressure. In cases where the PAWP is <15 mm Hg but there is a history and echocardiogram suggestive of "left" heart disease and/or diuretic treatment, the use of an acute fluid challenge may unmask LV diastolic dysfunction and discriminate between pulmonary arterial hypertension (PAH) and left heart disease.[10,11] Although this approach is intuitively appealing (ie, seems to make sense), evidence on optimal fluid volume and timing, as well as the clinical relevance of a particular response, is still sparse.

Vasoreactivity testing has multiple uses in PH. In idiopathic PAH, a positive vasoreactivity response, defined as a reduction of the mPAP $\geq$10 mm Hg to

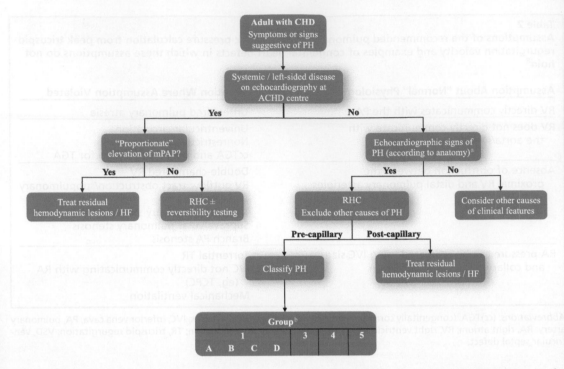

Fig. 1. Approach to the patient with congenital heart disease and features of pulmonary hypertension. In the presence of systemic/left-sided disease, clinical judgment is required to decide whether a small increase in pulmonary pressure is reflective of and proportionate to the degree of disease. [a] Refer to Dimopoulos and colleagues.[8] [b] See **Table 3** for pulmonary arterial hypertension associated with congenital heart disease (PAH-CHD) classification. (A)CHD, (adult) congenital heart disease; HF, heart failure; mPAP, mean pulmonary artery pressure; PH, pulmonary hypertension; RHC, right heart catheterization.

reach an absolute mean value of ≤40 mm Hg with an increased or unchanged cardiac output, carries prognosis and management implications (treatment with calcium-channel blockers).[6] Vasoreactivity testing is also performed in patients with unrepaired CHD and borderline hemodynamics, that is, a PVR index between 4 and 8 WU · m², to assess "reversibility" of the pulmonary vascular disease and aid the decision to operate. The absence of evidence-based thresholds for deciding operability[12] and uncertainty about the prognostic relevance of preoperative vasoreactivity testing is, however, reflected in the latest American Heart association/American College of Cardiology ACHD guidelines, which do not advocate vasoreactivity testing in this context.[13] Of note, independent from any impact on clinical decision making, the degree of response to acute pulmonary vasodilator administration seems to carry some prognostic insight.

A different type of vasoreactivity testing is integral to heart transplant assessment. In patients with systemic ventricular dysfunction (or other left-sided disease) and combined precapillary and postcapillary PH, response to milrinone and/ or sodium nitroprusside can help identify patients who may be eligible for heart versus heart-lung transplantation. In patients with low cardiac index, any medication that increases transpulmonary flow may decrease PVR via recruitment and distension of the pulmonary vasculature. This subset of patients does not have pulmonary vascular disease as a cause of elevated PVR, and the increase in flow unmasks preserved pulmonary vascular reserve. Patients with a fixed precapillary component may benefit from mechanical circulatory support, for example, LV assist device implantation, as a bridge to reassessment and heart transplantation.[14,15]

Complementary Imaging

Multimodality noninvasive imaging of the heart and lungs, including cardiovascular magnetic resonance (CMR), computed tomography, and ventilation-perfusion (V/Q) scanning, is helpful to diagnose incidental CHD and exclude other forms of PH, for example, connective tissue disease-related or chronic thromboembolic PH. CMR-augmented cardiac catheterization (in a

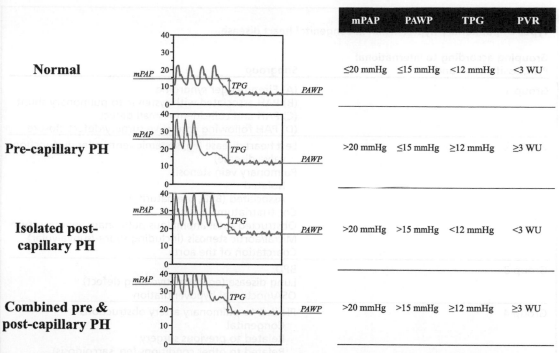

	mPAP	PAWP	TPG	PVR
Normal	≤20 mmHg	≤15 mmHg	<12 mmHg	<3 WU
Pre-capillary PH	>20 mmHg	≤15 mmHg	≥12 mmHg	≥3 WU
Isolated post-capillary PH	>20 mmHg	>15 mmHg	<12 mmHg	<3 WU
Combined pre & post-capillary PH	>20 mmHg	>15 mmHg	≥12 mmHg	≥3 WU

Fig. 2. Patients with precapillary pulmonary hypertension (PH) have a raised mean pulmonary artery pressure (mPAP) with a normal pulmonary artery wedge pressure (PAWP), hence a raised pulmonary vascular resistance (PVR). Postcapillary PH is characterized by an abnormally elevated PAWP. Isolated or combined pre- and postcapillary PH are differentiated on the basis of PVR and/or diastolic pressure gradient (DPG = diastolic pulmonary artery pressure − PAWP).[6,31,60] dPAP, diastolic pulmonary artery pressure.

hybrid laboratory) may be useful in accurately assessing hemodynamics in patients with complex CHD and/or multiple sources of pulmonary blood flow, combinations of shunts, or significant valvular regurgitation, in whom estimates of PVR by cardiac catheterization may be inaccurate.[16]

TYPES OF PULMONARY HYPERTENSION OBSERVED IN ADULTS WITH CONGENITAL HEART DISEASE
Precapillary Pulmonary Hypertension in Patients with Congenital Heart Disease

PH is not a single disease, and different forms are best approached with entirely distinct management strategies. Classifying the type of PH is essential in the management of all patients, including those with CHD, because it directs management. **Table 3** describes types of PH that can be encountered in ACHD patients. Group 1, namely, PAH-CHD, has attracted the most attention, especially since the introduction of PAH therapies. The histologic changes seen in the pulmonary circulation are indistinguishable from what is seen in other types of PAH, including idiopathic disease. The histologic classification of pulmonary vascular disease, which is still used in a modified form, was first proposed by Heath and Edwards in 1958[17] describing a cohort of patients predominantly with PAH-CHD. The initial, potentially reversible changes of arterial muscular hypertrophy and intimal thickening (grades I–III) progress to plexiform lesions and necrotizing arteritis (grade IV), which are deemed irreversible. Even though an increasing PVR is observed in progressive histologic grades, a clear correlation between the two is lacking. Moreover, neither histology nor cardiac catheterization can dependably foresee the outcome of reparative surgery. Nowadays, lung biopsies are rarely performed in clinical practice.[18,19]

A clinical classification has been developed for PAH-CHD (group 1), aimed mainly at simple defects (see **Table 3**). Groups A and B are patients with Eisenmenger syndrome (A) and those with systemic-to-pulmonary shunts (B). These 2 groups reside at different points along a continuum in terms of both hemodynamics and histologic changes, with Eisenmenger syndrome at the severe end of the spectrum. Eisenmenger syndrome is defined by patients born with a

Table 3
Types of pulmonary hypertension in congenital heart disease

Grouping according to International PH Classification and WS	Subgroup
Group 1	(A) Eisenmenger syndrome (B) PAH associated with systemic-to-pulmonary shunt (C) PAH and coincidental/small defect (D) PAH following corrective surgery/defect closure

Group 2	Left heart disease (eg, systemic ventricular dysfunction, valve disease)
	Pulmonary vein stenosis
	  Isolated
	  Associated (BPD, prematurity)
	Cor triatriatum
	Obstructed total anomalous pulmonary venous return
	Mitral/aortic stenosis (including supra-/subvalvular)
	Coarctation of the aorta

Group 3	BPD Lung disease (eg, restrictive lung defect) OSA/nocturnal hypoventilation

Group 4	PH due to pulmonary artery obstructions
	  Congenital
	  Related to previous surgery
	  Related to other conditions (eg, sarcoidosis)

Group 5 (complex CHD)	Segmental PH
	Isolated pulmonary artery of ductal origin
	Absent pulmonary artery
	Pulmonary atresia with VSD and MAPCAs
	Hemitruncus
	Other
	Single ventricle
	  Unoperated
	  Operated
	Scimitar syndrome

Based on the updated clinical classification of pulmonary hypertension from the Proceedings of the 6th World Symposium on Pulmonary Hypertension.[9,59]

Abbreviations: BPD, bronchopulmonary dysplasia; CHD, congenital heart disease; MAPCA, major aortopulmonary collateral artery; PAH, pulmonary arterial hypertension; PH, pulmonary hypertension; VSD, ventricular septal defect; WS, 6th World Symposium on Pulmonary Hypertension.

systemic-to-pulmonary shunt who eventually develop severe pulmonary vascular disease with consequent shunt reversal (now pulmonary-to-systemic or bidirectional shunting). PAH-CHD patients with left-to-right shunting have less severe pulmonary vascular disease, and some may be eligible for defect closure if the histologic changes can be deemed reversible. Defects that are more likely to lead to the development of pulmonary vascular disease include large central shunts (eg, truncus arteriosus, an aortopulmonary window, or large surgical shunts such as central, Potts, or Waterston shunts), large ventricular septal defects (VSDs) present in isolation or as part of complex cardiac anatomy (eg, univentricular hearts without pulmonary stenosis—an unprotected pulmonary circulation), or a large patent ductus arteriosus.[20–23] Improvements in diagnosis and surgical and interventional treatment have led to a decrease in the incidence and prevalence of Eisenmenger syndrome in developed countries, but it remains prevalent in developing countries.[24] Despite advances in treatment, Eisenmenger syndrome is associated with significant morbidity and mortality, related to PAH, chronic cyanosis, and the underlying cardiac defect (**Table 4**).

Group C PAH includes patients with only small or seemingly coincidental congenital defects. The presence of pulmonary vascular disease alongside a small cardiac defect, usually a VSD of less than 1 cm or an ASD of less than 2 cm in

Table 4
Multisystem complications of Eisenmenger syndrome

Cardiac	Hematologic	Other
Heart failure	Bleeding	Renal failure
Arrhythmias	Thrombosis	Hepatic dysfunction
Infective endocarditis	Hyperviscosity	Cerebral abscess
	Thrombocytopenia	Cholelithiasis
		Gout
		Paraganglioma

diameter, cannot be readily explained only by the small hemodynamic burden placed on the pulmonary vasculature by the defect itself, and likely reflects a separate process similar to idiopathic PAH.[6,9]

The fourth subgroup of PAH-CHD, namely postoperative PAH (which persists, recurs, or develops after CHD surgery), forms a growing proportion patients, currently about 20% of cases.[25] Following simple shunt repair, the prevalence of PH on echocardiographic screening is 3% to 5.7%.[2,26,27] In many patients, residual PAH after surgery or intervention is expected based on preoperative hemodynamics, whereas in others it may be unexpected and can develop years after the procedure. Certain genetic variants, such as the SOX17 and BMPR2 risk genes, have been documented in patients with PAH-CHD and may explain some of the phenotypic variation and the predisposition to PAH observed in these patients.[28,29] The presence of PAH significantly affects prognosis in these patients.

Other types of precapillary PH can be encountered in CHD, including PH resulting from pulmonary artery obstruction, coexisting bronchopulmonary dysplasia (often encountered in patients with Down syndrome), and "segmental" PH (currently classified under group 5, PH with unclear and/or multifactorial mechanisms, see **Table 3**). The latter group encompasses "any condition with abnormal underlying cardiac or vascular anatomy, usually including varied sources of pulmonary blood supply, which results in distal pulmonary vascular disease that affects various lung segments to differing degrees."[30] In this situation, the degree of V/Q mismatch determines the severity of symptoms and relates to differences in the perfusion of various lung segments and physiologic dead space (caused by collateral supply to the lung from the aorta, and coexisting intracardiac shunting). Segmental PH is typical of patients with tetralogy of Fallot with pulmonary atresia and major aortopulmonary collateral arteries. Cardiac catheterization to confirm segmental PH should only be performed in centers with expertise, because measurement of pressures and calculation of PVR in each lung segment can be difficult.

Another precapillary form of PH in CHD patients, classified under group 5 PH, is pulmonary vascular disease in Fontan patients. This rarely fulfills the classic definition of PH, because the low pulmonary blood flow and absence of a subpulmonary ventricle means that a relative and mild elevation in PVR can occur with low or normal PA pressures, but even this modest increase in resistance to flow has a large negative consequence in the absence of a subpulmonary pump.

Postcapillary Pulmonary Hypertension in Patients with Congenital Heart Disease

Postcapillary PH, which is PH with an increase in left-sided filling pressures (group 2 PH),[6] is common in ACHD patients and can occur as a result of left-sided lesions, including valve or outflow tract obstruction, valve regurgitation, and systolic or diastolic systemic ventricular dysfunction. Indeed, long-term sequelae involving the systemic ventricle and valves are common in ACHD patients with significant hemodynamic lesions and those who have undergone corrective surgery, especially when operated on in earlier surgical eras with higher rates of ventriculotomy and ischemic or reperfusion injury. Pulmonary venous obstruction, either congenital or as a complication of prior repair, can also contribute to PH in this group.

PH secondary to left heart disease reflects an increase in left atrial/pulmonary venous pressures, and can be isolated (with normal PVR) or combined with a precapillary component (and hence higher than normal PVR, see **Fig. 1**). The latter may be the result of chronic changes in the pulmonary vasculature, with endothelial dysfunction, infiltration of inflammatory cells, vasoconstriction, and vascular remodeling,[31] which leads to a further increase in mPAP and an increase in PVR. Careful study of hemodynamics is required when assessing patients for heart transplantation, for example, individuals with impaired systemic right ventricles and/or systemic atrioventricular valve regurgitation with advanced heart failure refractory to treatment.

MANAGEMENT OF PULMONARY HYPERTENSION IN ADULT CONGENITAL HEART DISEASE
Management of Pulmonary Arterial Hypertension-Congenital Heart Disease

The management strategy and role of PAH therapies depends on the presence and type of PAH-CHD. The distinct features of Eisenmenger syndrome (group A), particularly the presence of long-standing cyanosis and the underlying cardiac defect, result in a range of systemic complications, which require regular contact with specialists in PAH-CHD working within a wider multidisciplinary team.[6,13] Expert-led supportive management and the avoidance of historical practices (such as routine venesection) are an essential part of the management of Eisenmenger syndrome.[32] Endocarditis prophylaxis around high-risk dental procedures, immunization against influenza and *Pneumococcus*, contraception (not containing estrogen), and screening for and treatment of iron deficiency are recommended. Pregnancy should be avoided and adequate contraception prescribed. General anesthesia and sedation carry significant risks and nonessential surgery should be avoided, and essential surgery should be performed in specialist centers with adequate expertise. Randomized controlled trials (RCTs) have shown a benefit of the endothelin receptor antagonist (ERA) bosentan and the phosphodiesterase inhibitors sildenafil and tadalafil on hemodynamics, exercise capacity, and quality of life.[33–36] The recent MAESTRO trial, which assessed the effect of macitentan (an ERA) versus placebo in patients with Eisenmenger syndrome (including those with Down syndrome and those in New York Heart Association functional class II) did not meet the prespecified primary end point of change in exercise capacity over a 16-week period, but was associated with a decrease in B-type natriuretic peptide and improved hemodynamics compared with placebo.[37] The prognostic implications of PAH therapy in this patient group have been in contemporary populations are supported by evidence from several retrospective studies.[4,38–40]

For patients with PAH-CHD with systemic-to-pulmonary shunts (group B), the degree of elevation of PVR at cardiac catheterization, along with other metrics such as ratio of pulmonary to systemic resistance ($R_p:R_s$), is used to identify patients who could benefit from repair of the defect, with or without preceding PAH therapy. In patients with established pulmonary vascular disease (PVR index >8 WU · m^2 or $R_p:R_s$ >2/3 and/or net right-to-left shunt), defect closure shortens survival and should be avoided.[41] Conversely, in patients with a sizable shunt and normal pulmonary vascular physiology (PVR index <4 WU · m^2, $R_p:R_s$ <1/3), repair is strongly indicated and can be associated with an improved exercise tolerance, lower risk of atrial tachyarrhythmia, and better long-term outcome.[42,43] In patients with borderline hemodynamics (PVR index 4–8 WU · m^2, 2/3 > $R_p:R_s$ > 1/3), who fall within the "gray zone" of guideline recommendations, a trial of PAH therapy with reassessment of hemodynamics and possible repair of the defect has been advocated (the so-called "treat-and-repair" strategy). This approach remains controversial and should only be considered in selected patients following review in expert centers.[21,44–46] The use of fenestrated devices or surgical patches, which allow decompression of the right heart,[47] have also been described.

Experts often use PAH therapies in patients with PAH and small or coincidental defects (group C), even though evidence is lacking. However, some of these patients (idiopathic PAH with small atrial communications) were included with other idiopathic PAH patients in major RCTs.[48,49] Patients who develop PAH following CHD repair were also included in small numbers in most RCTs of PAH therapies. Although underpowered for formal subgroup analysis, these trials have allowed the use of PAH therapies in this patient cohort.[41]

Management of Other Types of Pulmonary Hypertension in Adult Congenital Heart Disease

There is little evidence to guide management of segmental PH and abnormal pulmonary resistance in Fontan patients. Expert centers do occasionally trial PAH therapies in these patients, on a case-by-case basis, after careful synthesis of available information from the clinical history and underlying physiology. In patients with a "failing Fontan" circulation, PAH therapies have been used to optimize hemodynamics, especially when refractory to other treatments. In those with stable Fontan physiology, some short-term physiologic studies have suggested modest benefit, but findings are mixed and long-term effects remain unexplored.[50–56]

In contrast to precapillary PH, there is no role for PAH therapies in the management of postcapillary PH, which requires the identification and management of active hemodynamic lesions. There are few empiric data to guide the use of conventional heart failure medication, such as angiotensin-converting enzyme inhibitors and angiotensin receptor blockers, and these medications are usually reserved for patients with systemic ventricular dysfunction, including those with systemic right ventricle. β-Blockers are used by some centers for patients with severe systemic ventricular dysfunction or in the presence of arrhythmias, but caution is required in the presence of RV dysfunction or conduction abnormalities. Mineralocorticoid receptor antagonists are used for right-sided congestive symptoms, and sometimes in higher doses for their renin-angiotensin-aldosterone system blocking effects. Loop diuretics are frequently used to control congestive heart failure. Despite a true absence of any evidence or experience in CHD, there is increasing interest for the use of newer heart failure therapies, such as sacubitril-valsartan,[57] GLP1 receptor agonists, and SGLT2 inhibitors, in this population.

FUTURE PERSPECTIVES

There has been significant progress in the understanding and management of PH related to ACHD over the past several decades, but numerous questions still remain. The epidemiology of PAH-CHD is changing and so should its management. As clinicians' understanding of the genetic basis of PH improves, personalized phenotyping and treatment is likely to improve outcomes. New tools to allow better assessment of operability in patients with borderline pulmonary vascular disease are sorely needed. It also remains unclear whether goal-oriented therapy (with specific targets aimed at optimizing outcome), as used in idiopathic disease, is effective for the management of PAH-CHD, and what the treatment targets should be. Indeed, risk-assessment tools specific to PAH-CHD are lacking, although multicenter efforts have allowed the identification of prognostic markers in Eisenmenger syndrome.[58] Finally, the role of PAH therapies in complex ACHD remains unclear.

SUMMARY

International collaboration and study designs that address the small sample size available at individual centers, heterogeneity of the population, and relatively low event rates are required to improve the understanding and treatment of CHD PH. In the absence of definitive evidence, expert multidisciplinary care[13] and education for patients and nonspecialist physicians is paramount in achieving wider engagement, preventing loss to follow-up, and supporting appropriate referrals to specialist services.

FUNDING

None.

ACKNOWLEDGMENTS

None.

DISCLOSURE

Professor K. Dimopoulos has received unrestricted educational support from Actelion and has been a consultant to and received grants and personal fees from Actelion (United Kingdom), Pfizer, United States, GlaxoSmithKline, United Kingdom, and Bayer/MSD, Germany. Dr A. Constantine has received a personal educational grant from Actelion (a Janssen Pharmaceutical Company of Johnson & Johnson). Professor A.R. Opotowsky has grants from Actelion and Roche Diagnostics and has served on an Independent Data Monitoring Board for Actelion.

REFERENCES

1. Duffels MGJ, Engelfriet PM, Berger RMF, et al. Pulmonary arterial hypertension in congenital heart disease: an epidemiologic perspective from a Dutch registry. Int J Cardiol 2007;120(2):198–204.
2. van Riel ACMJ, Schuuring MJ, van Hessen ID, et al. Contemporary prevalence of pulmonary arterial hypertension in adult congenital heart disease following the updated clinical classification. Int J Cardiol 2014;174(2):299–305.
3. Engelfriet PM, Duffels MGJ, Möller T, et al. Pulmonary arterial hypertension in adults born with a heart septal defect: the Euro Heart Survey on adult congenital heart disease. Heart 2007;93(6):682–7.
4. Dimopoulos K, Inuzuka R, Goletto S, et al. Improved survival among patients with Eisenmenger syndrome receiving advanced therapy for pulmonary arterial hypertension. Circulation 2010;121(1):20–5.
5. Galiè N, Saia F, Palazzini M, et al. Left main coronary artery compression in patients with pulmonary arterial hypertension and angina. J Am Coll Cardiol 2017;69(23):2808–17.
6. Galiè N, Humbert M, Vachiery J-L, et al. 2015 ESC/ERS guidelines for the diagnosis and treatment of

pulmonary hypertension: the Joint Task Force for the diagnosis and treatment of pulmonary hypertension of the European Society of Cardiology (ESC) and the European Respiratory Society (ERS) Endorsed by: Association for European Paediatric and Congenital Cardiology (AEPC), International Society for Heart and Lung Transplantation (ISHLT). Eur Respir J 2015;46(4):903–75.

7. Koestenberger M, Apitz C, Abdul-Khaliq H, et al. Transthoracic echocardiography for the evaluation of children and adolescents with suspected or confirmed pulmonary hypertension. Expert consensus statement on the diagnosis and treatment of paediatric pulmonary hypertension. The European Paediatric Pulmonary Vascular Disease Network, endorsed by ISHLT and DGPK. Heart 2016;102(Suppl 2):ii14–22.

8. Dimopoulos K, Condliffe R, Tulloh RMR, et al. Echocardiographic screening for pulmonary hypertension in congenital heart disease. J Am Coll Cardiol 2018;72(22):2778–88.

9. Simonneau G, Montani D, Celermajer DS, et al. Haemodynamic definitions and updated clinical classification of pulmonary hypertension. Eur Respir J 2019;53(1):1801913.

10. Fujimoto N, Borlaug BA, Lewis GD, et al. Hemodynamic responses to rapid saline loading: the impact of age, sex, and heart failure. Circulation 2013; 127(1):55–62.

11. Robbins IM, Hemnes AR, Pugh ME, et al. High prevalence of occult pulmonary venous hypertension revealed by fluid challenge in pulmonary hypertension. Circ Heart Fail 2014;7(1): 116–22.

12. Balzer DT, Kort HW, Day RW, et al. Inhaled nitric oxide as a preoperative test (INOP test I): the INOP test study group. Circulation 2002;106(12 Suppl 1): I76–81.

13. Stout KK, Daniels CJ, Aboulhosn JA, et al. 2018 AHA/ACC guideline for the management of adults with congenital heart disease: a report of the American College of Cardiology/American Heart Association Task Force on clinical practice guidelines. J Am Coll Cardiol 2018;25255. https://doi.org/10.1016/j.jacc.2018.08.1029.

14. Etz CD, Welp HA, Tjan TDT, et al. Medically refractory pulmonary hypertension: treatment with nonpulsatile left ventricular assist devices. Ann Thorac Surg 2007;83(5):1697–705.

15. Nair PK, Kormos RL, Teuteberg JJ, et al. Pulsatile left ventricular assist device support as a bridge to decision in patients with end-stage heart failure complicated by pulmonary hypertension. J Heart Lung Transplant 2010;29(2):201–8.

16. Muthurangu V, Taylor A, Andriantsimiavona R, et al. Novel method of quantifying pulmonary vascular resistance by use of simultaneous invasive pressure monitoring and phase-contrast magnetic resonance flow. Circulation 2004;110(7):826–34.

17. Heath D, Edwards JE. The pathology of hypertensive pulmonary vascular disease. Circulation 1958; 18(4):533–47.

18. Rabinovitch M, Haworth SG, Castaneda AR, et al. Lung biopsy in congenital heart disease: a morphometric approach to pulmonary vascular disease. Circulation 1978;58(6):1107–22.

19. Haworth SG. Pulmonary vascular disease in ventricular septal defect: structural and functional correlations in lung biopsies from 85 patients, with outcome of intracardiac repair. J Pathol 1987; 152(3):157–68.

20. Simonneau G, Galiè N, Rubin LJ, et al. Clinical classification of pulmonary hypertension. J Am Coll Cardiol 2004;43(12 Supplement):S5–12.

21. Dimopoulos K, Peset A, Gatzoulis MA. Evaluating operability in adults with congenital heart disease and the role of pretreatment with targeted pulmonary arterial hypertension therapy. Int J Cardiol 2008;129(2):163–71.

22. Collins-Nakai RL, Rabinovitch M. Pulmonary vascular obstructive disease. Cardiol Clin 1993; 11(4):675–87.

23. Hoffman JI, Rudolph AM. The natural history of ventricular septal defects in infancy. Am J Cardiol 1965; 16(5):634–53.

24. Hjortshøj CS, Jensen AS, Sørensen K, et al. Epidemiological changes in Eisenmenger syndrome in the Nordic region in 1977-2012. Heart 2017; 103(17):1353–8.

25. van Dissel AC, Mulder BJM, Bouma BJ. The changing landscape of pulmonary arterial hypertension in the adult with congenital heart disease. J Clin Med 2017;6(4). https://doi.org/10.3390/jcm6040040.

26. van Riel ACMJ, Blok IM, Zwinderman AH, et al. Lifetime risk of pulmonary hypertension for all patients after shunt closure. J Am Coll Cardiol 2015;66(9): 1084–6.

27. Lammers AE, Bauer LJ, Diller G-P, et al. Pulmonary hypertension after shunt closure in patients with simple congenital heart defects. Int J Cardiol 2020. https://doi.org/10.1016/j.ijcard.2019.12.070.

28. Zhu N, Welch CL, Wang J, et al. Rare variants in SOX17 are associated with pulmonary arterial hypertension with congenital heart disease. Genome Med 2018;10(1):56.

29. Roberts KE, McElroy JJ, Wong WPK, et al. BMPR2 mutations in pulmonary arterial hypertension with congenital heart disease. Eur Respir J 2004;24(3): 371–4.

30. Dimopoulos K, Diller G-P, Opotowsky AR, et al. Definition and management of segmental pulmonary hypertension. J Am Heart Assoc 2018;7(14). https://doi.org/10.1161/JAHA.118.008587.

31. Vachiéry J-L, Adir Y, Barberà JA, et al. Pulmonary hypertension due to left heart diseases. J Am Coll Cardiol 2013;62(25 Suppl):D100–8.

32. Dimopoulos K, Wort SJ, Gatzoulis MA. Pulmonary hypertension related to congenital heart disease: a call for action. Eur Heart J 2014;35(11):691–700.

33. Galiè N, Beghetti M, Gatzoulis MA, et al. Bosentan therapy in patients with Eisenmenger syndrome: a multicenter, double-blind, randomized, placebo-controlled study. Circulation 2006;114(1):48–54.

34. Iversen K, Jensen AS, Jensen TV, et al. Combination therapy with bosentan and sildenafil in Eisenmenger syndrome: a randomized, placebo-controlled, double-blinded trial. Eur Heart J 2010;31(9):1124–31.

35. Mukhopadhyay S, Nathani S, Yusuf J, et al. Clinical efficacy of phosphodiesterase-5 inhibitor tadalafil in Eisenmenger syndrome—a randomized, placebo-controlled, double-blind crossover study. Congenit Heart Dis 2011;6(5):424–31.

36. D'Alto M, Romeo E, Argiento P, et al. Bosentan-sildenafil association in patients with congenital heart disease-related pulmonary arterial hypertension and Eisenmenger physiology. Int J Cardiol 2012;155(3):378–82.

37. Gatzoulis MA, Landzberg M, Beghetti M, et al. Evaluation of macitentan in patients with Eisenmenger syndrome. Circulation 2019;139(1):51–63.

38. Diller G-P, Körten M-A, Bauer UMM, et al. Current therapy and outcome of Eisenmenger syndrome: data of the German National Register for congenital heart defects. Eur Heart J 2016;37(18):1449–55.

39. Hascoet S, Fournier E, Jaïs X, et al. Outcome of adults with Eisenmenger syndrome treated with drugs specific to pulmonary arterial hypertension: a French multicentre study. Arch Cardiovasc Dis 2017;110(5):303–16.

40. Arnott C, Strange G, Bullock A, et al. Pulmonary vasodilator therapy is associated with greater survival in Eisenmenger syndrome. Heart 2017. https://doi.org/10.1136/heartjnl-2017-311876.

41. Manes A, Palazzini M, Leci E, et al. Current era survival of patients with pulmonary arterial hypertension associated with congenital heart disease: a comparison between clinical subgroups. Eur Heart J 2014;35(11):716–24.

42. Attie F, Rosas M, Granados N, et al. Surgical treatment for secundum atrial septal defects in patients >40 years old. A randomized clinical trial. J Am Coll Cardiol 2001;38(7):2035–42.

43. Humenberger M, Rosenhek R, Gabriel H, et al. Benefit of atrial septal defect closure in adults: impact of age. Eur Heart J 2011;32(5):553–60.

44. Yao A. "Treat-and-repair" strategy for atrial septal defect and associated pulmonary arterial hypertension. Circ J 2016;80(1):69–71.

45. Bradley EA, Ammash N, Martinez SC, et al. "Treat-to-close": non-repairable ASD-PAH in the adult: results from the North American ASD-PAH (NAAP) multicenter registry. Int J Cardiol 2019. https://doi.org/10.1016/j.ijcard.2019.03.056.

46. Constantine A, Dimopoulos K. Evaluating a strategy of PAH therapy pre-treatment in patients with atrial septal defects and pulmonary arterial hypertension to permit safe repair ("treat-and-repair"). Int J Cardiol 2019;291:142–4.

47. Talwar S, Keshri VK, Choudhary SK, et al. Unidirectional valved patch closure of ventricular septal defects with severe pulmonary arterial hypertension: hemodynamic outcomes. J Thorac Cardiovasc Surg 2014;148(6):2570–5.

48. Pulido T, Adzerikho I, Channick RN, et al. Macitentan and morbidity and mortality in pulmonary arterial hypertension. N Engl J Med 2013;369(9):809–18.

49. Sitbon O, Channick R, Chin KM, et al. Selexipag for the treatment of pulmonary arterial hypertension. N Engl J Med 2015;373(26):2522–33.

50. Giardini A, Balducci A, Specchia S, et al. Effect of sildenafil on haemodynamic response to exercise and exercise capacity in Fontan patients. Eur Heart J 2008;29(13):1681–7.

51. Ovaert C, Thijs D, Dewolf D, et al. The effect of bosentan in patients with a failing Fontan circulation. Cardiol Young 2009;19(4):331–9.

52. Goldberg DJ, French B, McBride MG, et al. Impact of oral sildenafil on exercise performance in children and young adults after the Fontan operation: a randomized, double-blind, placebo-controlled, crossover trial. Circulation 2011;123(11):1185–93.

53. Schuuring MJ, Vis JC, van Dijk APJ, et al. Impact of bosentan on exercise capacity in adults after the Fontan procedure: a randomized controlled trial. Eur J Heart Fail 2013;15(6):690–8.

54. Rhodes J, Ubeda-Tikkanen A, Clair M, et al. Effect of inhaled iloprost on the exercise function of Fontan patients: a demonstration of concept. Int J Cardiol 2013;168(3):2435–40.

55. Hebert A, Mikkelsen UR, Thilen U, et al. Bosentan improves exercise capacity in adolescents and adults after Fontan operation: the TEMPO (Treatment with Endothelin receptor antagonist in Fontan patients, a randomized, placebo-controlled, double-blind study Measuring Peak Oxygen Consumption) study. Circulation 2014;130(23):2021–30.

56. Goldberg DJ, Zak V, Goldstein BH, et al. Results of the Fontan Udenafil Exercise Longitudinal (FUEL)

trial. Circulation 2019. https://doi.org/10.1161/CIRCULATIONAHA.119.044352.

57. Maurer SJ, Pujol Salvador C, Schiele S, et al. Sacubitril/valsartan for heart failure in adults with complex congenital heart disease. Int J Cardiol 2020;300:137–40.

58. Kempny A, Hjortshøj CS, Gu H, et al. Predictors of death in contemporary adult patients with Eisenmenger syndrome: a multicenter study. Circulation 2017;135(15):1432–40.

59. Rosenzweig EB, Abman SH, Adatia I, et al. Paediatric pulmonary arterial hypertension: updates on definition, classification, diagnostics and management. Eur Respir J 2019;53(1). https://doi.org/10.1183/13993003.01916-2018.

60. Dimopoulos K, Ernst S, McCabe C, et al. Pulmonary artery denervation: a new, long-awaited interventional treatment for combined pre- and post-capillary pulmonary hypertension? JACC Cardiovasc Interv 2019;12(3):285–8.

Heart Failure in Adult Congenital Heart Disease

Luke J. Burchill, MBBS, PhD[a,b,*], Melissa G.Y. Lee, MBBS, PhD[a,c,d], Vidang P. Nguyen, MD[e], Karen K. Stout, MD[f]

KEYWORDS

- Cardiac defects • Cardiopulmonary exercise testing • Congenital heart disease • Fontan procedure
- Heart failure • Right ventricle • Tetralogy of Fallot • Ventricular remodeling

KEY POINTS

- The burden of heart failure in adult congenital heart disease (ACHD) continues to grow and remains a formidable complication with high morbidity and mortality.
- Risk stratification and prognostication of heart failure in ACHD is challenging for many reasons including but not limited to the significant clinical heterogeneity within the ACHD population.
- Multi-modality investigations are indicated in all ACHD patients with suspected heart failure.
- Treatment of ACHD-related heart failure is guided by heart failure classification with early referral for advanced heart failure assessment.

CASE STUDY

Mr D is a 47-year-old man with D-transposition of the great arteries treated with a Mustard repair at age 2 years and transcatheter stenting of a superior vena cava baffle stenosis at age 35 years. He now presents to clinic with New York Heart Association (NYHA) functional class III symptoms, including fatigue, breathlessness with minimal exertion, weight gain, and poor sleep. Examination confirms a comfortable looking gentleman in no acute distress. He has a midline sternotomy scar and a body mass index of 30 kg/m² with 7-kg weight gain in the preceding 6 months. Blood pressure is 120/70 mm Hg, regular pulse at 70 beats per minute, and oxygen saturations 98% on room air. Jugular venous pulsation is 7 cm above the sternal angle. He has a 3/6 pansystolic murmur at the left lower sternal edge. Lung fields are clear to auscultation. His liver edge is palpable 3 cm below the right costal margin, and he has mild pitting edema of both legs extending to the knees. Electrocardiogram and Holter monitor show sinus node dysfunction with intact atrioventricular conduction. Transthoracic echocardiogram demonstrates a hypertrophied and dilated systemic right ventricle with moderately reduced ejection fraction (35%–40%) and moderately severe regurgitation of the tricuspid (systemic atrioventricular) valve, both rated as mild and stable 1 year earlier. There is no evidence of residual baffle stenosis or leak. The following questions arise: (1) What investigations are indicated in cases where adult congenital heart disease (ACHD)-related heart failure (HF) is suspected? (2) How do we classify ACHD-related HF and evaluate prognosis? (3) Which evidence-based treatments should be considered in this case?

[a] Department of Cardiology, The Royal Melbourne Hospital, Grattan Street, Parkville, Melbourne, VIC 3050, Australia; [b] Department of Medicine, The University of Melbourne, Melbourne, Australia; [c] Heart Research, Clinical Sciences, Murdoch Children's Research Institute, Melbourne, Australia; [d] Department of Paediatrics, The University of Melbourne, Melbourne, Australia; [e] Department of Cardiology, Cedars-Sinai Heart Institute, 127 S San Vicente Boulevard a3600, Los Angeles, CA 90048, USA; [f] Division of Cardiology, Department of Medicine, University of Washington, Seattle, WA 98195, USA
* Corresponding author. Department of Cardiology, The Royal Melbourne Hospital, Grattan Street, Parkville, Melbourne, VIC 3050, Australia.
E-mail address: blj@unimelb.edu.au

Cardiol Clin 38 (2020) 457–469
https://doi.org/10.1016/j.ccl.2020.04.010
0733-8651/20/© 2020 Elsevier Inc. All rights reserved.

INTRODUCTION

ACHD-related HF has often defied description or understanding leading to uncertainty surrounding the best approach to treatment. In recent years, research and clinical guidelines for ACHD-related HF have started to address these knowledge gaps leading to greater consensus on how to best assess and treat those presenting with ACHD-related HF. Even so, fundamental questions about ACHD-related HF remain. In this article we examine recent contributions to the field with a focus on ACHD-related HF research that translates into clinical practice.

HOW COMMON IS ADULT CONGENITAL HEART DISEASE–RELATED HEART FAILURE?

HF is a leading cause of mortality and morbidity in ACHD accounting for 21% to 40% of all ACHD deaths in large cohort and registry studies.[1–4] In a large study of 6969 ACHD patients, HF mortality increased exponentially over two decades while other causes of death remained relatively unchanged.[3] Among ACHD subgroups, HF is consistently reported as the leading cause of death in patients with moderate or complex congenital heart disease (CHD),[1,3,5–7] particularly in patients with Eisenmenger syndrome, systemic right ventricle, and single ventricle with Fontan palliation. ACHD-related morbidity also continues to rise with time. Population-based studies have demonstrated a dramatic increase in hospitalizations for ACHD-related HF in recent years.[8–10] Burchill and colleagues[8] analyzed data from approximately 8 million adult HF admissions in the United States between 1998 and 2011 and demonstrated a 91% increase in ACHD-versus a 21% increase in non-ACHD-related HF. ACHD-related HF hospitalizations resulted in significantly higher costs and procedural burden compared with non-ACHD HF hospitalizations.[8] Despite advances in care for the ACHD population, long-term survival and freedom from hospitalization remains significantly compromised by HF, particularly in those with more complex types of CHD.

DEVELOPING A COMMON LANGUAGE FOR CLASSIFYING AND REPORTING ADULT CONGENITAL HEART DISEASE–RELATED HEART FAILURE

The lack of a uniform definition for ACHD-related HF poses challenges not only for epidemiologic studies but also for developing clinical care and treatment guidelines. There is also a limited capacity to develop quality care indicators by which to track, compare, and harmonize ACHD-related HF care. Many, if not all, patients with ACHD meet criteria for having or being at increased risk of ACHD-related HF. The 2016 American Heart Association (AHA) Scientific Statement regarding Chronic HF in CHD defined CHD-related HF as a "syndrome characterized by either or both pulmonary and systemic venous congestion and/or inadequate peripheral oxygen delivery, at rest or during stress, caused by cardiac dysfunction…."[11] Most people born with complex congenital heart defects meet this definition for CHD-related HF at birth. Many have surgeries to repair their heart defects; however, they are not cured and late-onset complications are common. The ACHD AP classification system, first described in 2019, is intended to capture the complexity of ACHD anatomy and physiology, which are not always correlated.[12] Although not strictly for HF, the AP system offers a more integrated approach for classifying the severity of ACHD. Anatomic complexity is graded as I (simple), II (moderate), or III (great) and physiologic state is graded as stage A to D according to NYHA functional class, arrhythmia history, ventricular and valvular function, and the presence of end-organ dysfunction (see Table 4 of the 2018 AHA/American College of Cardiology [ACC] ACHD guidelines[12]). By making explicit the anatomic and physiologic variables at play, the AP classification system facilitates a more integrated and holistic approach to treatment.

NYHA classification is embedded within the ACHD AP classification system. It is worth noting that NYHA functional class alone has been found to predict disease severity and mid- to long-term ACHD mortality.[13] However, large cohort studies have shown that reduced exercise capacity and oxygen delivery (on cardiopulmonary testing [CPET]) is not uncommon in NYHA functional class I ACHD patients.[14,15] Thus, a combination of subjective (NYHA functional class) and objective (CPET) evaluation is important for identifying patients with asymptomatic ACHD-related HF.

Clinical stages of HF can also be classified using the ACC/AHA staging system (**Table 1**).[16] Largely for patients with acquired (ie, non-congenital forms) HF, the system purposefully guides clinicians on how to escalate treatment as HF progresses. Stage A patients are considered at risk of HF caused by comorbid conditions (e.g. hypertension, diabetes) and/or family history of HF. Stage B patients are those with existing structural heart disease or left ventricular systolic dysfunction. As such, most patients with ACHD fall into stage B and are considered pre-HF. Many patients with ACHD meet criteria for stage C because of the presence of clinical HF symptoms and a smaller

Table 1
Clinical stages and treatment of heart failure

ACC/AHA HF Classification System	Treatment Recommendations

Stage A
Pre-HF. Family history of HF or increased HF risk based on the presence of the following medical conditions:
Hypertension
Diabetes
CAD
Metabolic syndrome
History of alcohol abuse
History of rheumatic fever
Family history of cardiomyopathy
Medications associated with cardiomyopathy
	Regular exercise
	Stop smoking
	Low-sodium diet
	Treatment of hypertension
	Treatment of high cholesterol
	Abstinence of alcohol or recreational drugs
	Consideration of:
	  ACE-I or an ARB for patients with CAD, diabetes, or hypertension
	  β-Blocker for hypertension

Stage B
Pre-HF. Left (systemic) ventricular systolic dysfunction on cardiac imaging (ie, echocardiogram or cardiac MRI) but without HF symptoms
	Treatments as listed in stage A plus:
	  Consideration of ACE-I/ARB
	  β-Blocker if EF <40% or a history of MI
	  Aldosterone antagonist if history of MI, diabetes, and EF ≤35%
	  Exclusion of significant CAD, valvular or residual CHD requiring intervention

Stage C
Diagnosis of HF with current or prior symptoms of HF
	Treatments listed in stage A and B plus:
	  Diuretics
	  Daily weight
	  Fluid restriction
	  Consideration of device therapy, CRT, and/or ICD in selected patients

Stage D
Advanced HF symptoms unresponsive to treatment
	Treatments listed in stages A to C plus evaluation of candidacy for:
	  High-risk heart surgery in a specialized CHD center
	  Heart transplant
	  Mechanical circulatory support
	  Palliative care

Abbreviations: ACE-I, angiotensin-converting enzyme inhibitor; ARB, angiotensin II receptor blocker; CAD, coronary artery disease; CHD, congenital heart disease; CRT, cardiac resynchronization therapy; EF, ejection fraction; HF, heart failure; ICD, implantable cardiac defibrillator; MI, myocardial infarction; MRI, magnetic resonance imaging.

Adapted from Yancy CW, Jessup M, Bozkurt B, Butler J, Casey DE, Jr., Drazner MH, et al. 2013 ACCF/AHA guideline for the management of heart failure: a report of the American College of Cardiology Foundation/American Heart Association Task Force on Practice Guidelines. J Am Coll Cardiol. 2013;62:e147-239.

subset of ACHD patients are classified as stage D based on advanced HF symptoms not responsive to treatment. Stage D HF describes advanced progression of HF characterized by structural abnormalities of the heart and severe resting symptoms despite optimal medical, surgical, and device therapy. The ACC/AHA classification system guides clinicians on which HF treatments to consider across each stage of HF.[16] Despite the lack of evidence for standard HF treatments in ACHD, certain treatments (β-blockers, renin-angiotensin aldosterone system antagonists, device therapies) may be justified according to ventricular function, blood pressure, hemodynamic profile (ie, systemic vascular resistance and ventricular afterload determined at the time of cardiac catheterization), and comorbidities (e.g, hypertension, diabetes, kidney impairment). It is important to ensure there are no other contributors to HF for which treatment would improve symptoms or ventricular function. Considerations include physiologic abnormalities such as valve dysfunction and residual shunts, or anatomic abnormalities such as coarctation of the aorta which increase afterload. Rhythm abnormalities are common in ACHD and also need to be assessed, because tachyarrhythmias or bradycardia can contribute to HF symptoms.

CLINICAL PRESENTATION OF ADULT CONGENITAL HEART DISEASE–RELATED HEART FAILURE

Many patients with ACHD have adapted to their underlying condition and consider reduced functional capacity to be their baseline.[14,15] A significant number of ACHD patients subjectively report having no limitations despite objective (CPET) evidence to the contrary. As such, worsening of NYHA functional class in patients with ACHD is significant and should prompt further evaluation, particularly given the association between NYHA functional class and worse clinical outcomes in this population.[17]

The clinical presentation of ACHD-related HF is highly variable and atypical. It is difficult to distinguish whether the symptoms are a cause or a manifestation of HF. Examples include atrial arrhythmias in patients with atrial switch for transposition of the great arteries or ventricular arrhythmia in patients with tetralogy of Fallot. In fact, in patients with tetralogy of Fallot, ventricular arrhythmia has been associated with myocardial fibrosis, elevated left ventricular end-diastolic pressure, and diastolic dysfunction on echocardiographic parameters.[18–20] These are all examples of the significant overlap between HF and arrhythmia in ACHD.

Other HF manifestations are idiosyncratic and manifest in patients with a Fontan circulation. These distinctive manifestations may include abdominal pain and diarrhea with protein-losing enteropathy and dyspnea with plastic bronchitis. Although the development of protein-losing enteropathy and plastic bronchitis is rare affecting up to 11%[21,22] and less than 5%[23,24] of patients with a Fontan circulation, respectively, these complications are extremely debilitating and carry high rates of hospitalization and mortality.[25,26] Because of the variety in manifestations, clinicians should have a low degree of suspicion for initiating investigation for ACHD-related HF, even in patients reporting subtle changes in functional capacity or other HF symptoms.

PROGNOSTICATION IN ADULT CONGENITAL HEART DISEASE–RELATED HEART FAILURE

Risk stratification and prognostication of HF in ACHD is challenging for many reasons. Significant clinical heterogeneity within the ACHD population makes it difficult to translate research findings from one subgroup to another. For reasons that are unclear, there is also significant variation in the clinical trajectory of HF, even among patients with the same CHD subtype and surgical repair.

Ventricular Dysfunction

ACHD HF may not be directly related to ventricular dysfunction and is reflected in the weaker association between ventricular dysfunction and B-type natriuretic peptide (BNP) or N-terminal pro-B-type natriuretic peptide (NT-proBNP) in ACHD compared with HF in acquired heart disease. Importantly, the risk of ventricular dysfunction varies according to CHD lesion complexity. Patients with a systemic right ventricle, such as those who have undergone an atrial switch procedure for transposition of the great arteries,[27,28] are at high risk of systemic ventricular systolic dysfunction. In contrast, patients with single ventricle physiology may manifest clinical features of systemic venous congestion as a reflection of the inherent limitations of the Fontan circulation rather than a direct reflection of ventricular systolic dysfunction.[29] Regardless, the finding of ventricular dysfunction is prognostically important and at least moderate ventricular dysfunction indicates a higher risk of sudden cardiac death in the ACHD population[30] and in subgroups including those with a systemic right ventricle[27,31–33] and in patients with repaired tetralogy of Fallot.[34]

Cardiopulmonary Exercise Testing

CPET includes assessment of exercise capacity and ventilatory gas exchange during exercise and is widely used in the follow-up of patients with ACHD.[35] It is essential that results obtained during CPET are referenced against patients with the same underlying ACHD lesion subtype because of inherent differences in baseline exercise tolerance between different subgroups.[14,15] A summary of CPET measurements and thresholds for predicting mortality and/or adverse outcomes by ACHD subtype is presented in **Table 2**. Peak oxygen consumption (Vo_2 max) is of prognostic importance because lower peak Vo_2 has been independently associated with hospitalization and mortality in mixed ACHD patient cohorts[14] and within certain ACHD subtypes.[15] A recent systematic literature review reported peak Vo_2 to be an inconsistent predictor for mortality in the Fontan population.[36] Peak Vo_2 has also been proposed for the assessment of perioperative risk and early mortality in patients with tetralogy of Fallot undergoing surgical pulmonary valve replacement.[37] Although peak Vo_2 is widely used at the time of ACHD and HF assessment, CPET provides further important information. This includes measures of ventilatory efficiency, exercise oscillatory ventilation (EOV), heart rate reserve, and peak exercise blood pressure. Ventilatory efficiency is expressed as the minute

Table 2
CPET thresholds for predicting mortality and/or adverse outcomes by ACHD subtypes

ACHD Subtype	Outcome
Tetralogy of Fallot	Peak Vo_2 predictor of early mortality after surgical pulmonary valve replacement[37] VE/VCO$_2$ slope >31 predictor of all-cause mortality[38]
Systemic right ventricle	VE/VCO$_2$ slope ≥35.4 and peak Vo_2% ≤52.3% associated with an increased 4-y risk of death/hospitalization (cohort of d-TGA with Mustard/Senning repairs)[39] Lower peak exercise SBP, especially <180 mm Hg, associated with adverse clinical events (d-TGA with Mustard/Senning repairs and cc-TGA)[44]
Ebstein anomaly	Peak Vo_2 (<60% of predicted) and heart rate reserve (<25 bpm) predictors of death/hospitalization/cardiac surgery[43]

Fontan physiology	Peak Vo_2 inconsistent predictor for mortality in systematic literature review[36]
	 Available cutoffs suggestive to be predictive of mortality:
	     Peak Vo_2 <21.0 mL/kg/min[69]
	     Peak Vo_2 <16.6 mL/kg/min[40]
	     VE/VCO$_2$ slope >33.5[40]
	     Peak heart rate <122.5 bpm[40]
	 Change in peak Vo_2 (−3% points/y) and change in peak heart rate (−4% points/y) predictor of 5-y risk of cardiovascular adverse events[70]
	 Presence of EOV associated with higher risk of death or transplant[45]

Abbreviations: EOV, exercise oscillatory ventilation; SBP, systolic blood pressure; TGA, transposition of the great arteries; VCO$_2$, volume of exhaled carbon dioxide; VE, minute ventilation; Vo_2, maximal oxygen uptake.

ventilation carbon dioxide production relationship (VE/VCO$_2$ slope). An elevated VE/VCO$_2$ slope greater than 30 is a powerful prognostic marker of HF. An elevated VE/VCO$_2$ slope is inversely related to cardiac output at peak exercise and is at least partly explained by a decrease in pulmonary perfusion. ACHD patient studies have demonstrated VE/VCO$_2$ slope to be independently predictive of hospitalization and/or mortality.[38–40] In fact, the combined use of VE/VCO$_2$ and peak Vo_2 has been demonstrated to have a higher predictive value than the use of either measurement alone.[39] Measures of heart rate and blood pressure response to exercise can also be assessed by CPET. Failure to achieve at least 80% of the heart rate reserve (the difference between the resting and maximum heart rate) is widely viewed as a cutoff for chronotropic incompetence or the inability of the heart to respond to exercise.[41] Chronotropic Incompetence is seen in up to two-thirds of patients with ACHD and has been associated with NYHA functional class, hospitalization, and mortality.[42] In patients with Ebstein anomaly, heart rate reserve has been demonstrated to be a significant predictor of adverse outcomes.[43] In addition, lower peak exercise systolic blood pressure, especially less than 180 mm Hg, has been associated with clinical events in patients with systemic right ventricle.[44] Although all CPET measurements require maximal effort tests for accuracy, EOV is assessed on submaximal CPET tests. EOV signifies regular oscillations in minute ventilation during exercise and is thought to be caused by abnormal respiratory autoregulation. EOV is a common phenomenon in patients with Fontan physiology affecting more than a third of patients and has been demonstrated to be an independent predictor of mortality or transplantation in the Fontan population.[45]

Natriuretic Peptides

Although BNP and NT-proBNP are often elevated at baseline in asymptomatic patients with ACHD, there is growing evidence that these biomarkers may be helpful for evaluating disease severity. Studies exploring NT-proBNP and survival outcome have demonstrated worse survival in patients with higher versus lower NT-proBNP.[46,47] Among 595 ACHD outpatients followed for a median of 42 months, those in the highest quartile of NT-proBNP values (>33.3 pmol/L) had event- and heart-failure-free survival of only 35% and 72% at 50 months, respectively, compared with 87% and 99% in patients in the lowest NT-proBNP quartile (<6.8 pmol/L).[47] A normal NT-proBNP (<14 pmol/L) had a high negative predictive value thereby making it a useful screening tool for ruling out HF and death.[47] The risk of an adverse event could be further categorized with the addition of additional biomarkers, namely high-sensitivity troponin-T and growth-differentiation factor 15.[47] Patients who had elevated levels of all three biomarkers were at highest risk of cardiovascular events.[47] In another prospective study, red cell distribution width was associated with adverse cardiovascular outcome in patients with ACHD independent of NT-proBNP.[48]

Heart Failure Prediction Models

There are scarce studies exploring prediction models for HF in ACHD. One of the earliest HF prediction models used in ACHD is the Seattle HF Model. The Seattle HF Model combines age, sex, weight, cardiac medication use, NYHA functional class, systolic blood pressure, systemic ejection fraction, laboratory values, and presence of a device to predict mean, 1-, 2-, and 3-year survival.[49] Seattle HF Model is used to identify patients at risk for adverse events in the ACHD population but the predicted mortality risks have been shown not to be representative of actual ACHD survival.[50] Baggen and colleagues[51] published a prediction model for a composite end point of mortality, HF, or arrhythmia in 602 patients with moderate or complex ACHD and were able to distinguish between high- and low-risk patients by incorporating similar clinical variables including age, body mass index, congenital lesion, NYHA functional class, cardiac medication use, reinterventions, and NT-proBNP. The prediction model was then externally validated in a different ACHD population of 402 patients and was able to discriminate between patients with and without an adverse outcome within 4 years of follow-up.[51] A systematic review exploring risk factors for adverse outcomes in ACHD-related HF[17] confirmed the literature for risk factors and prediction models in ACHD-related HF is scant. Not surprisingly, CHD lesion characteristics, NYHA functional class, and BNP were predictive of adverse outcome in ACHD-related HF.[17] Further research that includes large populations with well-defined clinical HF phenotypes is needed before prediction models are used to reliably guide ACHD HF care in daily clinical practice.

INVASIVE HEMODYNAMIC EVALUATION

Because of the unique and highly complex anatomy of patients with CHD, invasive cardiac catheterization is an integral part in the diagnosis and management. Information that is gathered from an invasive catheterization includes filling pressures; measures of vascular resistance; shunt fraction; and angiographic assessment of arterial and venous anatomy, anastomoses, and collateral vessels.

Pulmonary hypertension is common in patients with ACHD with and without HF. Pulmonary arterial hypertension is defined as mean pulmonary artery pressure by right heart catheterization greater than or equal to 25 mm Hg, pulmonary capillary wedge pressure less than or equal to 15 mm Hg, and pulmonary vascular resistance (PVR) greater than or equal to 3 Wood units. To calculate PVR one must first determine the transpulmonary gradient, the difference between the mean pulmonary artery pressure and the pulmonary capillary wedge pressure. By dividing transpulmonary gradient by cardiac output one can estimate the PVR. A common pitfall in patients with ACHD is to rely on automatically derived estimates of PVR without accounting for intracardiac shunting or careful consideration of the accuracy of cardiac output and the methods being used to derive it.

Cardiac output is most commonly determined by two methods: the Fick calculation and thermodilution. The Fick calculation is based on the principles that oxygen content diffuses through an area at a rate that depends on the difference in concentration between two points. However, in the presence of intracardiac shunting the flow for the pulmonary circuit (Qp) and the flow of the systemic circuit (Qs) must be calculated. The Qp assesses the difference between the pulmonary venous and arterial blood and Qs assess the difference between the systemic and mixed venous blood. The degree of shunting is typically expressed as the ratio between the Qp and Qs. A shunt is considered hemodynamically significant when Op/Qs ratio is greater than 1.5:1.[11] However, a normal Qp/Qs ratio does not rule out the presence of shunting because bidirectional blood flow can make this value look normal. When shunt closure is being considered, it is important to first determine the PVR. Although a patient may be hypoxic from right-to-left shunting, those with a PVR greater than 6 Wood units are not suitable for shunt closure because it may predispose them to right ventricular failure caused by the lack of a "pop off." Certain tools, such as automatic cardiac flow monitors, are less likely to be accurate in the CHD population.[52]

Invasive hemodynamic assessment is informative in patients with a Fontan circulation presenting with features of systemic venous congestion or other HF symptoms. Failing Fontan physiology is characterized by high central filling pressures and low cardiac output.[53] The lack of a contractile subpulmonic ventricle leads to a reliance on pre-load and passively pulmonary flow to propel blood to the systemic ventricle. Any increase in PVR leads to a decline in cardiac output. Long-standing nonpulsatile flow in the pulmonary bed leads to endothelial dysfunction and nitric oxide dysregulation, which increases the risk of developing pulmonary vascular disease.[54] Chronically reduced preload also leads to remodeling and diastolic dysfunction of the systemic ventricle. With the lack of validated noninvasive testing, routine cardiac catheterization remains necessary in the assessment of PVR and cardiac output in patients with Fontan physiology.[55] Although echocardiography is important in the surveillance of cardiac structure and function, Doppler cardiac output has only been shown to have a moderate correlate with the Fick cardiac output.[56]

ADVANCED HEART FAILURE TREATMENT

A growing number of patients with ACHD are presenting with advanced stage D HF.[7,57] With the lack of evidence-based methods of prognostic surveillance, clinical deterioration is rapid and unexpected. Because of patient complexity, the unpredictable clinical course of ACHD-related and the need for extensive multidisciplinary review and discussion, early referral for advanced HF is recommended.[11,58] The clinical flow of patients with CHD presenting with HF is provided in **Fig. 1**. This should occur before the development of irreversible end-organ dysfunction.

In addition to requiring more time for invasive hemodynamic assessment, imaging, and subspecialist review, patients with ACHD and families often need more time to align their expectations with those of the advanced HF team. Many patients with ACHD report being told they would not survive beyond childhood or following a major surgery. The sense that they have already "defied the odds," can feed into an altered perception of risk and mortality. Additionally, the transition from a pediatric to an adult medicine care team restarts the process of establishing trust between providers, the patient, and their family. Difficult conversations frequently arise at the time of

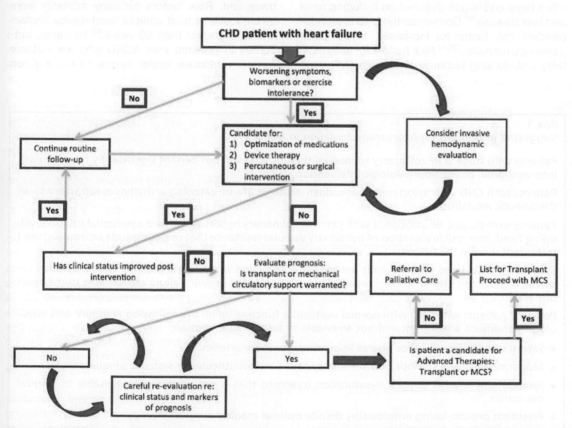

Fig. 1. Clinical flow of patients with CHD presenting with symptomatic and advanced HF. CHD, congenital heart disease; MCS, mechanical circulatory support. (*Reprinted with permission from Ross HJ, Law Y, Book WM, Broberg CS, Burchill L, Cecchin F, et al. Transplantation and Mechanical Circulatory Support in Congenital Heart Disease: A Scientific Statement from the American Heart Association. Circulation. 2016;133:802-20 ©2016 American Heart Association, Inc.*)

advanced HF assessment including whether to pursue high-risk interventions or proceed with advanced HF treatment options, such as mechanical circulatory support (MCS) or transplantation. Time is needed to introduce to patients and families the option of palliative and symptom-driven care as an alternative to high-risk treatments.

Heart transplantation remains the treatment of choice for eligible patients with severe advanced HF including those with end-stage ACHD-related HF. Suggested indications for heart transplantation in CHD are given in **Box 1**. Over time, the proportion of heart transplantations performed in patients with ACHD has increased.[58–60] Between 1999 and 2010 the prevalence of heart transplantation among patients with ACHD increased 41%.[61] Between 2015 and 2018, more than 200 adult patients with CHD were transplanted in the United States[59] with approximately 40% having univentricular anatomy.[60] Patients with ACHD are a high-risk group for transplant because they have undergone multiple prior sternotomies, have a significantly higher risk of allosensitization, may have occult pulmonary hypertension, and often have end-organ dysfunction including renal and liver disease.[62] Consequently, CHD is an independent risk factor for increased 1-year post-transplant mortality.[63,64] Risk factors for early mortality include long ischemic time, high PVR, redo

transplantation, and Fontan physiology.[61,65,66] For those who survive the high-risk early postoperative period, survival is actually superior to those without CHD with a median survival of more than 20 years compared with 14 years in those with ischemic heart disease.[67] This may be caused by the lower incidence of cardiovascular comorbidities, such as diabetes and atherosclerotic disease, in this younger population.

The use of MCS devices for patients with advanced stage HF has also increased over time.[60] Given the anatomic complexity of ACHD, this group of patients may not experience similar benefits from durable MCS as patients without ACHD. This is in large part caused by a greater need for biventricular support[68] but other factors also increase mortality risk. Using the Interagency Registry for Mechanically Assisted Circulatory Support (INTERMACS) database to compare patients with and without ACHD undergoing MCS, VanderPluym and colleagues[68] found patients with ACHD had significantly higher mortality post-MCS exclusively during the first 5 months after implant and a lower probability of receiving a transplant. Risk factors for early mortality were biventricular or total artificial heart device implant and age greater than 50 years.[68] However, outcomes in patients with ACHD who are suitable for left ventricular assist device (LVAD) support

---

Box 1
Suggested indications for heart transplantation in ACHD

Patients with stage D HF refractory to medical therapy who will not benefit significantly from surgical, interventional, or electrophysiologic intervention

Patients with CHD with associated near-sudden death or life-threatening arrhythmias refractory to all therapeutic modalities

Patients with stage C HF associated with reactive pulmonary hypertension and a potential risk of developing fixed, irreversible elevation of pulmonary vascular resistance that could preclude orthotopic heart transplantation in the future

Stage C HF associated with systemic ventricular dysfunction in pediatric patients with previously repaired or palliated CHD when HF is associated with significant growth failure attributable to the heart disease

Pediatric patients with CHD with normal ventricular function when the following anatomic and physiologic conditions are present and not amenable to surgical intervention:

• Severe stenosis (stenoses) or atresia in proximal coronary arteries

• Moderate-to-severe stenosis or insufficiency of the atrioventricular or systemic semilunar valves

• Symptomatic arterial oxygen desaturation (cyanosis) that is not considered amenable to surgical correction

• Persistent protein-losing enteropathy despite optimal medical-surgical therapy

Abbreviations: CHD, congenital heart disease; HF, heart failure.

Reprinted with permission from Ross HJ, Law Y, Book WM, Broberg CS, Burchill L, Cecchin F, et al. Transplantation and Mechanical Circulatory Support in Congenital Heart Disease: A Scientific Statement from the American Heart Association. Circulation. 2016;133:802-20 ©2016 American Heart Association, Inc.

seem to be comparable with patients without ACHD. The finding of equivalent survival among patients with ACHD treated with LVAD support, regardless of ventricular morphology, suggests LVAD is an option for those with end-stage HF, biventricular anatomy, and predominant systemic ventricular systolic dysfunction. Careful surgical planning is warranted because most modern day LVADs were designed for a morphologic left (systemic) ventricle.

In contrast, little is known about the use of temporary MCS, such as the intra-aortic balloon pump and Impella (Abiomed, Danvers, MA), in patients with ACHD who present with cardiogenic shock. With the unique anatomic challenges and lack of evidence to their use, most centers refrain from using short-term mechanical support. This proves to be a disadvantage in patients considered for heart transplantation in the United States, where listing status is based on the degree of hemodynamic support needed with higher priority given to those with temporary MCS devices (status 1 and 2). The new allocation system changes by United Network of Organ Sharing in 2018 addressed this disadvantage by giving higher priority to patients with CHD (status 4). However, the added challenges of allosensitization, elevated surgical risk from prior sternotomies, and need for CHD expertise at the transplant center makes the path to heart transplantation arduous and difficult for patients and providers alike. The key to success is an early referral to an advanced HF team so that a multidisciplinary care team can address many of these risk factors early.

RETURN TO CASE STUDY

Returning to Mr D, the 47-year-old man with D-transposition of the great arteries treated with a Mustard repair at age 2 years and transcatheter stenting of a superior vena cava baffle stenosis now presenting with NYHA functional class III symptoms with fatigue, dyspnea, and poor sleep, with clinical features of volume overload.

What Investigations Are Indicated When Adult Congenital Heart Disease–Related Heart Failure Is Suspected?

The following investigations are indicated in all patients with ACHD presenting with suspected HF: electrocardiogram, transthoracic echocardiogram, chest radiograph, and blood tests assessing for modifiable factors that may aggravate HF and/or indicate end-organ damage. Measurement of NT-proBNP or BNP and cardiopulmonary exercise testing (including respiratory function tests) further assist in guiding disease severity and

prognostication. Modifiable factors that are evaluated with blood tests include anemia, iron deficiency, thyroid dysfunction, infection, ischemia, and vitamin deficiencies (ie, vitamin D, thiamine) when indicated. Blood tests for end-organ dysfunction includes kidney and liver function tests. Elevated NT-proBNP or BNP confirms significant ventricular dysfunction, provides prognostic information,[46,47] and may be helpful in tracking response to treatment in some patients with HF. In this case, Mr D had evidence of end-organ dysfunction with mild kidney impairment (glomerular filtration rate 70 mL/min/1.73 m^2) and a congestive hepatopathy with normal bilirubin but mildly elevated glutamyl transpeptidase, and alkaline phosphatase. NT-proBNP was moderately elevated at 400 pg/mL (normal <125 pg/mL). Mr D underwent a sleep study that confirmed moderate to severe obstructive sleep apnea. On CPET, Mr D exercised for 10 minutes, 11 seconds with anaerobic threshold achieved early. Blood pressure response and oxygen saturations were normal throughout. Peak oxygen uptake (Vo_2) was reduced at 19 mL/kg/min (52% predicted) with a blunted peak heart rate response (127 bpm [65% predicted]) indicating chronotropic incompetence. The O_2 pulse response was blunted and plateaued at 69% predicted indicating reduced stroke volume response to exercise. The VE/VCO_2 slope was abnormal at 33.

How Do We Classify Adult Congenital Heart Disease–Related Heart Failure?

To promote consistent classification and communication, we support the use of the ACHD AP classification system and the ACC/AHA classification systems (**Fig. 2**). Using our case study as an example, Mr D would be classified as ACHD AP classification IIIC and ACC/AHA HF classification stage C. Alignment between the staging systems is evident and the use of both systems enables consistent communication with ACHD and HF specialists.

Which Evidence-Based Treatments Should Be Considered in This Case?

HF classification guides treatment of ACHD-related HF. As previously discussed (see section on developing a common language for classifying and reporting ACHD-related HF and **Table 1**), all patients with ACC/AHA HF classification stage C HF should be given lifestyle and dietary advice with commencement of diuretics for fluid retention and consideration of afterload reducing angiotensin-converting enzyme inhibitors or angiotensin II receptor blockers and β-blockaders.

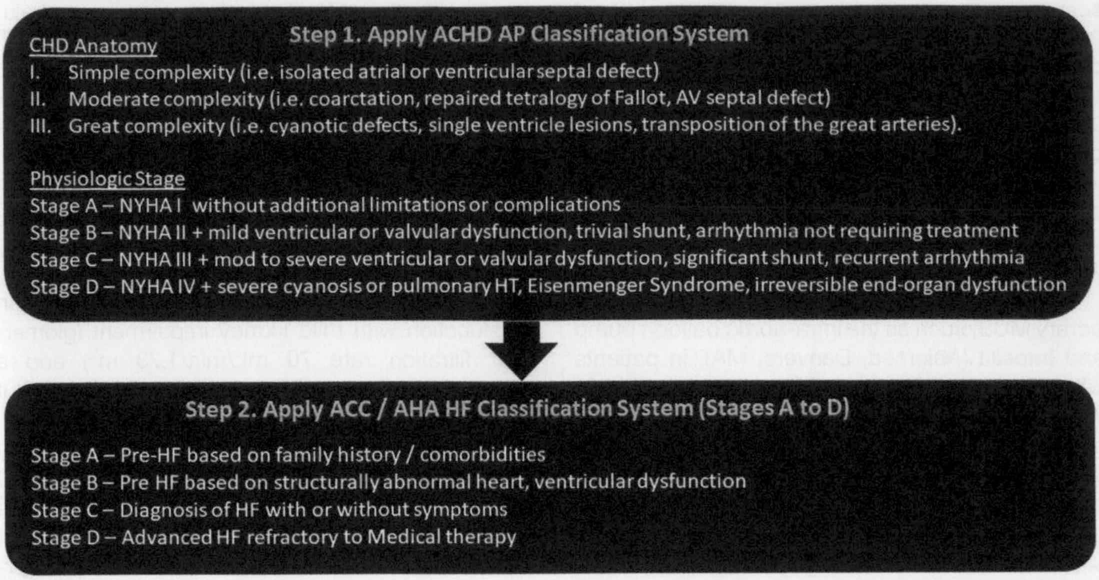

Step 1. Apply ACHD AP Classification System

CHD Anatomy
I.   Simple complexity (i.e. isolated atrial or ventricular septal defect)
II. Moderate complexity (i.e. coarctation, repaired tetralogy of Fallot, AV septal defect)
III. Great complexity (i.e. cyanotic defects, single ventricle lesions, transposition of the great arteries).

Physiologic Stage
Stage A – NYHA I without additional limitations or complications
Stage B – NYHA II + mild ventricular or valvular dysfunction, trivial shunt, arrhythmia not requiring treatment
Stage C – NYHA III + mod to severe ventricular or valvular dysfunction, significant shunt, recurrent arrhythmia
Stage D – NYHA IV + severe cyanosis or pulmonary HT, Eisenmenger Syndrome, irreversible end-organ dysfunction

Step 2. Apply ACC / AHA HF Classification System (Stages A to D)

Stage A – Pre-HF based on family history / comorbidities
Stage B – Pre HF based on structurally abnormal heart, ventricular dysfunction
Stage C – Diagnosis of HF with or without symptoms
Stage D – Advanced HF refractory to Medical therapy

Fig. 2. Two-step application of the ACHD AP and ACC/AHA HF classification systems is recommended when evaluating patients with ACHD-related HF. AV, atrioventricular; CHD, congenital heart disease; HT, hypertension; NYHA, New York Heart Association.

Aldosterone antagonists may also be considered. Mr D was enrolled in cardiac rehabilitation and provided with a written HF action plan that included recommendations for physical activity, daily weights, and fluid and salt restriction. Oral frusemide 40 mg daily and oral ramipril 2.5 mg daily were commenced with initial weekly followed by monthly and then 3-monthly review of kidney function. A low-dose long-acting β-blocker was trialed but ceased because of worsening chronotropic incompetence and fatigue. He has been scheduled for a full heart study to exclude pulmonary hypertension and to guide optimization of medical therapy. Progression to refractory stage D HF will prompt early referral for advanced HF assessment and review of treatment options including MCS, heart transplantation, advanced care planning, and palliative care.

SUMMARY

As the population of patients with ACHD ages and grows, so too does the burden of ACHD-related HF. Despite the advances in medical and surgical therapies over the last decades, ACHD-related HF remains a formidable complication with high morbidity and mortality. There are ongoing challenges in determining the true burden of ACHD-related HF because of a lack of consensus definition of HF and an absence of population-based registries with clearly defined ACHD and HF cohorts. This challenge is further compounded by

inherent differences in the natural course and outcomes of ACHD-related HF within and across its subtypes. In recent years, research and clinical guidelines for ACHD-related HF have started to address these knowledge gaps leading to greater consensus on how to best assess and treat those presenting with ACHD-related HF. High-quality studies focused on ACHD-related HF are required to better identify predictors of HF and to improve surveillance and management of this challenging condition.

DISCLOSURE

The authors have nothing to disclose.

REFERENCES

1. Oechslin EN, Harrison DA, Connelly MS, et al. Mode of death in adults with congenital heart disease. Am J Cardiol 2000;86:1111–6.
2. Nieminen HP, Jokinen EV, Sairanen HI. Causes of late deaths after pediatric cardiac surgery: a population-based study. J Am Coll Cardiol 2007; 50:1263–71.
3. Diller GP, Kempny A, Alonso-Gonzalez R, et al. Survival prospects and circumstances of death in contemporary adult congenital heart disease patients under follow-up at a large tertiary centre. Circulation 2015;132:2118–25.
4. Norozi K, Wessel A, Alpers V, et al. Incidence and risk distribution of heart failure in adolescents and

adults with congenital heart disease after cardiac surgery. Am J Cardiol 2006;97:1238–43.

5. Engelings CC, Helm PC, Abdul-Khaliq H, et al. Cause of death in adults with congenital heart disease: an analysis of the German National Register for Congenital Heart Defects. Int J Cardiol 2016;211:31–6.

6. Verheugt CL, Uiterwaal CS, van der Velde ET, et al. Mortality in adult congenital heart disease. Eur Heart J 2010;31:1220–9.

7. Yu C, Moore BM, Kotchetkova I, et al. Causes of death in a contemporary adult congenital heart disease cohort. Heart 2018;104:1678–82.

8. Burchill LJ, Gao L, Kovacs AH, et al. Hospitalization trends and health resource use for adult congenital heart disease-related heart failure. J Am Heart Assoc 2018;7:e008775.

9. Lal S, Kotchetkova I, Cao J, et al. Heart failure admissions and poor subsequent outcomes in adults with congenital heart disease. Eur J Heart Fail 2018;20:812–5.

10. Zomer AC, Vaartjes I, van der Velde ET, et al. Heart failure admissions in adults with congenital heart disease; risk factors and prognosis. Int J Cardiol 2013;168:2487–93.

11. Stout KK, Broberg CS, Book WM, et al. Chronic heart failure in congenital heart disease: a scientific statement from the American Heart Association. Circulation 2016;133:770–801.

12. Stout KK, Daniels CJ, Aboulhosn JA, et al. 2018 AHA/ACC guideline for the management of adults with congenital heart disease: a report of the American College of Cardiology/American Heart Association Task Force on clinical practice guidelines. Circulation 2019;139:e698–800.

13. Bredy C, Ministeri M, Kempny A, et al. New York Heart Association (NYHA) classification in adults with congenital heart disease: relation to objective measures of exercise and outcome. Eur Heart J Qual Care Clin Outcomes 2018;4:51–8.

14. Diller GP, Dimopoulos K, Okonko D, et al. Exercise intolerance in adult congenital heart disease: comparative severity, correlates, and prognostic implication. Circulation 2005;112:828–35.

15. Kempny A, Dimopoulos K, Uebing A, et al. Reference values for exercise limitations among adults with congenital heart disease. Relation to activities of daily life–single centre experience and review of published data. Eur Heart J 2012; 33:1386–96.

16. Yancy CW, Jessup M, Bozkurt B, et al. 2013 ACCF/AHA guideline for the management of heart failure: a report of the American College of Cardiology Foundation/American heart association Task Force on practice guidelines. J Am Coll Cardiol 2013;62:e147–239.

17. Wang F, Harel-Sterling L, Cohen S, et al. Heart failure risk predictions in adult patients with congenital heart disease: a systematic review. Heart 2019; 105:1661–9.

18. Babu-Narayan SV, Kilner PJ, Li W, et al. Ventricular fibrosis suggested by cardiovascular magnetic resonance in adults with repaired tetralogy of Fallot and its relationship to adverse markers of clinical outcome. Circulation 2006;113:405–13.

19. Khairy P, Harris L, Landzberg MJ, et al. Implantable cardioverter-defibrillators in tetralogy of Fallot. Circulation 2008;117:363–70.

20. Aboulhosn JA, Lluri G, Gurvitz MZ, et al. Left and right ventricular diastolic function in adults with surgically repaired tetralogy of Fallot: a multi-institutional study. Can J Cardiol 2013;29:866–72.

21. Feldt RH, Driscoll DJ, Offord KP, et al. Protein-losing enteropathy after the Fontan operation. J Thorac Cardiovasc Surg 1996;112:672–80.

22. Atz AM, Zak V, Mahony L, et al. Longitudinal outcomes of patients with single ventricle after the Fontan procedure. J Am Coll Cardiol 2017;69: 2735–44.

23. Caruthers RL, Kempa M, Loo A, et al. Demographic characteristics and estimated prevalence of Fontan-associated plastic bronchitis. Pediatr Cardiol 2013; 34:256–61.

24. Allen KY, Downing TE, Glatz AC, et al. Effect of Fontan-associated morbidities on survival with intact Fontan circulation. Am J Cardiol 2017;119: 1866–71.

25. Schumacher KR, Singh TP, Kuebler J, et al. Risk factors and outcome of Fontan-associated plastic bronchitis: a case-control study. J Am Heart Assoc 2014; 3:e000865.

26. Johnson JN, Driscoll DJ, O'Leary PW. Protein-losing enteropathy and the Fontan operation. Nutr Clin Pract 2012;27:375–84.

27. Roos-Hesselink JW, Meijboom FJ, Spitaels SE, et al. Decline in ventricular function and clinical condition after Mustard repair for transposition of the great arteries (a prospective study of 22-29 years). Eur Heart J 2004;25:1264–70.

28. Gelatt M, Hamilton RM, McCrindle BW, et al. Arrhythmia and mortality after the Mustard procedure: a 30-year single-center experience. J Am Coll Cardiol 1997;29:194–201.

29. Gewillig M. The Fontan circulation. Heart 2005;91: 839–46.

30. Koyak Z, Harris L, de Groot JR, et al. Sudden cardiac death in adult congenital heart disease. Circulation 2012;126:1944–54.

31. Schwerzmann M, Salehian O, Harris L, et al. Ventricular arrhythmias and sudden death in adults after a Mustard operation for transposition of the great arteries. Eur Heart J 2009;30:1873–9.

32. Diller GP, Radojevic J, Kempny A, et al. Systemic right ventricular longitudinal strain is reduced in adults with transposition of the great arteries, relates to

subpulmonary ventricular function, and predicts adverse clinical outcome. Am Heart J 2012;163: 859–66.

33. Piran S, Veldtman G, Siu S, et al. Heart failure and ventricular dysfunction in patients with single or systemic right ventricles. Circulation 2002;105: 1189–94.

34. Ghai A, Silversides C, Harris L, et al. Left ventricular dysfunction is a risk factor for sudden cardiac death in adults late after repair of tetralogy of Fallot. J Am Coll Cardiol 2002;40:1675–80.

35. Guazzi M, Arena R, Halle M, et al. 2016 focused update: clinical recommendations for cardiopulmonary exercise testing data assessment in specific patient populations. Circulation 2016;133:e694–711.

36. Udholm S, Aldweib N, Hjortdal VE, et al. Prognostic power of cardiopulmonary exercise testing in Fontan patients: a systematic review. Open Heart 2018;5: e000812.

37. Babu-Narayan SV, Diller GP, Gheta RR, et al. Clinical outcomes of surgical pulmonary valve replacement after repair of tetralogy of Fallot and potential prognostic value of preoperative cardiopulmonary exercise testing. Circulation 2014;129:18–27.

38. Muller J, Hager A, Diller GP, et al. Peak oxygen uptake, ventilatory efficiency and QRS-duration predict event free survival in patients late after surgical repair of tetralogy of Fallot. Int J Cardiol 2015;196: 158–64.

39. Giardini A, Hager A, Lammers AE, et al. Ventilatory efficiency and aerobic capacity predict event-free survival in adults with atrial repair for complete transposition of the great arteries. J Am Coll Cardiol 2009; 53:1548–55.

40. Fernandes SM, Alexander ME, Graham DA, et al. Exercise testing identifies patients at increased risk for morbidity and mortality following Fontan surgery. Congenit Heart Dis 2011;6:294–303.

41. Brubaker PH, Kitzman DW. Chronotropic incompetence: causes, consequences, and management. Circulation 2011;123:1010–20.

42. Diller GP, Dimopoulos K, Okonko D, et al. Heart rate response during exercise predicts survival in adults with congenital heart disease. J Am Coll Cardiol 2006;48:1250–6.

43. Radojevic J, Inuzuka R, Alonso-Gonzalez R, et al. Peak oxygen uptake correlates with disease severity and predicts outcome in adult patients with Ebstein's anomaly of the tricuspid valve. Int J Cardiol 2013; 163:305–8.

44. van der Bom T, Winter MM, Groenink M, et al. Right ventricular end-diastolic volume combined with peak systolic blood pressure during exercise identifies patients at risk for complications in adults with a systemic right ventricle. J Am Coll Cardiol 2013;62:926–36.

45. Nathan AS, Loukas B, Moko L, et al. Exercise oscillatory ventilation in patients with Fontan physiology. Circ Heart Fail 2015;8:304–11.

46. Miyamoto K, Takeuchi D, Inai K, et al. Prognostic value of multiple biomarkers for cardiovascular mortality in adult congenital heart disease: comparisons of single-/two-ventricle physiology, and systemic morphologically right/left ventricles. Heart Vessels 2016;31:1834–47.

47. Baggen VJ, van den Bosch AE, Eindhoven JA, et al. Prognostic value of N-Terminal Pro-B-type natriuretic peptide, troponin-T, and growth-differentiation factor 15 in adult congenital heart disease. Circulation 2017;135:264–79.

48. Baggen VJM, van den Bosch AE, van Kimmenade RR, et al. Red cell distribution width in adults with congenital heart disease: a worldwide available and low-cost predictor of cardiovascular events. Int J Cardiol 2018;260:60–5.

49. Levy WC, Mozaffarian D, Linker DT, et al. The Seattle Heart Failure Model: prediction of survival in heart failure. Circulation 2006;113:1424–33.

50. Stefanescu A, Macklin EA, Lin E, et al. Usefulness of the Seattle Heart Failure Model to identify adults with congenital heart disease at high risk of poor outcome. Am J Cardiol 2014;113:865–70.

51. Baggen VJM, Venema E, Zivna R, et al. Development and validation of a risk prediction model in patients with adult congenital heart disease. Int J Cardiol 2019;276:87–92.

52. Seckeler MD, Typpo K, Deschenes J, et al. Inaccuracy of a continuous arterial pressure waveform monitor when used for congenital cardiac catheterization. Congenit Heart Dis 2017;12:815–9.

53. Gewillig M, Brown SC. The Fontan circulation after 45 years: update in physiology. Heart 2016;102: 1081–6.

54. Zongtao Y, Huishan W, Zengwei W, et al. Experimental study of nonpulsatile flow perfusion and structural remodeling of pulmonary microcirculation vessels. Thorac Cardiovasc Surg 2010;58: 468–72.

55. Baumgartner H, Bonhoeffer P, De Groot NM, et al. ESC Guidelines for the management of grown-up congenital heart disease (new version 2010). Eur Heart J 2010;31:2915–57.

56. Egbe AC, Connolly HM, Taggart NW, et al. Invasive and noninvasive hemodynamic assessment in adults with Fontan palliation. Int J Cardiol 2018; 254:96–100.

57. Greutmann M, Tobler D, Kovacs AH, et al. Increasing mortality burden among adults with complex congenital heart disease. Congenit Heart Dis 2015;10:117–27.

58. Ross HJ, Law Y, Book WM, et al. Transplantation and mechanical circulatory support in congenital heart

disease: a scientific statement from the American Heart Association. Circulation 2016;133:802–20.

59. Nguyen VP, Dolgner SJ, Dardas TF, et al. Improved outcomes of heart transplantation in adults with congenital heart disease receiving regionalized care. J Am Coll Cardiol 2019;74:2908–18.

60. Maxwell BG, Wong JK, Sheikh AY, et al. Heart transplantation with or without prior mechanical circulatory support in adults with congenital heart disease. Eur J Cardiothorac Surg 2014;45:842–6.

61. Karamlou T, Hirsch J, Welke K, et al. A United Network for Organ Sharing analysis of heart transplantation in adults with congenital heart disease: outcomes and factors associated with mortality and retransplantation. J Thorac Cardiovasc Surg 2010;140:161–8.

62. Stewart GC, Mayer JE Jr. Heart transplantation in adults with congenital heart disease. Heart Fail Clin 2014;10:207–18.

63. Doumouras BS, Alba AC, Foroutan F, et al. Outcomes in adult congenital heart disease patients undergoing heart transplantation: a systematic review and meta-analysis. J Heart Lung Transplant 2016; 35:1337–47.

64. Burchill LJ, Edwards LB, Dipchand AI, et al. Impact of adult congenital heart disease on survival and mortality after heart transplantation. J Heart Lung Transplant 2014;33:1157–63.

65. Besik J, Szarszoi O, Hegarova M, et al. Non-Fontan adult congenital heart disease transplantation survival is equivalent to acquired heart disease transplantation survival. Ann Thorac Surg 2016; 101:1768–73.

66. Lamour JM, Kanter KR, Naftel DC, et al. The effect of age, diagnosis, and previous surgery in children and adults undergoing heart transplantation for congenital heart disease. J Am Coll Cardiol 2009; 54:160–5.

67. Khush KK, Cherikh WS, Chambers DC, et al. The International Thoracic Organ Transplant Registry of the International Society for Heart and Lung Transplantation: thirty-fifth adult heart transplantation report-2018; focus theme: Multiorgan transplantation. J Heart Lung Transplant 2018;37:1155–68.

68. VanderPluym CJ, Cedars A, Eghtesady P, et al. Outcomes following implantation of mechanical circulatory support in adults with congenital heart disease: an analysis of the Interagency Registry for Mechanically Assisted Circulatory Support (INTERMACS). J Heart Lung Transplant 2018;37:89–99.

69. Ohuchi H, Negishi J, Noritake K, et al. Prognostic value of exercise variables in 335 patients after the Fontan operation: a 23-year single-center experience of cardiopulmonary exercise testing. Congenit Heart Dis 2015;10:105–16.

70. Egbe AC, Driscoll DJ, Khan AR, et al. Cardiopulmonary exercise test in adults with prior Fontan operation: the prognostic value of serial testing. Int J Cardiol 2017;235:6–10.

Moving?

Make sure your subscription moves with you!

To notify us of your new address, find your **Clinics Account Number** (located on your mailing label above your name), and contact customer service at:

Email: journalscustomerservice-usa@elsevier.com

800-654-2452 (subscribers in the U.S. & Canada)
314-447-8871 (subscribers outside of the U.S. & Canada)

Fax number: 314-447-8029

Elsevier Health Sciences Division
Subscription Customer Service
3251 Riverport Lane
Maryland Heights, MO 63043

ELSEVIER

Printed and bound by CPI Group (UK) Ltd, Croydon, CR0 4YY

03/10/2024

01040307-0020